AMBULATORY CARE PROCEDURES FOR THE NURSE PRACTITIONER

SECOND EDITION

AMBULATORY CARE PROCEDURES FOR THE NURSE PRACTITIONER

SECOND EDITION

Margaret R. Colyar, DSN, APRN, C-FNP/C-PNP
Family Nurse Practitioner
University of Utah
Salt Lake City, Utah

Cynthia R. Ehrhardt, RN, ARNP, MSN, FNP-CS
Ocala, Florida

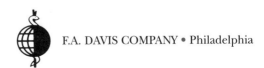

F.A. DAVIS COMPANY • Philadelphia

F. A. Davis Company
1915 Arch Street
Philadelphia, PA 19103
www.fadavis.com

Printed in the United States of America

Last digit indicates print number: 10 9 8 7 6 5

Acquisitions Editor: Joanne Patzek DaCunha, RN, MSN
Developmental Editor: Alan Sorkowitz
Cover Designer: Louis J. Forgione

As new scientific information becomes available through basic and clinical research, recommended treatments and drug therapies undergo changes. The author(s) and publisher have done everything possible to make this book accurate, up to date, and in accord with accepted standards at the time of publication. The author(s), editors, and publisher are not responsible for errors or omissions or for consequences from application of the book, and make no warranty, expressed or implied, in regard to the contents of the book. Any practice described in this book should be applied by the reader in accordance with professional standards of care used in regard to the unique circumstances that may apply in each situation. The reader is advised always to check product information (package inserts) for changes and new information regarding dose and contraindications before administering any drug. Caution is especially urged when using new or infrequently ordered drugs.

Library of Congress Cataloging-in-Publication Data

Colyar, Margaret R., 1948-
   Ambulatory care procedures for the nurse practitioner/Margaret R.
Colyar, Cynthia R. Ehrhardt.– 2nd ed.
   p. ; cm.
Includes bibliographical references and index.
   ISBN 10: 0-8036-1123-4   ISBN 13: 978-0-8036-1123-8
1. Nurse practitioners. 2. Ambulatory medical care. 3. Nursing.
   [DNLM: 1. Ambulatory Care–methods. 2. Nursing Process. 3. Nurse Practitioners.
WY 150 C727a 2004] I. Ehrhardt, Cynthia R., 1951- II. Title.
RT82.8.C64 2004
610.73–dc22

2003019743

This book is lovingly dedicated to Shirley and Don Jones and Stephen Colyar.
The encouragement from these family members made this book possible.

Preface

Expectations for the new nurse practitioner and the practicing nurse practitioner in the ambulatory care setting have changed. They must be prepared to perform an increasing array of skills competently to meet patient care needs. The inspiration for this book came when, on graduating from a nurse practitioner program, I found no procedural resources directed toward the needs of the nurse practitioner in ambulatory care. The need to perform many procedures—those not taught in my nurse practitioner program—was apparent. The physician I practiced with required a knowledge base in procedural skills greater than the one I possessed. Fortunately, this physician was willing to teach me the necessary procedures. This improved care to our patients and decreased the necessity to refer many patients for procedures easily performed in the ambulatory care (outpatient) setting.

There are many demands on the newly graduated nurse practitioner and the nurse practitioner currently in practice. This text was developed to assist these two groups. We believe the procedures outlined will improve the marketability of the nurse practitioner and serve as a good reference tool for family and/or adult nurse practitioners in an ambulatory care setting. Prerequisites for this book are basic anatomy and physiology, microbiology, pharmacology, principles of aseptic technique, and basic nursing skills. This book would be an appropriate text for incorporation of procedural techniques throughout a family or an adult nurse practitioner curriculum. It also would be appropriate for an elective on minor surgery and diagnostic procedures and interpretation. Another potential use for this book would be as part of the protocol/guidelines in the nurse practitioner's practice.

Many procedures performed by primary care physicians are not currently appropriate for the nurse practitioner to perform. The procedures in this book were chosen based on a comprehensive study of types of procedures currently used in the nurse practitioner's practice. Many of the procedures can be used in any ambulatory setting. Twelve new procedures have been added to this edition—blood culture collection; capillary blood collection; central venous access; cervical cap insertion; chest tubes for emergency transport; circumcision; Dermabond application; dislocation reduction, shoulder, no anesthesia; IUD insertion; lumbar puncture; occipital nerve block; and thin preparation Pap smear.

Some of the procedures need specialized equipment, and some use equipment commonly found in any office. A few of the procedures—flexible chest tube insertion, circumcision, colposcopy, endometrial biopsy, IUD insertion and removal, lumbar puncture, occipital nerve block, paracentesis, sigmoidoscopy, and thrombosed hemorrhoid removal—require additional training. They are included for reference only. Check with your State Board of Nursing if you are unsure whether or not a certain procedure may be performed by nurse practitioners in the state in which you practice.

The major theme of this book is clinical application of knowledge and clinical skills. There are seven sections in the book. These sections are based on body systems for ease of classification. Each major section begins with diagnostic procedures the nurse practitioner performs with the basis for their interpretation. Next in each section, listed in alphabetical order, are procedures performed in an ambulatory care setting.

Each procedure contains seven parts. First, an *Overview* is presented, outlining causes, incidence, and other specific information intrinsic to each procedure. The *Health Promotion/Prevention* section gives tips to the nurse practitioner to pass on to the client to help promote health or prevent the need for the procedure in the future. *Options* lists one to four methods of performing the procedure and gives a choice of how to perform the procedure. The *Rationale* section gives reasons to perform the procedure. *Indications* tell the nurse practitioner when the procedure should be performed, and *Contraindications* tells the nurse practitioner when not to perform the procedure. The *Procedure* section lists the necessary equipment and gives step-by-step instructions for performing each procedure listed under Options. *Client Instructions* assist the nurse practitioner with postprocedure instructions, listing what the client must and must not do to have an optimal recovery period. At the end of each chapter is the Bibliography for further information gathering.

We hope you will find this text to be a good learning tool and a great resource in your practice.

Acknowledgments

We acknowledge the following people for their contributions, assistance, and patience while compiling this book: Joanne DaCunha, RN, MSN, Nursing Acquisitions Editor at F. A. Davis, for believing in the merits of this book, and Denise Melomo, artist, for her expertise in sketching the line drawings from which the illustrations in this book were made.

Many colleagues at Tri County Family Health Care in Madison, Florida, and Family Health Service in Ocala, Florida, were instrumental in this book. Colleagues at Rapides Regional Medical Center, Alexandria, Louisiana; Jackson Parish Hospital, Jonesboro, Louisiana; and Stansbury Medical Center, Stansbury Park, Utah, posed for the photographs in the book. These models include Linda Alby, Steve Colyar, Hugh Gentry, Cindy Grappe, Aleene Hale, Lane Helm, Debra Lefler, Anne Martin, and Shaneal Wright.

Contributors

Tracy Call-Schmidt, MS, C-FNP
Pain Management Specialist
Assistant Professor
University of Utah
Salt Lake City, Utah

Margaret Colyar, DSN, APRN,
C-FNP/C-PNP
Associate Professor
Director, NP Specialty Program
University of Utah
Salt Lake City, Utah

Angela Deneris, CNM, PhD
Associate Professor, Clinical
Nurse-Midwifery and Women's
Health Nurse Practitioner Programs

Jane M. Dyer, CNM, FNP, MS, MBA
Associate Professor, Clinical
Director, Nurse-Midwifery and
Women's Health Nurse Practitioner
Programs

Cynthia Ehrhardt, RN, ARNP, MSN,
FNP-CS
Adjunct Faculty
University of Central Florida
Ocala, Florida

Ann Green, RN, FNP
Rural practice
Louisiana

Sandy Kuhn, RN, WHNP
Rural practice
Florida

Geeta Maharaj, MS, C-PNP
Instructor, Clinical
University of Utah
Salt Lake City, Utah

CONSULTANTS

Colleen Grebus, ARNP, MS, FNP
Family Nurse Practitioner
Foundation Medical Partners—Primary Care of Milford
Milford, New Hampshire

Margo Packheiser, RN, MSN, APRN-BC, ANP/GNP
Clinical Associate Professor
University of North Carolina at Greensboro
Greensboro, North Carolina

Wendy L. Wright, MS, RN, ARNP, FNP
Adult/Family Nurse Practitioner
Merrimack Village Family Practice
Merrimack, New Hampshire

CONTENTS

S E C T I O N ➤ *Two*
Musculoskeletal Procedures <small>123</small>

DIAGNOSTIC TESTING

PROCEDURES

S E C T I O N ➤ *Three*
Genitourinary and Breast Procedures <small>205</small>

DIAGNOSTIC TESTING

SECTION ➤ *Four*

Head: Eyes, Ears, Nose, and Mouth   287

PROCEDURES

Dermatologic Procedures

1

PUNCH BIOPSY

MARGARET R. COLYAR

CPT Code

21550	Biopsy of soft tissue of neck or thorax
21920	Biopsy of soft tissue of back or flank, superficial
23066	Biopsy of soft tissue of shoulder, superficial
24065	Biopsy of upper arm and elbow area
23066	Biopsy of soft tissue of forearm or wrist, superficial
27040	Biopsy of soft tissue of pelvis and hip area
27323	Biopsy of soft tissue of thigh or knee
27613	Biopsy of soft tissue of leg and ankle area
11100	Skin lesion

Depends on the site, technique, and if benign or malignant lesions

Biopsy is the removal of a small piece of tissue from the skin for microscopic examination. Partial or full thickness of skin over the lesion is removed for evaluation.

OVERVIEW

➤ Incidence unknown

USES

Full and partial dermal lesions such as
➤ **Basal cell carcinoma**
➤ **Squamous cell carcinoma**
➤ **Actinic keratoses**
➤ **Seborrheic keratoses**
➤ **Lentigo**
➤ Lipomas
➤ Melanomas
➤ Nevi
➤ Warts—**verruca vulgaris**

3

RATIONALE

➤ To confirm etiology of lesion for treatment
➤ To establish or confirm a diagnosis for treatment and/or intervention

INDICATIONS

➤ Partial- or full-dermal-thickness lesion not on the face, eye, lip, or penis

CONTRAINDICATIONS

➤ Lesion on eyelid, lip, or penis, REFER to a physician
➤ Infection at the site of the biopsy
➤ Bleeding disorder
➤ Lesions that are deep or on the face, REFER to a physician

🗹 *Informed consent required*

PROCEDURE

Punch Biopsy

Equipment

➤ Antiseptic skin cleanser
➤ Drape—sterile
➤ Gloves—sterile
➤ Disposable biopsy punch (Fig. 1–1)
➤ Pickups—sterile

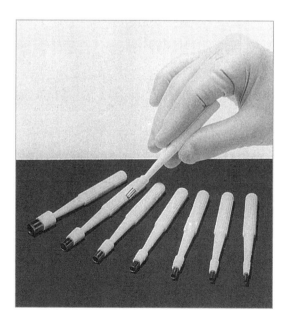

FIGURE 1 • 1 Disposable biopsy punches.

➤ Scissors—sharp for the fine tissue—sterile
➤ 3-mL syringe
➤ 27- to 30-gauge, $\frac{1}{2}$-inch needle
➤ 1% lidocaine
➤ Container with 10% **formalin**
➤ 4 × 4 gauze
➤ Nonstick dressing (Adaptic or Telfa)
➤ Kling
➤ Tape
➤ **Steri strips** (if biopsy will be greater than 4 mm)

Procedure

➤ Position the client so that the area to be biopsied is easily accessible.
➤ Cleanse the skin with antiseptic skin cleanser.
➤ Put on gloves.
➤ Drape the area to be biopsied.
➤ Anesthetize with 1% lidocaine.
➤ With the thumb and index finger, spread the skin to apply tension opposite natural skin tension lines.
➤ Apply biopsy punch to skin, rotate per manufacturer's directions, and remove the punch (Fig. 1–2).
➤ With pickups, pull up loosened skin.
➤ Cut with scissors, and place tissue in tissue container of 10% formalin (Fig. 1–3).
➤ If less than 2 to 3 mm, apply nonstick dressing and pressure dressing.
➤ If greater than 4 mm, apply Steri strips and cover with 4 ×4 gauze.
➤ Apply Kling and secure with tape.

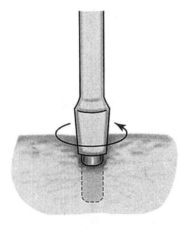

FIGURE 1 • 2 Apply biopsy punch to skin and rotate.

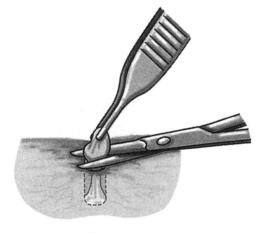

FIGURE 1 • 3 Cut with scissors.

Client Instructions

➤ Keep dressing clean, dry, and in place for 48 hours to decrease the chance of bleeding and oozing.
➤ Avoid touching or contaminating the area biopsied.
➤ To prevent the chance of infection, take cephalexin (Keflex) 500 mg three times per day or cefadroxil (Duricef) 500 mg twice a day for 5 days.
➤ Some redness, swelling, and heat are normal. Return to the office if symptoms of infection occur, such as
  ➢ Yellow or green drainage
  ➢ Red streaks
  ➢ Pain
  ➢ Elevated temperature
➤ Take acetaminophen (Tylenol) or ibuprofen (Motrin) every 4 to 6 hours as needed for pain.

BIBLIOGRAPHY
De Vries, H.J., et al (1995). Reduced wound contraction and scar formation in punch biopsy wounds. Native collagen dermal substitutes. A clinical study. *Br J Dermatol*, 132(5), 690–697.

2

SKIN BIOPSY

MARGARET R. COLYAR

CPT Code	
11300–303	Shaving of epidermal or dermal lesion; single lesion—trunk, arms, or legs
11305–308	Shaving of epidermal or dermal lesion; single lesion—scalp, neck, hands, feet, or genitalia
11400–406	Excision benign lesions—trunk, arms, or legs
11420–426	Excision benign lesions—scalp, neck, hands, feet, or genitalia
11600–606	Excision malignant lesions—trunk, arms, or legs
11620–626	Excision malignant lesions—scalp, neck, hands, feet, or genitalia

Add modifier 22 or 09922 for unusual or complicated excision.

Skin **biopsy** is the excision of a small piece of living tissue for microscopic examination. The two major categories of skin biopsy are
➤ Partial dermal thickness—shave and **curettage**
➤ Full dermal thickness—punch and elliptical excision

OVERVIEW
➤ Incidence unknown

HEALTH PROMOTION/PREVENTION
➤ Inspect the skin periodically for lesions.
➤ Note lesions that change size or color, are irregular, or are painful.

OPTIONS
➤ *Method 1*—shave biopsy
  ➤ Use for elevated skin lesions such as
    • Skin tags
    • Benign **nevi** (interdermal)
    • Epithelial tags
    • Small **basal cell carcinomas**
    • **Condyloma acuminatum**
    • Cherry **angiomas**
    • **Actinic keratoses**
    • **Seborrheic keratoses**
    • **Lentigo**
    • **Verruca vulgaris** (warts)
➤ *Method 2*—curettage biopsy
  ➤ Use for
    • Seborrheic keratoses
    • Superficial basal cell carcinomas
    • Crusting actinic keratoses
➤ *Method 3*—elliptical excisional biopsy
  ➤ Use for full-dermal-thickness lesions such as
    • Basal cell carcinoma
    • **Squamous cell carcinoma**
    • Actinic keratoses
    • Seborrheic keratoses
    • Lentigo
    • Lipomas
    • **Melanomas**
    • Nevi
    • Verruca vulgaris (warts)

RATIONALE
➤ To confirm or make a diagnosis of a skin lesion
➤ To determine definitive treatment of a skin lesion
➤ To remove a disfiguring or painful lesion

INDICATIONS

➤ Nonmalignant skin lesions not on the eyelid, lip, face, or penis
➤ Superficial skin lesions

CONTRAINDICATIONS

➤ Infection is suspected at biopsy site
➤ Bleeding disorder
➤ If melanoma is suspected, do *not* use shave or curettage. Elliptical excision is preferred.
➤ If on eyelid, lip, face, or penis, REFER
➤ If deep lesions, REFER

☑ *Informed consent required*

PROCEDURE

Skin Biopsy

Equipment

➤ Methods 1, 2, and 3
  ➤ Antiseptic skin cleanser
  ➤ Drape—sterile
  ➤ Gloves—nonsterile
  ➤ 3-mL syringe
  ➤ 27- to 30-gauge, $^1/_2$-inch needle
  ➤ 1% lidocaine
  ➤ Container of 10% **formalin**
  ➤ Cautery or Monsel's solution
  ➤ Pickups—sterile (optional)
➤ Method 1 only
  ➤ No. 15 scalpel or sterile scissors
➤ Method 2 only
  ➤ Dermal **curette**
➤ Method 3 only
  ➤ Needle driver with scissors—sterile
  ➤ Suture (see Chapter 22 for information on choosing the appropriate type and size of suture)
  ➤ Tape
  ➤ Nonstick dressing (Adaptic or Telfa)
  ➤ 4 × 4 gauze
  ➤ Topical antibiotic (Bactroban, Neosporin, or Polysporin)

Procedure

METHOD 1—SHAVE BIOPSY

➤ Position the client for comfort with the area of the skin lesion easily accessible.

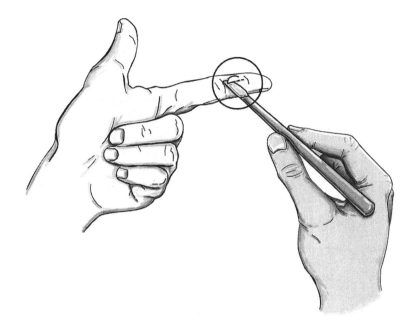

FIGURE 2 • 1 Shave biopsy. Incise parallel to the skin.

➤ Cleanse the skin lesion and a 3-inch-diameter circle around the lesion.
➤ Drape the area.
➤ Put on gloves.
➤ Inject 1% lidocaine under the lesion using a 27- to 30-gauge needle to create a wheal.
➤ Incise lesion parallel to the skin (Fig. 2–1).
➤ Place the tissue in a container of 10% formalin.
➤ Cauterize the base of the wound or apply Monsel's solution to retard bleeding.

METHOD 2—CURETTAGE BIOPSY

➤ Position the patient for comfort with the area of the skin lesion easily accessible.
➤ Cleanse the skin lesion and a 3-inch-diameter area around the lesion.
➤ Drape the area.
➤ Put on gloves.
➤ Inject 1% lidocaine under the lesion using a 27- to 30-gauge needle to create a wheal.
➤ Scrape the lesion with the curette (Fig. 2–2).
➤ Place the tissue in a container of 10% formalin.
➤ Cauterize the base of the wound or apply Monsel's solution to retard bleeding.

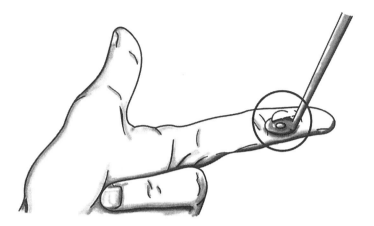

FIGURE 2 • 2 Curettage biopsy. Scrape the lesion with the curette.

METHOD 3—ELLIPTICAL EXCISIONAL BIOPSY (FULL DERMAL THICKNESS)

➤ Position the patient for comfort with the area of the skin lesion easily accessible.
➤ Draw an outline of the expected incision in the direction of the skin tension lines. The outline should be three times longer than it is wide.
➤ Cleanse the skin lesion and a 3-inch-diameter area around the lesion.
➤ Put on gloves.
➤ Inject 1% lidocaine under the lesion using a 27- to 30-gauge needle to create a wheal that covers the entire area of the proposed incision.
➤ Drape the area.
➤ Incise around the outline with the scalpel (Fig. 2–3).

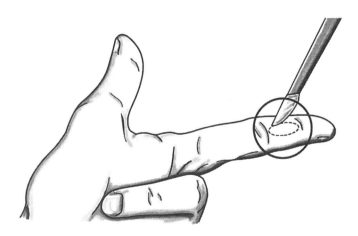

FIGURE 2 • 3 Elliptical excisional biopsy. Incise around the outline with the scalpel.

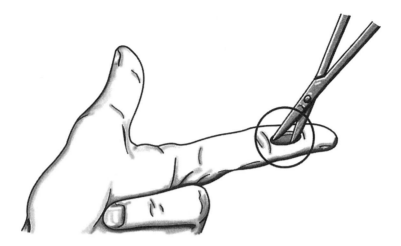

FIGURE 2 • 4 Undermine the edges of the wound to release tension.

➤ Pull up a corner of skin with pickups.
➤ Pull tissue as you excise just below full thickness of the tissue.
➤ Start at one corner and work to the center.
➤ Go to the other corner and work toward the center.
➤ Put all excised tissue in a container of 10% formalin.
➤ Closure
  ➢ If a small lesion, simple single-layer closure with nylon suture is appropriate (see Chapter 22).
  ➢ If lesion is larger with tension
    • Undermine the edges of the wound to release the tension (Fig. 2–4).
    • Incise the subcutaneous tissue the entire length of each side of the wound with the scalpel.
    • Spread the incised subcutaneous tissue with scissors (Fig. 2–5).
    • Suture using the simple single-layer technique.

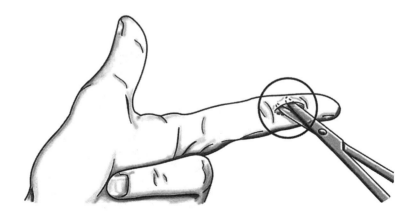

FIGURE 2 • 5 Spread the incised subcutaneous tissue with scissors.

- If a larger, deeper lesion with tension
  - Undermine the subcutaneous tissue as just described.
  - Close subcutaneous tissue with absorbable suture and **inverted** knot (see Chapter 22).
  - Close skin using simple closure technique.
  - Apply topical antibiotic, nonstick dressing, cover with 4 × 4 gauze, and secure with tape.

Client Instructions

- Some inflammation (redness, swelling, and pain) is normal.
- To prevent infection, keep the dressing in place for 24 hours, then remove the dressing and keep the area clean and dry. After the second day, you may wash the area gently with soap and water. Monitor for signs of infection, such as
  - Yellow and green drainage
  - Red streaks
  - Excessive pain
  - Elevated temperature
- Return to the office immediately if infection occurs.
- Some bleeding and oozing are normal for the first 24 to 48 hours. If your bandage becomes soaked with blood, reapply dry gauze and pressure. If the bleeding does not stop, notify your practitioner.
- Avoid tension to the wound area by limiting movement. Tension may cause the wound to pull apart. If the wound does pull apart, notify the practitioner.
- Take Tylenol No. 3 (acetaminophen with codeine) every 4 to 6 hours as needed for pain. When the pain lessens, take Tylenol or ibuprofen (Motrin) every 4 to 6 hours as needed.
- Return to the office (in _____) for stitch removal (depends on site sutured; see Table 22–1).

BIBLIOGRAPHY

Pfenninger, J.L., and Fowler, G.C. (1994). *Procedures for primary care physicians.* St. Louis: Mosby.

Surajachar, M.D. (1996). Principles of skin biopsies for the family physician. *Am Fam Physician,* 54(8), 2411–2418.

Walters, G.K. (1996). Managing soft tissue wounds. *Adv Nurse Practitioners,* 4(3), 37–40, 54.

Zuber, T.J., and Dewitt, D.E. (1994). The fusiform excision. *Am Fam Physician,* 49(2), 371–376.

3

WOOD'S LIGHT EXAMINATION

CYNTHIA R. EHRHARDT

CPT Code

None

The **Wood's light** is a useful and inexpensive tool in clinical practice. It is powered by alternating or direct current that converts ultraviolet light into visible light, and it usually has an accompanying magnification lens. It provides a simple diagnostic method in the evaluation of
➤ Many dermatologic problems
➤ **Fluorescein**-staining evaluation of eye injuries

OVERVIEW

➤ Incidence is unknown.
➤ Most common dermatologic lesions that fluoresce are listed in Table 3–1.
➤ Detection of chemicals applied to the skin. Affected areas are a different color than the surrounding skin.
  ➤ Prior cleansing of the area to be examined causes false-negative result.
  ➤ Certain skin lesions do not fluoresce.
  ➤ Systemic antibiotic therapy, such as with tetracyclines, can cause fluorescence in some lesions.
  ➤ Cosmetics present on the skin interfere with fluorescence.
➤ Detection of eye injuries with fluorescein. When applied to the eye, fluorescein has a higher concentration of uptake in areas where there has been disruption of the cornea or sclera. Under a Wood's light, the injured area fluoresces as a bright yellow-green.
➤ Detection of porphyrins in the urine. These appear bright red.

RATIONALE

➤ Skin—To allow the clinician to differentiate dermatologic presentation of types of bacterial, fungal, and pigmented lesions found on the skin
➤ Eye—To allow the visual assessment of injuries to the cornea and conjunctiva with fluorescein staining
➤ Urine—To screen for **porphyria**—a rare metabolic disorder
➤ Clinical evaluation of dermatitis, the eye, or urine by the unaided eye alone may result in an inappropriate assessment and render an unsuccessful treatment regimen.

TABLE 3•1 FLUORESCENCE OF LESIONS AND PARASITES WITH THE WOOD'S LIGHT

LEISON	FLUORESCENCE
Erythrasma	
Corynebacterium minutissimum	Varing shades of pink to coral red
Tinea Capitis (3 Varities)	
Microsporum audouinii	Brilliant green
M.canis	Brilliant green
Trichophyton schoenleinii	Pale green
Tinea Versicolor	Yellow to deep green
Pseudomonas Aeruginosa	Blue-green to green
Pigmentation Alterations	
Albinism	Cold bright white
Ash-leaf spot of tuberous sclerosis	Blue-white
Depigmentation	Cold bright white
Hypopigmentation	Blue-white
Hyperpigmentation	Purple-brown
Leprosy	Blue-white
Vitiligo	Blue-white
Squamous cell carcinoma[*]	Bright red
Common Parasitic Infestations	
Scabies	Magnification of track and/or mite
Pediculosis (*capitis, corporis, pubis*)	Visualization of louse

[*]The diagnosis of this dermatologic disorder should be made by pathologic assessment.

INDICATIONS

➤ Skin or hair lesions
➤ Corneal abrasion
➤ Suspicion of porphyria

CONTRAINDICATIONS

➤ None

PROCEDURE

Wood's Light—Skin

Equipment

➤ Wood's light
➤ Darkened room

Procedure

➤ Have the client position himself or herself comfortably.
➤ Explain to the client that the Wood's light has the same characteristics as

a typical black light; the room will be darkened, and the black light will be turned on to examine for fluorescence of the lesion in question.
➤ Have all lights turned off.
➤ Hold the Wood's light approximately 6 to 8 inches from the lesion in question, and observe the characteristics of the fluorescence of the lesion.

Bibliography

Green, C. (ed). (1987). *Handbook of adult primary care.* New York: John Wiley.
Driscoll, C., et al (1996) (3rd ed.). *The family practice desk reference.* St. Louis: Mosby.
Habif, T. (1996) (3rd ed.). *Clinical dermatology: A color guide to diagnosis and therapy.* St. Louis: Mosby.
Murtagh, J. (1995) (2nd ed.). *Practice tips.* New York: McGraw-Hill.
Pfenninger, J.L., and Fowler, G.C. (1994). *Procedures for primary care physicians.* St. Louis: Mosby.

Abscesses—Incision and Drainage
Furuncle, Felon, Paronychia, Pilonidal Cyst, Perianal Cyst

4

Margaret R. Colyar

CPT Code	
10060	Incision and drainage of abscess
10080	Incision and drainage of pilonidal cyst; simple
10081	Incision and drainage of pilonidal cyst; complicated
10140	Incision and drainage of hematoma or seroma or fluid collection

An abscess is a localized collection of pus surrounded by inflamed tissue in any part of the body. Types of abscess included in this chapter are
➤ **Furuncle** (boil)—an abscess of the hair follicle or sweat gland
➤ **Felon**—an abscess of the soft tissue of the terminal joint of the finger
➤ **Paronychia**—an abscess or cellulitis of the nail folds, usually the proximal and lateral edges

➤ **Pilonidal cyst**—an abscess located in the gluteal fold close to the anus, caused by an ingrown hair. One or more sinus openings may exist. Males are more prone than females to develop pilonidal cysts. Younger people have pilonidal cysts more often than the elderly.

➤ **Perianal cyst**—an abscess around or close to the anus

OVERVIEW

➤ Incidence unknown
➤ Causative organisms of most abscesses
  ➤ *Staphylococcus aureus*
  ➤ *Streptococcus* species
➤ Areas of most frequent occurrence of abscesses
  ➤ Extremities
  ➤ Under the breasts
  ➤ Axillae
  ➤ Buttocks
  ➤ Hair follicles

HEALTH PROMOTION/PREVENTION

➤ Cleanse skin daily with an antiseptic soap such as unscented Dial soap.
➤ Do not squeeze face lesions.
➤ Do not shave closely.
➤ Discourage nail biting and finger sucking.

RATIONALE

➤ To diminish pain
➤ To promote healing

INDICATIONS

➤ Collection of pus causing pain and/or not resolved by use of an antibiotic
➤ Small abscesses
➤ Small abscesses that enlarge
➤ Large abscesses

CONTRAINDICATIONS

➤ Abscesses on the face in the triangle of the bridge of the nose and corners of the mouth.
  ➤ Use conservative measures to decrease or prevent the chances for septic phlebitis and intracranial extension.
➤ Observe carefully and obtain a culture of the abscess from people with
  ➤ Debilitating disease
  ➤ Compromised immune system

▰ *Informed consent required*

PROCEDURE

Incision and Drainage—Furuncle

Equipment

➤ Antiseptic skin cleanser
➤ Topical anesthetic—ethyl chloride or verruca freeze kit
➤ 1% to 2% lidocaine with or without epinephrine
➤ 3- to 10-mL syringe
➤ 27- to 30-gauge, $^1/_2$-inch needle
➤ 4 × 4 gauze—sterile
➤ Tube gauze—optional for use on fingers
➤ No. 11 scalpel
➤ Drape—sterile
➤ Gloves—sterile
➤ Curved **hemostats**—sterile
➤ **Iodoform** gauze—$^1/_4$- to 1-inch
➤ Culture swab
➤ Scissors—sterile
➤ Tape

Procedure

➤ Position the client with the abscess easily accessible.
➤ Cleanse the abscess and a 3-inch-diameter area surrounding the abscess with antiseptic skin cleanser.
➤ Drape the abscess with a sterile drape.
➤ Put on gloves.
➤ Perform a field block by anesthetizing the perimeter around the abscess with 1% or 2% lidocaine with or without epinephrine. Do *not* inject lidocaine into the abscess because it does not work well in an acidic medium. If the client cannot tolerate a field block, topical anesthesia can be used to freeze the top of the abscess if desired.
➤ Using the No. 11 scalpel, incise the abscess deeply enough and long enough to allow easy drainage of the purulent material and to prevent premature closure of the wound (Fig. 4–1).
➤ Obtain a culture (Fig. 4–2) by inserting the culturette deeply into the wound cavity or by withdrawing purulent drainage with a syringe and 18-gauge needle. In case of a breast abscess that is not subareolar, a biopsy should be done.
➤ Explore the abscess cavity. Break down any sacs or **septa** using curved hemostats (Fig. 4–3).
➤ After expressing all purulent material, pack with iodoform gauze, leaving a small amount protruding from the wound (Fig. 4–4).
➤ Dress with sterile gauze.

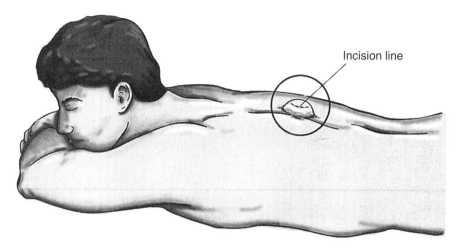

Incision line

FIGURE 4 • 1 Incise the abscess deep and wide to allow easy drainage and to prevent premature closure.

Incision and Drainage of Abscess—Paronychia

Additional Equipment for Paronychia

➤ 1% to 2% lidocaine without epinephrine
➤ If **subungual,** sterile paperclip or cautery tip

Procedure

➤ Position client with the abscess easily accessible.
➤ Cleanse the abscess and a 3-inch-diameter area around the abscess with antiseptic skin cleanser.

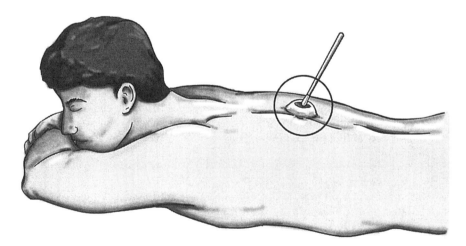

FIGURE 4 • 2 Obtain a culture from deep inside the wound cavity.

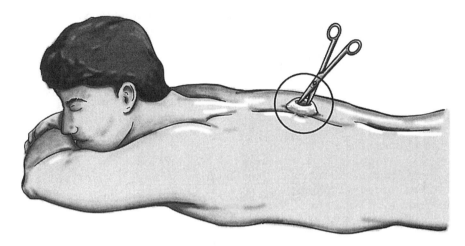

FIGURE 4 • 3 Break down any sacs or septa using hemostats.

➤ Drape the abscess with a sterile drape.
➤ Put on gloves.
➤ Perform a field block by anesthetizing the perimeter around the abscess with 1% or 2% lidocaine without epinephrine. Do *not* inject lidocaine into the abscess because it does not work well in an acidic medium. If the client cannot tolerate a field block, topical anesthesia can be used to freeze the top of the abscess if desired.

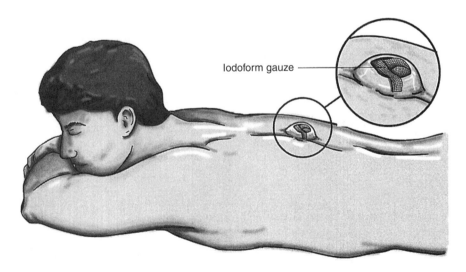

Iodoform gauze

FIGURE 4 • 4 Pack the wound with iodoform gauze, leaving a small amount protruding from the wound.

➤ If the matrix is involved and an abscess has formed a subungual (under the fingernail) tract, use a hot paperclip or cautery tip to bore through the nail to drain pus and blood.
  ➢ Partial removal of nail plate may be needed (see Chapter 10).
➤ Lift the proximal nail fold. If purulent material is not released freely, incise the skin at the point of highest tension using the No. 11 scalpel.
➤ Obtain a culture by inserting the culturette deeply into the wound cavity or by withdrawing purulent drainage with a syringe and 18-gauge needle.
➤ Explore the abscess cavity. Break down any sacs or septa using curved hemostats.
➤ After expressing all purulent material, pack with iodoform gauze, leaving a small amount protruding from the wound.
➤ Dress with sterile gauze.
➤ Cover with tube gauze.

Incision and Drainage—Pilonidal Cyst

Additional Equipment for Pilonidal Cyst

➤ Cotton-tipped applicator

Procedure

➤ Same as incision and drainage of furuncle except
  ➢ Position patient in left lateral or lithotomy position.
  ➢ Leave wound open to drain and heal by secondary intention (delayed closure 8 to 12 weeks).
  ➢ Probe sinus tracts with cotton-tipped applicator. If deep, REFER to a surgeon.
  ➢ If superficial (less than 5 mm), perform elliptical excision for pilonidal sinus.

Incision and Drainage—Perianal Abscess

Can be done if perianal or ischiorectal; if supralevator or intersphincteric, REFER to a surgeon.

Additional Equipment for Perianal Abscess

➤ 0.9% sodium chloride
➤ Peripads

Procedure

➤ Position patient in left lateral or lithotomy position.
➤ Perform a digital examination and/or anoscopy (see Chapter 89) to look for internal opening (i.e., fistula; usually 50% incidence).
➤ If a fistula is not present
  ➢ Drape the abscess with sterile drapes.
  ➢ Cleanse the area with an antiseptic skin cleanser.

- ➤ Use topical anesthetic to freeze the top of the abscess. Local anesthetic is not practical because an acidic environment does not respond well to anesthesia.
- ➤ Using the No. 11 scalpel, incise over the area of greatest tension.
- ➤ Obtain a culture by inserting the culturette deeply into the wound cavity or by withdrawing purulent drainage with a syringe and 18-gauge needle.
- ➤ After expressing all purulent material, irrigate with 0.9% sodium chloride.
- ➤ Pack with iodoform gauze, leaving a small amount hanging from the wound.
- ➤ Dress with sterile gauze or peripad.
➤ To relieve pain when fistula is present, insert a 16- to 18-gauge needle into the abscess and withdraw purulent material. REFER to a surgeon.

Client Instructions

➤ Return to the office in 2 days to have dressing changed.
➤ Observe for signs and symptoms of infection, such as
  - ➤ Yellow or green drainage
  - ➤ Red streaks
  - ➤ Increasing pain
  - ➤ Elevated temperature
➤ If symptoms of infection occur, return to the office.
➤ Prevent recurrence of the abscess by taking an antibiotic—dicloxacillin 250 mg four times a day, cefadroxil 500 mg twice a day, or cephalexin 500 mg three times a day.
➤ Contrary to popular belief, incised abscesses are painful and usually require narcotic analgesia for the first 24 hours. For pain relief, take Tylenol No. 3 every 4 to 6 hours for the first 24 hours, then take ibuprofen.
➤ If you had a pilonidal or perianal cyst drained, take a sitz bath with warm water three or four times per day. You may cleanse the area by using the shower or irrigating the area with a squeeze bottle.
➤ If the abscess recurs, return to the office for evaluation.
➤ If the abscess was in an extremity, observe for cellulitis and/or gangrene.

BIBLIOGRAPHY

Armstrong, J.H., and Barcia, P.J. (1994). Pilonidal sinus disease. The conservative approach. *Arch Surg,* 129, 914–917.
Johnson, R.A. (1995). Cyst removal. Punch, push, pull. *Skin,* 1(1), 14–15.
Pfenninger, J.L., and Fowler, G.C. (1994). *Procedures for primary care physicians.* St. Louis: Mosby.
Tosti, A., et al (1992). Role of foods in the pathogenesis of chronic paronychia. *J Am Acad Dermatol,* 27(11), 706–710.

BITES
ANTS, ARTHROPODS (SPIDERS), BEES, AND WASPS

5

CYNTHIA R. EHRHARDT

CPT Code	
989.5	Fire ant bite
919.4	Superficial bite without mention of infection (includes nonvenomous spider bites, non–fire ant bites, bee bites, and wasp bites)
919.5	Superficial nonvenomous infected bite
989.5	Bee sting (allergic or shock)
989.5	Spider bite, venomous

Bites are puncture wounds and tears in the skin, with injection of a **proteolytic,** venomous chemical, by an insect. Treatment of a bite depends on the type of offending organism, depth of the puncture, and extent of the tear in the skin.

OVERVIEW

➤ Incidence—In the Southeastern United States, at least 60% of the population has been stung by these insects.
➤ **Hemolysis** and **cutaneous** infarct lead to necrosis of tissue at the site over a period of hours to days. Extent of the hemolysis and cutaneous infarct determines treatment regimen.
➤ Severe reactions present with symptoms such as
  ➤ Generalized urticaria
  ➤ Angioedema
  ➤ Respiratory difficulty
  ➤ Change in level of consciousness
➤ Clinical manifestations of insect bites (Table 5–1)
➤ Identification of type of spider (Table 5–2)
➤ Medications used with insect bites (Table 5–3)

HEALTH PROMOTION/PREVENTION

➤ Use natural organic and pesticide chemical controls.
➤ Observe for and avoid anthills.

TABLE 5•1 CLINICAL MANIFESTATIONS OF INSECT BITES

Fire Ant and Harvester Ant Bite
➤ Reactions of a mild-to-moderate nature will present as a localized response (urticaria wheal, localized induration, and erythema) and initially be painful, but decrease over time.
➤ Have small whitish pustule, central core with minimal erythema after the first 24 hr. After 48 hr, the white pustule remains but erythema subsides.

Brown Recluse and Black Window
➤ Brown recluse bites
  ➤ Painful
  ➤ Blue cyanotic center surrounded by pallor and erythema
  ➤ Necrotic ulcers within hours to days
➤ Black window bites
  ➤ Sharp stinging
  ➤ Easy to overlook— white center with trace erythema
  ➤ Necrotic ulcers within hours to days

TABLE 5•2 IDENTIFICATION OF TYPE OF SPIDER

Brown Recluse Spiders
➤ Rarely exceed 5 mm in size
➤ Fiddle shape on back — 0.5 to 2 cm in length
➤ Hairy

Black Widow Spiders
➤ Black to dark brown with a characteristic "red hourglass" on the ventral surface of the body

---

TABLE 5•3 OVERVIEW OF MEDICATIONS USED WITH INSECT BITES

Antibiotic Therapy
Topical or oral antibiotics have not been found to be effective with fire ant, spider, bee, or wasp bites unless evidence of secondary infection is present.

Antihistamines
May be of benefit in fire ant, bee, and wasp bites. Use of antihistamines such as diphenhydramine (Benadryl) appears to reduce localized reactions and **pruritus**. Use with brown recluse and black widow bites has not been of benefit.

Oral Steroids
Have been occasionally beneficial with brown recluse and black widow bites in reducing localized inflammation if greater than 2 cm in diameter. Use in lesions greater than 14 cm is recommended. Dosage: 1 mg/kg body weight. Oral dapsone 50 to 100 mg/day has been effective in reducing the incidence of **latrodectism** (abdominal rectus spasm) and hemolytic anemia resulting from black widow bites.

➤ Avoid going barefoot in grassy areas.
➤ Thoroughly check all stored clothing for spiders.
➤ Before entering bed, inspect bedding for spiders.
➤ Avoid bright colors, perfumes, and scented products that can attract and agitate bees and wasps.
➤ Carry "bee-sting kit" if there is a known history of moderate-to-severe reaction to bee and wasp stings when out in known environmental habitat of these insects.

RATIONALE

➤ To prevent infection
➤ To diminish inflammation
➤ To diminish discomfort

INDICATIONS

➤ Bite by ant, spider, bee, or wasp

CONTRAINDICATIONS

➤ None

PROCEDURE

Bites

Equipment

➤ Basin—sterile
➤ Povidone-iodine (Betadine) soak or antibacterial soap
➤ Gloves—sterile
➤ Meat tenderizer paste—1 part water mixed with 1 part meat tenderizer
➤ Epinephrine 1:1000 vial(s)
➤ 1-mL syringe (tuberculin) with needle
➤ Ice pack
➤ Magnifying lens—optional
➤ Adhesive bandage (Band-Aid) or dressing if indicated

Procedure

➤ Inspect area for puncture wound. (In early spider bites, it is possible to visualize the two-fang puncture bite.)
➤ Avoid warm compresses to the bite area. Heat causes vasodilation, allowing bite venom to be circulated more quickly.

Bee or Wasp Stings

➤ If bite has occurred within 5 minutes, apply a paste of meat tenderizer (which is a proteolytic agent).

Fire Ant and Spider Bites

➤ Gently clean the bite area and soak in cool, soapy water for 10 to 15 minutes.
➤ Dry gently.
➤ No dressing is required unless open, exudative, and gaping wound.
➤ Apply an ice pack for 12 to 24 hours.

Client Instructions

➤ Keep the wound clean and dry.
➤ Apply cool compresses to the bite for 12 to 24 hours to lessen localized inflammation.
➤ Antibiotics are not required.
➤ Observe for signs and symptoms of infection, such as
  ➤ Increase in pain after 24 hours
  ➤ Increase in temperature
  ➤ Redness or swelling
  ➤ Yellow or greenish drainage
  ➤ Foul odor
➤ If any of the signs and symptoms of infection are found, return to the office.
➤ To relieve pain
  ➤ Acetaminophen may be taken every 4 to 6 hours as needed for mild pain for first 24 hours.
  ➤ Ibuprofen or other nonsteroidal anti-inflammatory drugs should be avoided for the first 24 hours to lessen bleeding.
  ➤ After 24 hours, alternating nonsteroidals with acetaminophen may be beneficial.
  ➤ Tylenol No. 3 may be used for severe pain.
➤ Wound cleaning—The primary goal is to prevent secondary infection. Topical antibiotic ointment has not shown benefit or harm when applied to the bite.
  ➤ Use hydrogen peroxide to remove any crusts.
  ➤ Wash gently with soapy water and blot area dry.
  ➤ Unless the wound is oozing, do not cover.
  ➤ Return to the office in 2 days for moderately severe brown recluse and black widow spider bites. If mild bite, return to the office in 5 to 7 days.

BIBLIOGRAPHY

American Family Physician Tips. (1992). *Brown recluse spider bites in pregnant women.* 45(6), 652–659.
American Family Physician Tips. (1992). *Black widow envenomation.* 46(6), 193–204.
American Medical Association. (1996). *Physicians' current procedural terminology.* Chicago: Author.
Habif, T. (1996) (3rd ed.). *Clinical dermatology: A color guide to diagnosis and therapy.* St. Louis: Mosby.
Matzen, R., and Lang, R. (1993). *Clinical preventive medicine.* St. Louis: Mosby.
Miller, T. (1992). Latrodectism. Bite of black widow spider. *Am Fam Physician,* 45(1), 45–56.
Murtagh, J. (1995) (2nd ed.). *Practice tips.* New York: McGraw-Hill.
Pfenninger, J.L., and Fowler, G.C. (1994). *Procedures for primary care physicians.* St. Louis: Mosby.

6

BITES
CATS, DOGS, AND HUMANS

CPT Code	
12001–07	Simple repair of superficial wounds of scalp, neck, axillae, external genitalia, trunk, or extremities
12031–37	Layer closure of wounds of scalp, axillae, trunk, or extremities (not hands or feet)
12041–47	Layer closure of wounds of neck, hands, feet, or external genitalia

Bites include punctures, tearing wounds, crush injuries, or lacerations into the skin caused by the teeth of animals or humans. Children ages 5 to 14 years account for 30% to 50% of victims of all mammalian bites.

OVERVIEW

➤ Incidence—1% of all emergency department visits
  ➤ Cat and dog bites—0.5 to 1 million per year
  ➤ Human bites—incidence unknown
➤ Complicating factors
  ➤ Cat and dog bites—Saliva contains gram-negative bacteria—*Pasteurella multocida*
  ➤ Human bites—Saliva contains 10 bacteria per milliliter, including the gram-positive bacteria *Staphylococcus aureus* (3% are resistant to antibiotics) and streptococci and the gram-negative bacteria *Proteus* species, *Escherichia coli*, *Pseudomonas* species, *Neisseria* species, and *Klebsiella* species.

HEALTH PROMOTION/PREVENTION

➤ Teach appropriate behavior around animals.
➤ Do *not* provoke attacks.

RATIONALE

➤ To prevent bacterial infection in the wound
➤ To promote wound healing

INDICATIONS

➤ Necrosis

CONTRAINDICATIONS

➤ Bite on the face, REFER to plastic surgeon or emergency department.
➤ Blood supply has been disrupted, REFER to emergency department.

☑ *Informed consent required*

Determine the following
➤ Origin of the bite
➤ Patient (if younger than 4 years old and older than 50 years old, there is a greater risk of infection)
➤ Severity
➤ Location
➤ Size
➤ Depth
➤ Amount of contamination (puncture wound has greatest risk of infection) and amount of time that has elapsed between the bite and treatment. Keep in mind that an area of poor vascularity is at greater risk for infection and poor healing. Do a culture and Gram's stain of the wound.

PROCEDURE

Bites

Equipment

➤ Basin—sterile
➤ Povidone-iodine (Betadine) soak—povidone-iodine solution and 0.9% sterile sodium chloride mixed 50/50
➤ Gloves—sterile
➤ Syringe—20 to 60 mL
➤ 2 needles—27- to 30-gauge and 18- to 20-gauge
➤ 1% lidocaine
➤ Scissors—sterile
➤ Curved hemostats—sterile
➤ Forceps—sterile
➤ Suture—No. 3-0 to 5-0 nylon
➤ 4 × 4 gauze—sterile
➤ Culture swab
➤ Topical antibiotic—Bactroban or Polysporin
➤ Iodoform gauze—$^1/_4$- to 1-inch

Procedure

➤ Culture the wound if the bite is 72 hours old. If the client has an elevated temperature, get a complete blood count, erythrocyte sedimentation rate, and possibly blood cultures.

➤ If area of bite was on hands or feet, soak in povidone-iodine soak (50% povidone-iodine and 50% 0.9% sodium chloride) for 10 to 15 minutes. If unable to soak, irrigate with 250 to 500 mL of povidone-iodine/sodium chloride solution.

➤ Anesthetize wound with 1% lidocaine.

➤ Position the patient for comfort with the injured part easily accessible.

➤ Cleanse the skin with antiseptic skin cleanser.

➤ Irrigate the wound with 100 to 500 mL of sterile sodium chloride vigorously, using the syringe and 18-gauge needle.

➤ Put on gloves.

➤ Remove any devitalized tissue or foreign objects.

➤ Insert iodoform gauze snugly with $1/2$-inch protruding from the wound.

➤ Suture if the wound is clean and not a puncture.

➤ Apply topical antibiotic.

➤ Apply gauze dressing.

Client Instructions

➤ To prevent infection, abscess, cellulitis, septicemia, or osteomyelitis, take oral antibiotics (pencillin, amoxicillin/clavulanate [Augmentin], or erythromycin as prescribed) for 5 to 7 days.

➤ Observe for signs and symptoms of infection, such as
  ➣ Increase in pain after 24 hours
  ➣ Increase in temperature
  ➣ Redness or swelling
  ➣ Yellow or greenish drainage
  ➣ Foul odor

➤ If any of these symptoms develop, return to the office immediately.

➤ To relieve pain
  ➣ Take Tylenol No. 3 every 4 to 6 hours for 24 hours, then acetamino-phen or ibuprofen every 4 to 6 hours for mild pain relief.
  ➣ If fingers or toes are involved, exercise (wiggle) them frequently.
  ➣ Elevate the wounded part above the heart for 48 hours as much as possible.
  ➣ Immobilize the wounded part for 48 hours.
  ➣ Apply ice pack intermittently for the first 24 hours.

➤ Rabies—Consider rabies prophylaxis if the bite was from an animal.

➤ Tetanus—Tetanus prophylaxis is needed if not received within 10 years.

➤ Return to the office in 2 days for a recheck.

BIBLIOGRAPHY

Brandenberg, M.A., et al (1995). Hand injuries. Assessing the damage, closing the wound, preventing infection. *Consultant,* December, 1777–1786.

Lewis, K.T., and Stiles, M. (1995). Management of cat and dog bites. *Am Fam Physician,* 52(2), 479–485.

O'Boyle, C.M., et al (1985). *Emergency care, the first 24 hours.* Norwalk, CT: Appleton-Century-Crofts.
Swartz, G.R. (1992). *Principles and practice of emergency medicine.* Philadelphia: Saunders.
Wiley, J.F. (1990). Mammalian bites. Review of evaluation and management. *Clin Pediatr,* 29(5), 283–287.

7 BURNS—DEBRIDEMENT

CYNTHIA R. EHRHARDT

CPT Code

16000	Initial treatment of first-degree burn when no more than local treatment is required
16010	Dressing and/or debridement, initial or subsequent, under anesthesia
16015	Dressing and/or major debridement, initial or subsequent, under anesthesia—medium or large area
16020	Dressing and/or debridement, without anesthesia, of a small area
16025	Dressing and/or debridement, without anesthesia, of a medium area (whole extremity)
16030	Dressing and/or debridement, without anesthesia, of a large area (more than one extremity)

Document percentage of body surface area and depth of burn.

A burn is trauma to skin from exposure to heat, flame, radiation, chemicals (acid or alkali), or other agent that results in a loss of skin integrity. Burns can be described in two ways:
➤ The extent of body surface area (BSA) involved (Fig. 7–1)
➤ The depth or amount of tissue destroyed (Table 7–1)

OVERVIEW

➤ Incidence
  ➤ An estimated 2 million burns occur per year, with 25% of these requiring medical attention.

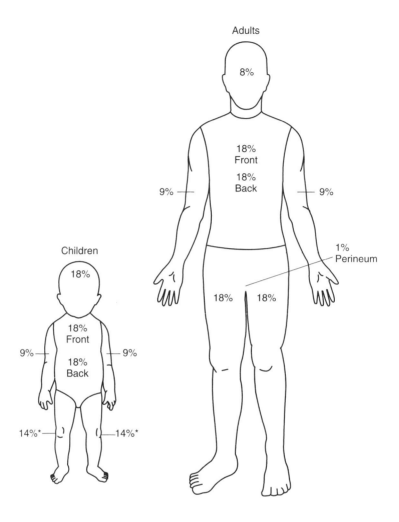

Adults

8%

18%
Front
18%
Back

9%   9%

1%
Perineum

18%   18%

Children

18%

18%
Front

9%   9%

18%
Back

14%*   14%*

* Subtract 1% from head for each year over one.
* Add 1/2% to each leg for each year over one.

FIGURE 7 • 1 Rule of nines.

> An estimated 100,000 burn patients require hospitalization, and 10,000 die from their burn injuries each year.
► Complications
  > Death
  > Temporary or permanent disfigurement
  > Temporary or permanent loss of function
  > Temporary or permanent disability
  > Psychosocial trauma

TABLE 7•1 DEPTH OF BURN INJURY

➤ First degree
  ➤ Superficial injection and redness of skin that blanches with pressure and has intact sensation
  ➤ Varying depth of involvement of the epidermal and dermal layers of skin with intact dermal appendages such as hair and sweat and sebaceous glands
➤ Second degree
  ➤ Superficial partial-thickness burn
    • Varying depth, but more involvement of dermal layer.
    • Intact dermal appendages such as hair and sweat and sebaceous glands.
    • Vascular dilation with accompanying blisters and bullae are common.
  ➤ Deep partial-thickness burn
    • Some vasodilation of deep blood vessels
    • Wet or dry and red or waxy-appearing skin that has decreased sensation
    • Vasodilation of the blood vessels resulting in red, weepy, and painful skin that can be easily wiped away
    • Painful sensation with or without pressure to the tissue
  ➤ Third degree
    • Loss of all anatomic structures of skin
    • Thrombosis and coagulation of blood vessels with or without involvement of deeper anatomic structures of muscle, ligament, and bone
    • White and charred tissue with absence of blanching
    • Sensation intact only to deep pressure

➤ Common causes are exposure to
  ➤ Hot liquids
  ➤ Steam
  ➤ Flames
  ➤ Flash electricity
  ➤ Radiation, including sunlight
  ➤ Hot solid materials
  ➤ Caustic chemicals
  ➤ Explosions resulting from chemical mixtures
  ➤ Severe cold
➤ Burn assessment includes systemic and skin systems
  ➤ Location and percentage of BSA involvement
    Rule of nines (see Fig. 7–1)
  ➤ Observation for evidence of respiratory distress
    Nasal flaring
    Intercostal retractions
    Dyspnea
    Chest pain
    Pale and/or **cyanotic**
    Evaluation of cardiovascular status (blood pressure and pulse)

HEALTH PROMOTION/PREVENTION

Health promotion is focused on eliminating situations that can result in injury to the skin. These measures include
➤ Promotion of safety habits
➤ Use of protective clothing when working with agents that can traumatize skin
➤ Promotion of a safe environment
Prevention includes
➤ Avoiding sunburn by use of sunscreens, generally skin protection factor (SPF) 15 or greater
➤ Turning hot water heaters to less than 120° F
➤ Keeping cooking pot handles pointed away from stove edge so that children cannot reach up and pull hot liquids onto themselves
➤ Keeping curling irons, irons, and hair dryers out of reach of children
➤ Buying stove guards, automatic coffeemakers, and fireproof portable heaters
➤ Using full-glove pot holders
➤ Temperature-testing all food
➤ Wearing gloves and goggles when mixing and using household chemicals
➤ Keeping all chemicals and caustic agents (e.g., batteries) stored in an elevated location and locked away from children
➤ Disposing of oily rags properly
➤ Storing flammables, including cigarette lighters and matches, properly and not smoking around flammable items or in bed
➤ Ensuring that protective equipment is selected, maintained, and used properly when working around chemical and/or caustic agents
➤ Using electrical outlet covers and ground-fault interrupter plugs to protect children from electrical shock
➤ Installing smoke detectors
➤ Having a planned fire evacuation route for home and work
➤ Having access to fire extinguishers and knowing how to use them
➤ Being cautious when using chemicals

OPTIONS

➤ First-degree burns—Treat in the office with
  ➤ Analgesics
  ➤ Antipyretics
  ➤ Skin lubricants
➤ Second-degree burns—superficial—Treat in the office with
  ➤ Thorough cleansing
  ➤ Removal of blisters
  ➤ Topical antibiotics
  ➤ Observation for secondary infection
➤ Second-degree burns—deep partial thickness—REFER to emergency department of nearest hospital
➤ Third-degree burns—Stabilize and transport patient to an emergency facility

Emergency Treatment for Stabilization and Transportation

➤ If symptoms of hypovolemia are present, establish two intravenous lines using large-bore angiocaths (16-gauge preferred in adults and 18-gauge in children) with an intravenous solution of Ringer's lactate. Rate is based on the following formula: (2 to 4 mL of Ringer's lactate per kg of body weight) $\times$ (percentage of BSA burned) = the amount of fluid replacement in the first 24 hours (2 mL $\times$ 70 kg $\times$ 50 BSA = 7000 mL); 50% of the solution should be given over the first 8 hours.
➤ Insert nasogastric tube and Foley catheter.
➤ Keep client warm.
➤ Apply sterile or clean sheets over the burned area.
Hospitalization is required based on burn center referral criteria
➤ Second-degree to third-degree burns, more than 10% of BSA burned if the patient is younger than age 10 or older than age 50
➤ Second-degree to third-degree burns with more than 20% of BSA damaged
➤ Second-degree to third-degree burns with a serious possibility of functional or cosmetic impairment (face, hands, feet, genitalia, perineum, major joints)
➤ Third-degree burns over greater than 5% of BSA
➤ Inhalation, electrical burns, and chemical burns that impair function or cause cosmetic damage

RATIONALE

➤ To minimize scarring and contractures
➤ To prevent infection
➤ To provide pain relief
➤ To decrease the extent of the burn
➤ To diminish the complications caused by the burn
➤ To promote optimal healing

INDICATIONS

➤ First-degree burns
➤ Second-degree superficial partial-thickness burns over less than 20% of BSA

CONTRAINDICATIONS

➤ Suspected deep second-degree or third-degree burn
➤ Suspected tendon, muscle, or bone involvement
➤ Meets criteria for hospitalization
  ➤ Circumferential burns of the neck, trunk, arms, or legs
  ➤ All but minimal burns of the eyes, ears, feet, perineum, genitalia, or hands
  ➤ Presence of other trauma unless minor
  ➤ Presence of any condition that may compromise wound healing, such as diabetes mellitus, cardiovascular disease, or immunodeficiency disorders

> Wounds for which the estimated time for closure is greater than
  3 weeks
> Poor social situations, such as child abuse or poor compliance with
  wound care instructions
> Younger than 2 years of age or extremely elderly (frail elderly)
> Suspected inhalation exposure

PROCEDURE

Burn—Debridement

Equipment

- Towels or sheets—sterile
- Gloves—sterile
- 3-mL syringe
- 25- or 27-gauge, $^1/_2$-inch needle
- 30- to 60-mL irrigation syringe
- 1% or 2% lidocaine without epinephrine
- 0.09% sodium chloride—sterile
- 4 × 4 gauze—sterile
- Gauze wrap—sterile
- Tape
- Topical antimicrobial cream, ointment, or medicated gauze (Table 7–2)
- Sterile suture set (prepackaged or self-made) should include
  - Curved and straight hemostats
  - Needle holders ($4^1/_2$- and 6-inch)
  - Forceps with teeth
  - Scalpel (No. 11 or 15 blade)
  - Iris scissors
  - Cup to hold sterile sodium chloride solution
  - 4 × 4 sterile gauze

Procedure

- Put on gloves.
- Anesthetize the wound by local or digital block.

TABLE 7•2 TOPICAL ANTIMICROBIALS

NAME	SPECTRUM	COST
Silver sulfadiazine (Silvadene)	Good broad spectrum; covers *Staphylococcus*	Expensive
Furacin	Good broad bactericidal; covers *Pseudomonas* and Enterobacteriaceae	Expensive
Povidone-iodine (Betadine)	Superficial; can easily become skin irritant; cannot be mixed with silver sulfadiazine	Reasonable
Silver nitrate	Poor penetration; used primarily when sensitive to other therapy agents; prone to stain skin	Reasonable

➤ Irrigate the wound sufficiently with 0.09% sodium chloride (usually 150 mL) to clean any cellular debris or residue.
➤ Blot the wound dry with sterile 4 × 4 gauze.
➤ Remove excess tissue, and drain any bullae or blisters present using iris scissors or scalpel blade.
➤ Apply liberal amount of antimicrobial ointment to the wound.
➤ Cover with 4 × 4 and dressing gauze wrap without restriction of range of motion or function.

Client Instructions

➤ Observe for signs of infection including
  ➤ Increased redness and warmth at the site
  ➤ Red streaks
  ➤ Swelling with yellow or green drainage
➤ Keep the area as clean as possible
➤ Topical antimicrobials, cream or ointment, usually are recommended for the first 7 days of treatment. Oral antibiotic therapy is required if secondary infection has occurred.
➤ Change the dressing twice a day for the first 7 days, then every 24 hours.
  ➤ When redressing the wound, if the dressing adheres to the wound, saturate the dressing with 0.09% sodium chloride and remove.
➤ If an arm, leg, hand, or foot is involved
  ➤ Keep elevated above the heart for 24 to 48 hours to reduce swelling.
  ➤ Perform range of motion exercises three to four times per day.
➤ Pain medication
  ➤ Avoid nonsteroidal drug usage because these drugs tend to retard healing.
  ➤ Take Tylenol No. 3 every 4 hours as needed initially, then acetaminophen.
➤ The deeper the burn, the greater the risk of permanent skin color changes.
➤ Receive a tetanus injection if none has been given in the last 5 years.
➤ Avoid sunburn to the burned area for 6 months to 1 year because of increased risk of reinjury.
➤ Return to the office in 2 days for recheck, then weekly.

BIBLIOGRAPHY

American Medical Association (1996). *Physician's current procedural terminology.* Chicago: Author.
Calistro, A. (1993). Burn care basics and beyond. *RN,* 56(3), 26–32.
Dlugasch, L. (1996). Emergency burn care for the first 24 hours. *Bert Rodgers school of continuing education home study courses for Florida nurses.* Sarasota, FL: Bert Rodgers.
Peate, W. (1992). Outpatient management of burns. *Am Fam Physician,* 45(3), 1321–1332.
Pfenninger, J.L., and Fowler, G.C. (1994). *Procedures for primary care physicians.* St. Louis: Mosby.
Trott, A. (1991). *Wounds and lacerations: Emergency care and closure.* St. Louis: Mosby.
Thelan, L., et al (1994). *Critical care nursing: Diagnosis and management.* St. Louis: Mosby.

8 DIGITAL NERVE BLOCK

MARGARET R. COLYAR

CPT Code	
01460	Anesthesia for all procedures on integumentary system of lower leg, ankle, and foot
01800	Anesthesia for all procedures on integumentary system of the forearm, wrist, and hand

Digital nerve blocks produce sensory anesthesia to selected toes and fingers before surgical repair, suture application, dislocation reduction, and nail procedures.

OVERVIEW
- ➤ Incidence is unknown.
- ➤ Understanding of the neuroanatomy of the digit is necessary to perform the digital block correctly (Fig. 8–1).

RATIONALE
- ➤ To diminish pain during invasive procedures

INDICATIONS
- ➤ Nail removal
- ➤ Ingrown toenail procedures
- ➤ Felon
- ➤ **Paronychia**
- ➤ Sutures to fingers or toes
- ➤ Dislocation reduction
- ➤ Removal of foreign body from fingers or toes

CONTRAINDICATIONS
- ➤ None

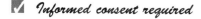 *Informed consent required*

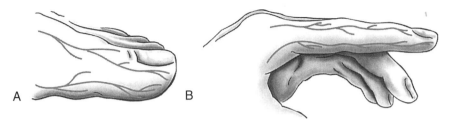

Figure 8 • 1 Neuroanatomy of the toe (A) and finger (B).

PROCEDURE
Digital Nerve Block

Equipment

➤ Antiseptic skin cleanser
➤ Gloves—nonsterile
➤ 3-mL syringe
➤ 27- to 30-gauge, $^1/_2$- to 1-inch needle
➤ 1% lidocaine—2 to 3 mL—*No* epinephrine should be used on digits.
➤ 4 × 4 gauze—sterile

Procedure

➤ Position the client supine with digit easily accessible.
➤ Cleanse the hand or foot with topical antiseptic skin cleanser.
➤ Put on gloves.

FINGERS

➤ Insert needle at 45-degree angle.
  ➤ Along the palmar crease on either side of the digit
  ➤ On anterior surface of the digit close to the bone (Fig. 8–2)

TOES

➤ Insert the needle toward the plantar surface on both sides of the toe.
➤ Injection sites are below the nail on the outer edges of the toe. Be careful not to pierce the plantar skin surface.
➤ Do not forget to aspirate the syringe before injecting lidocaine. If no blood returns in the syringe, lidocaine can be injected safely.
➤ Inject 1 to 2 mL of lidocaine while withdrawing the needle. Do not withdraw the needle from the skin.
➤ Redirect the needle across the extensor surface, and insert the needle further. Inject 0.5 mL of lidocaine while withdrawing needle.
  ➤ Repeat procedure on opposite side of the toe.
➤ Massage gently.
➤ Wait 5 to 10 minutes.

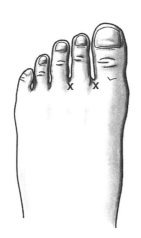
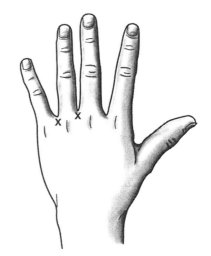

Figure 8 • 2 Injection sites.

Client Instructions

➤ Sensation to the finger or toe should return within 1 to 2 hours. If this does not occur, call the practitioner's office.

BIBLIOGRAPHY

Brandenberg, M.A., Hawkins, L., and Quick, G. (1995). Hand injuries. Assessing the damage, closing the wound, preventing infection. *Consultant,* December, 1777–1786.

Kroop, K., Trott, A., and Syverud, S. (1994). Comparison of digital versus metacarpal blocks for repair of finger injuries. *Ann Emerg Med,* 23(6), 1296–1300.

Saunders, C.E., and Ho, M.T. (1992). *Current emergency diagnosis and treatment.* Norwalk, CT: Appleton & Lange.

Swartz, G.R. (1992). *Principles and practices of emergency medicine.* Philadelphia: Saunders.

FISHHOOK REMOVAL

MARGARET R. COLYAR • CYNTHIA R. EHRHARDT

CPT Code	
10120	Incision and removal of foreign body, subcutaneous tissues; simple
10121	Incision and removal of foreign body, subcutaneous tissues; complicated

The removal of a fishhook from subcutaneous tissue can be accomplished using one of three common methods or the angiocath method. The common methods include (1) pull-through, (2) barb sheath, and (3) angler's string-yank.

OVERVIEW

➤ Incidence
  ➤ Dependent on geographic location and season
  ➤ Estimated at approximately 0.5 million to 1 million incidents per year
➤ Most common organisms found with secondary infection
  ➤ Gram-positive: *Staphylococcus aureus,* streptococci
  ➤ Gram-negative: *Klebsiella, Proteus, Pseudomonas* (salt water)

HEALTH PROMOTION/PREVENTION

➤ Use good fishing technique.
➤ Handle all fishhooks carefully.
➤ Store all fishhooks properly.
➤ Do not reach blindly into poorly lighted tackle boxes.
➤ Do not fish close to another person casting a line.

OPTIONS

To remove fishhook with minimal local trauma
➤ *Method 1*—pull-through technique
  ➤ Use with a single- or a multiple-barbed fishhook when the angle of penetration is such that the hook can be pushed through the skin.
➤ *Method 2*—barb sheath method
  ➤ Use with a single-barbed fishhook that is large but not too deep in the skin.
➤ *Method 3*—angler's string-yank method
  ➤ Use with a single-barbed fishhook that is embedded in such a way that it cannot be removed with the pull-through method.

RATIONALE

➤ To relieve pain and anxiety
➤ To diminish bacterial infection
➤ To promote healing

INDICATIONS

➤ Fishhook lodged in any subcutaneous tissue
➤ Fishhook in or close to the eyes, REFER to a physician.
➤ Suspected ligament involvement, REFER to an orthopedic physician.
➤ Penetration into a large-bore artery, REFER to a surgeon.

✔ *Informed consent required*

PROCEDURE

Fishhook Removal

Equipment

- ➤ Methods 1, 2, and 3
  - ➤ Antiseptic skin cleanser
  - ➤ Gloves—nonsterile
  - ➤ 3-mL syringe
  - ➤ 27- to 30-gauge, $^1/_2$-inch needle
  - ➤ 1% lidocaine
- ➤ Method 1 only
  - ➤ Wire cutter—from a hardware store
  - ➤ Pliers or **hemostats**—nonsterile
- ➤ Method 2 only
  - ➤ 18-gauge, $1^1/_2$-inch needle
- ➤ Method 3 only
  - ➤ Silk suture or 2 to 3 feet of strong string or fishing line

Procedure

METHOD 1—PULL-THROUGH TECHNIQUE

- ➤ Position the client with fishhook easily accessible.
- ➤ Put on gloves.
- ➤ Cleanse skin around the fishhook with antiseptic.
- ➤ Inject 1% lidocaine using the 27- to 30-gauge needle at the point of the hook.
- ➤ Using pliers or hemostats, force the fishhook tip through the skin.
- ➤ Cut off the eye of the fishhook close to the skin with wire cutters.
- ➤ Attach pliers or hemostats to the sharp end of the hook and pull the hook out (Fig. 9–1).

METHOD 2—BARB SHEATH METHOD

- ➤ Position the client with fishhook easily accessible.
- ➤ Put on gloves.
- ➤ Cleanse the skin around the fishhook with antiseptic skin cleanser.
- ➤ Inject 1% lidocaine using the 27- to 30-gauge needle at the point of the hook.
- ➤ Insert the 18-gauge needle parallel to the hook with bevel toward the inside curve of the hook (Fig. 9–2). Attempt to cover the barb with the bevel of the needle.
- ➤ Back the hook and needle out as a unit.

METHOD 3—ANGLER'S STRING-YANK METHOD

- ➤ Position the client with fishhook easily accessible.
- ➤ Put on gloves.
- ➤ Cleanse the skin around the fishhook with antiseptic skin cleanser.

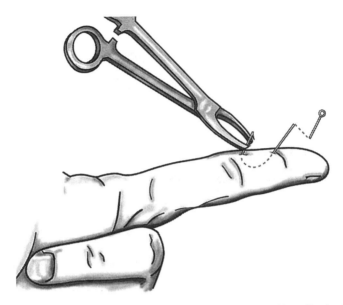

FIGURE 9 • 1 After cutting off the eye of the fishhook close to the skin, attach pliers or hemostats to the sharp end of the hook and pull the hook out.

➤ Inject 1% lidocaine using the 27- to 30-gauge needle at the point of the hook.
➤ Tie the string or suture around the hook where it enters the skin.
➤ With your finger, push the hook further into the skin, then lift the shank of the hook parallel to the skin (Fig. 9–3). The barb should be disengaged.

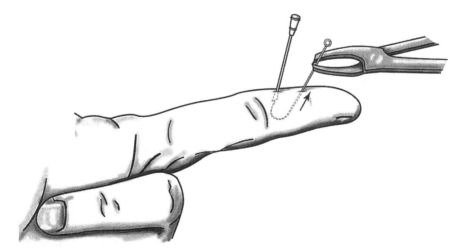

FIGURE 9 • 2 Cover the sharp end of the hook with an 18-gauge needle. Back the hook and needle out as a unit.

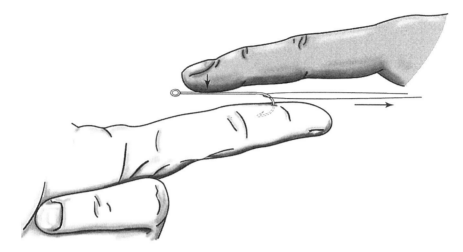

FIGURE 9 • 3 Push the fishhook downward with your finger. Using string or suture, quickly jerk the hook out.

➤ Using the string or suture, quickly jerk the hook out.

Client Instructions

➤ Tetanus prophylaxis is necessary if last tetanus injection was more than 5 years before the current incident.
➤ Observe for signs and symptoms of infection, such as
  ➤ Increase in pain after 24 hours
  ➤ Redness or swelling
  ➤ Yellow or greenish drainage
  ➤ Foul odor
➤ If any signs and symptoms of infection are found, return to the office.
➤ Take antibiotics as ordered for 5 days—cephalexin 500 mg three times per day or cefadroxil 500 mg twice per day—if infection is probable.
➤ Use pain medications as ordered. Take acetaminophen or ibuprofen every 4 to 6 hours as needed.
➤ Soak the affected part three times per day in warm salt water (1 teaspoon salt per 1 quart of water) for 2 days.
➤ Return to the office for a follow-up visit in 48 hours, then as needed.

BIBLIOGRAPHY

Brandenberg, M.A., Hawkins, L., and Quick, G.G. (1995). Hand injuries. Assessing the damage, closing the wound, preventing infection. *Consultant,* December, 1777–1786.
Pfenninger, J.L., and Fowler, G.C. (1994). *Procedures for primary care physicians.* St. Louis: Mosby.
Terrill, P. (1993). Fishhook removal. *Am Fam Physician,* 47(6), 1372.

10 NAIL REMOVAL

MARGARET R. COLYAR

CPT Code

11730–32   Nail removal, partial or complete

11750   Permanent nail removal, partial or complete

No code for cotton wick insertion—Use 11730–32 if part of the nail was removed.

An ingrown toenail occurs when the nail edge grows into the soft tissues, causing inflammation, erythema, pain, and, possibly, abscess formation (Fig. 10–1). Many times there is an offending nail **spicule** (small needle-shaped body) that must be removed.

OVERVIEW

➤ Incidence unknown
➤ Causes
  ➤ Curved nails
  ➤ Congenital malformation of the great toenail, an autosomal dominant trait
  ➤ Nails cut too short
  ➤ Nail trimmed round edges
  ➤ Poorly fitting or too-tight shoes
  ➤ High-heeled shoes
  ➤ Accumulation of debris under nail
  ➤ Poorly ventilated shoes
  ➤ Chronically wet feet

HEALTH PROMOTION/PREVENTION

➤ Cut nails straight across.
➤ Notch center of nail with a V.
➤ Wear absorbent socks.
➤ Wear shoes that allow proper ventilation.
➤ Wear shoes that fit properly.
➤ Avoid high-heeled shoes.
➤ Use good foot hygiene.

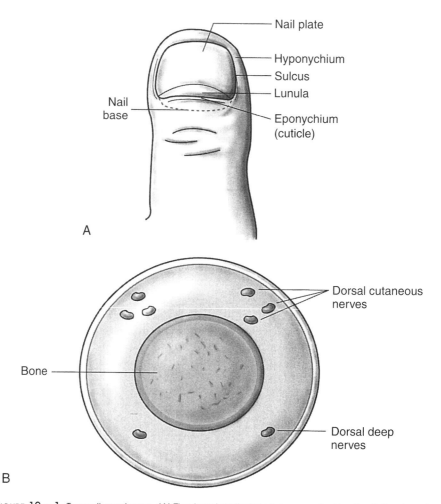

FIGURE 10 • 1 Toenail anatomy. *(A)* The hard *nail plate* is surrounded by the lateral and proximal folds of skin. The *cuticle*, or *eponychium*, formed by the ventral surface of the proximal nail fold, adheres to the newly formed nail plate. The *germinal matrix*, or *nail base*, lies under the cuticle. The *lunula*, or visible part of the nail-producing tissue, marks the distal border of the nail matrix. The *hyponychium* lies under the nail plate from the nailbed to the *sulcus*, or distal groove. *(B)* The blood supply to the nails is provided by the capillary branches of two digital arteries. Toenails are innervated by the dorsal and plantar digital nerve branches.

OPTIONS

➤ *Method 1*—cotton wick insertion
  ➤ A noninvasive technique to be used as the initial treatment. Six treatments may be required.
➤ *Method 2*—partial avulsion with phenolization
  ➤ For lesions lasting more than 2 months with significant infection and development of granulomatous tissue.

RATIONALE

- To diminish pain
- To prevent or relieve abscess formation
- To promote healing
- To prevent toenail regrowth

INDICATIONS

- Ingrown toenail without complicating medical history (onychocryptosis)
- Chronic, recurrent inflammation of the nail fold **(paronychia)**

CONTRAINDICATIONS

- Diabetes mellitus
- Peripheral vascular disease
- Peripheral neuropathy
- Anticoagulant therapy
- Bleeding abnormalities
- Immunocompromised state
- Pregnancy because of need to use phenol
- Allergy to local anesthetics

PROCEDURE

Nail Removal

Equipment

- Method 1 only
  - Antiseptic skin cleanser
  - Nail file or emery board
  - Cotton: 3 mm (1/8-inch) thick by 2.5 cm (1 inch) long
  - Gloves—nonsterile
  - Splinter forceps—sterile
  - Tincture of iodine
  - Silver nitrate stick
  - 4 × 4 gauze—sterile
  - Tape
- Method 2 only—digital nerve block
  - 5-mL syringe
  - 25- to 27-gauge, $^1/_2$- to 1-inch needle
  - 1% lidocaine without epinephrine
- Method 2—**avulsion**
  - Tourniquet
  - Gloves—sterile
  - Drape—sterile
  - **Hemostat**—sterile
  - Surgical scissors—sterile
  - Small straight hemostat—sterile
  - Cotton swabs—sterile
  - Silver nitrate stick

- 80% or 88% phenol
- Alcohol swabs
- Alcohol
- Antibiotic ointment (Bactroban, Neosporin, or Polysporin)
- Nonadherent dressing—Telfa or Adaptic
- Bandage roll (tube gauze)

Procedure

METHOD 1—COTTON WICK INSERTION

- Have the client lie supine with knees flexed and feet flat.
- Cleanse affected toe with antiseptic cleanser.
- File middle third of nail on the affected side with a nail file or emery board as illustrated (Fig. 10–2).
- Roll cotton to form a wick.
- Gently push the cotton wick under the distal portion of the lateral nail groove on the affected side using splinter forceps (Fig. 10–3).
- Identify the offending spicule and remove it.
- Continue to insert cotton wick to separate the nail from the nail groove (1 cm of cotton wick should remain free).
- Apply tincture of iodine to the cotton wick.
- Cauterize granulomatous tissue with silver nitrate stick.
- Bandage the toe.

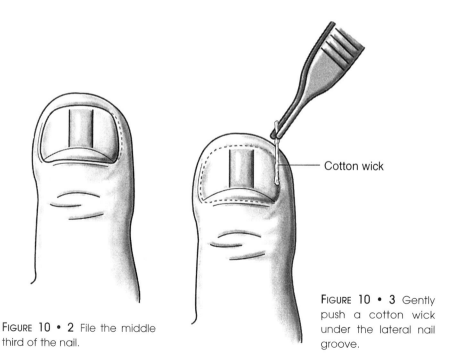

FIGURE 10 • 2 File the middle third of the nail.

FIGURE 10 • 3 Gently push a cotton wick under the lateral nail groove.

Client Instructions

➤ Change bandage daily, and apply tincture of iodine every other day.
➤ Return to the office weekly for cotton wick replacement.

METHOD 2—PARTIAL AVULSION WITH PHENOLIZATION

☑ *Informed consent required*

➤ Have the client lie supine with knees flexed and feet flat.
➤ For digital nerve block, prepare 3 to 5 mL of lidocaine without epinephrine to anesthetize the affected area.
➤ To anesthetize the nerves innervating the proximal phalanx (Fig. 10–4) on the extensor surface, insert the needle toward the plantar surface on the affected side.
➤ Injection sites are below the nail on the outer edges of the toe (Fig. 10–5). Be careful not to pierce the plantar skin surface.
➤ Inject 1 to 2 mL of lidocaine while withdrawing the needle. Do not withdraw the needle from the skin.
➤ Redirect the needle across the extensor surface, and insert the needle further. Inject 1 mL of lidocaine while withdrawing needle.
➤ Repeat procedure on opposite side of the digit.
➤ Allow 5 minutes for lidocaine to take effect before beginning procedure.
➤ Scrub the toe with antiseptic, rinse, dry, and drape with sterile drapes.

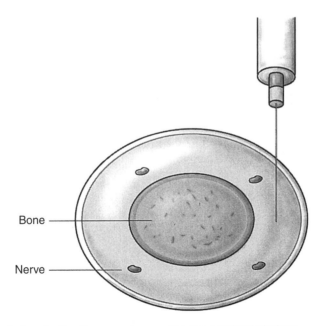

Bone

Nerve

FIGURE 10 • 4 Anesthetize the nerve innervating the proximal phalanx.

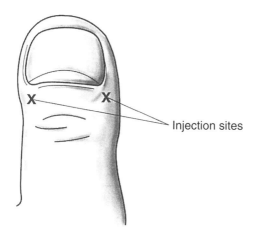

FIGURE 10 • 5 Inject the toe on the outer edges just below the nail.

➤ Place the tourniquet around the base of the toe. Perform procedure in 15 minutes or less to avoid ischemia.
➤ Insert a single blade of a small hemostat between the nailbed and the toe to open a tract (Fig. 10–6). Remove hemostat.
➤ Place the blade of the scissors in the tract, and cut the nail plate from distal edge to the proximal nail base (Fig. 10–7).
➤ Remove the nail with a small hemostat, using gentle rotation toward the affected nail (Fig. 10–8).

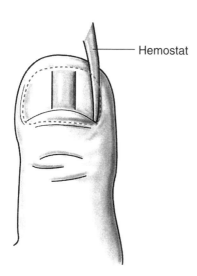

FIGURE 10 • 6 Insert a single blade of a hemostat between the nail bed and the toe to open a tract.

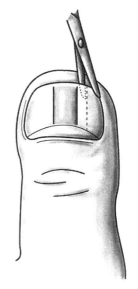

FIGURE 10 • 7 Cut the nail plate from distal edge to proximal nail base.

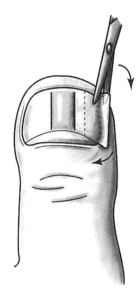

FIGURE 10 • 8 Remove the nail using gentle outward rotation toward the affected nail.

➤ Using a hemostat, inspect the nail groove for spicules.
➤ Dry the newly exposed nailbed.
➤ Rub cutton swab saturated with phenol on germinal matrix beneath the cuticle for 2 minutes.
➤ Cauterize granulomas with silver nitrate stick.
➤ Remove tourniquet and elevate foot for 15 minutes.
➤ Place a dressing in the toe.

Client Instructions

➤ Avoid ischemia of toe by loosening the bandage and hanging foot down.
➤ Notify the practitioner if pain or swelling increases or green or yellow discharge is present.
➤ If toes becomes cold and pale
  ➤ Elevate foot above heart level.
  ➤ Flex the toes.
  ➤ Check circulation by pressing on the toe and watching for return of redness when pressure is released.
  ➤ Call the practitioner if symptoms do not subside within 2 hours.
➤ Use pain medications as ordered. Take Tylenol No. 3 every 4 to 6 hours for the first 24 hours, then a nonsteroidal anti-inflammatory drug such as ibuprofen.
➤ Take ordered antibiotics for 5 days (cephalexin, tetracycline, trimethoprim-sulfamethoxazole, flucloxacillin).
➤ Return to the office for follow-up visit in 2 days.

B IBLIOGRAPHY

Barker, L.R., Burton, J.R., and Zieve, P.D. (1995) (4th ed.). *Principles of ambulatory medicine.* Baltimore: Williams & Wilkins.

Graber, R.F. (1987). Treatment of ingrown toenails. *Patient Care,* (3), 119–125.

Iseli, A. (1990). The management of ingrown toenails. *Aust Fam Physician,* 19(9), 1414–1419.

Pfenninger, J.L., and Fowler, G.C. (1994). *Procedures for primary care physicians.* St. Louis: Mosby.

Swartz, G.R. (1992). *Principles and practice of emergency medicine.* Philadelphia: Saunders.

11 RING REMOVAL

CYNTHIA R. EHRHARDT

CPT Code	
20670	Superficial removal of constricting metal band
20680	Deep removal of constricting metal band

Occasionally a ring must be removed from a digit. Whenever possible, a nondestructive method is preferred. Only when conservative methods have been exhausted should a ring cutter be used.

OVERVIEW

➤ Incidence unknown
➤ Complicating factors
  ➤ Swelling or **edema** to the digit
    • Increased pain and sensitivity to area
    • Embedding of metal filings into digit

General Principles

➤ Minimize the amount of pain.
➤ Smooth technique minimizes further trauma to area.
➤ Anesthesia may be necessary with severe pain.
➤ If skin integrity is compromised, treat as a puncture wound.
➤ Verify no ligamentous involvement.
➤ After ring is removed, re-evaluate vascular and motor functions.

HEALTH PROMOTION/PREVENTION

➤ Removal on a regular basis allows the wearer to be aware of ring size changes.

➤ Routinely remove the ring from the digit when working with hands.
➤ When trauma has occurred and the ring does not appear embedded, attempt to remove the ring immediately.
➤ If swelling has occurred, do not attempt removal without proper equipment.

OPTIONS

➤ *Method 1*—lubricant removal method
  ➤ Used if
    • No skin breakdown
    • Minimal edema to digit
    • No history of peripheral vascular disease
➤ *Method 2*—string-wrap method without tape anchor
  ➤ Used if
    • No skin breakdown
    • Minimal edema to digit
    • No suspected fracture or ligament damage
➤ *Method 3*—string method with tape anchor
  ➤ Used if
    • No skin breakdown
    • Minimal edema to digit
    • No suspected fracture or ligament damage
➤ *Method 4*—use of circular-blade ring cutter
  ➤ Used if
    • Suspected fracture or ligament injury
    • Ring embedded in the digit
    • Moderate-to-severe edema
    • Preservation of the ring not necessary

RATIONALE

➤ To prevent circulatory and nerve impairment to the digit

INDICATIONS

➤ Voluntary request for removal of the constricting ring
➤ Involuntary removal required because of circulatory compromise

CONTRAINDICATIONS

➤ Lack of patient cooperation
➤ Suspected open or closed fracture of the digit, REFER to orthopedic surgeon.
➤ Deep laceration with potential ligament involvement, REFER to orthopedic surgeon.
➤ Deeply embedded ring, REFER to orthopedic hand surgeon.

PROCEDURE

Ring Removal

Equipment

- ➤ Method 1 only
  - ➤ Liquid dishwashing soap or lubricant jelly
  - ➤ Windex—optional
  - ➤ Gloves—nonsterile
- ➤ Methods 2 and 3
  - ➤ Paper clips
  - ➤ Tape
  - ➤ Dental floss or 4-0 silk suture material
- ➤ Methods 2, 3, and 4
  - ➤ 1% lidocaine (no epinephrine)
  - ➤ 3-mL syringe
  - ➤ 27-gauge, $^1/_2$-inch needle
  - ➤ Needle-nose forceps or Kelly clamps—nonsterile
  - ➤ Topical antibiotic (Bactroban, Neosporin, or Polysporin)
  - ➤ Band-Aids or suitable dressing material
  - ➤ Gloves—nonsterile
  - ➤ Method 4 only
- ➤ Antiseptic skin cleanser
- ➤ 0.9% sodium chloride
- ➤ 20- to 30-mL syringe
- ➤ Circular-blade ring cutter
- ➤ Cool water

Procedure

METHOD 1—LUBRICANT REMOVAL METHOD

- ➤ Position the client comfortably.
- ➤ Soak affected digit in cool water for approximately 5 minutes with extremity elevated above the heart to decrease swelling.
- ➤ Apply a liberal coating of dishwashing liquid or lubricant jelly over the affected digit. If this fails, try spraying ring and finger with Windex.
- ➤ Rotate ring until ring slides off.

METHOD 2—STRING-WRAP METHOD WITHOUT TAPE ANCHOR

- ➤ Position the patient comfortably.
- ➤ If the patient is in moderate pain, consider anesthesia with lidocaine to the affected digit.
- ➤ Advance the ring to the narrowest part of the digit.
- ➤ Insert the thread (dental floss or 4-0 suture) under the ring using one of the following methods
  - ➤ *Straight thread technique*—Using forceps, slide the thread under the ring and pull through (Fig. 11–1).
  - ➤ *Paper-clip technique*—Bend paper clip to an approximately 45-degree angle.

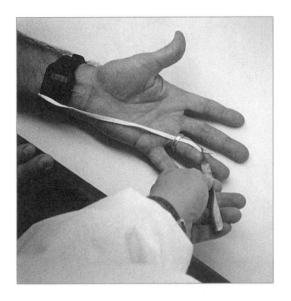

FIGURE 11 • 1 *Method 2—* String wrap method without tape anchor (straight thread technique). Using forceps, slide the thread underneath the ring and pull through.

- Insert the threaded paper clip between ring and digit; gently pull through with fingers or forceps and remove the paper clip (Fig. 11–2*A*).
➤ Apply a liberal coat of lubricant to distal part of digit.
➤ Wind thread with some tension around finger, beginning close to ring and continuing distally until six or eight single-layer wraps have been made (Fig. 11–2*B*).
➤ Holding distal part of thread firmly, begin pulling proximal end parallel to digit, causing the thread to unwind and removing the ring successfully (Fig. 11–2*C*).

METHOD 3—STRING METHOD WITH TAPE ANCHOR

➤ Same as Method 2 except
  ➤ Anchor the proximal end with tape at the base of the digit (Fig. 11–3), and begin to wind some tension around finger close to ring, continuing distally until six or eight single-layer wraps have been made.
  ➤ Release the anchored proximal end, and begin pulling with moderate tension toward the distal portion of the digit.

METHOD 4—USE OF THE CIRCULAR-BLADE RING CUTTER

➤ Position the client comfortably, palm up.
➤ If the client is in moderate pain, consider the use of digital block anesthesia with lidocaine.
➤ If possible, advance the ring to the narrowest part of the digit.
➤ Cleanse the area with antiseptic skin cleanser.
➤ Slip the small hook guide of the ring cutter.
➤ Position the ring cutter beneath the ring.

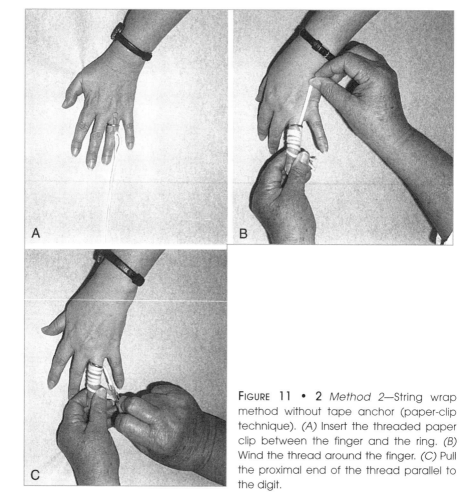

FIGURE 11 • 2 *Method 2*—String wrap method without tape anchor (paper-clip technique). *(A)* Insert the threaded paper clip between the finger and the ring. *(B)* Wind the thread around the finger. *(C)* Pull the proximal end of the thread parallel to the digit.

➤ When it is positioned, grip the saw handle and begin to apply a squeezing pressure to the ring while turning the circular blade until the cut is complete (Fig. 11–4).
➤ Release pressure, and remove the circular saw.
➤ Use needle-nose forceps or Kelly clamps to pull ring apart and remove ring.
➤ Use large syringe and flush area vigorously with 50 to 100 mL of 0.9% sodium chloride to remove any metal filings.
➤ Apply dressing as needed.

Client Instructions

➤ Observe for signs and symptoms of infection, such as
  ➤ Increase in pain after 24 hours

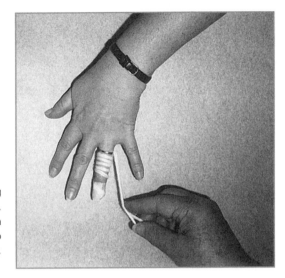

FIGURE 11 • 3 *Method 3*—String method with tape anchor. Anchor the proximal end with tape, wind the thread six to eight wraps, release the anchor, and pull.

- ➤ Increase in temperature
- ➤ Redness or swelling
- ➤ Yellow or greenish drainage
- ➤ Foul odor
- ➤ If any signs and symptoms of infection are found, return to the office.
- ➤ *Superficial skin abrasions*—Cleanse the abrasions with soapy water three times a day. Optional use of topical triple antibiotic (if no allergy).
- ➤ *To prevent infection*—Take oral antibiotics as prescribed for 7 to 10 days (cephalexin).
- ➤ *Pain and swelling*—Cool compresses to area for 5 to 10 min/hr for the first 24 hours. After 24 hours, apply heat for 5 to 10 minutes four to six times per day for 2 to 3 days.

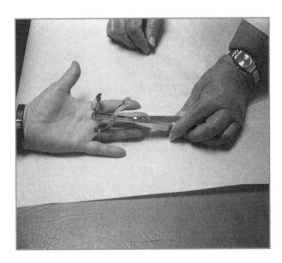

FIGURE 11 • 4 *Method 4*—Use of circular blade ring cutter. Position the ring cutter beneath the ring, apply pressure, and turn the circular blade.

> ➤ Tylenol No. 3 one or two tablets every 4 to 6 hours for 24 hours for severe pain, then use plain or extra-strength acetaminophen.
> ➤ *Tetanus*—Tetanus prophylaxis is needed if skin is broken and the patient has not had a booster in the past 5 years.
> ➤ Return to the office in 48 hours for recheck if there was a break in the skin, difficult removal, or moderate amount of edema to the finger; then, as needed.

BIBLIOGRAPHY

American Medical Association (1996). *Physician's current procedural terminology.* Chicago: Author.

Brandenburg, M.A., Hawkins, L., and Quick, G. (1995). Hand injuries. Assessing the damage, closing the wound, preventing infection. *Consultant,* December, 1777–1786.

Huss, C.D. (1988). Removing a ring from a swollen finger. *Patient care: Procedures for your practice.* Oradell, NJ: Medical Economics.

Murtagh, J. (1995) (2nd ed.). *Practice tips.* New York: McGraw-Hill.

Pfenninger, J.L., and Fowler, G.C. (1994). *Procedures for primary care physicians.* St. Louis: Mosby.

12

SEBACEOUS CYST REMOVAL

MARGARET R. COLYAR

CPT Code	
11400	Excision, benign lesion except skin tag, trunk, arms, or legs; lesion diameter 0.5 cm or less
11401-6	Differing lesion diameters
11420	Excision, benign lesion except skin tag, scalp, neck, hands, feet, genitalia; lesion diameter 0.5 cm or less
11421-26	Differing lesion diameters

A **sebaceous cyst** is not really an abscess by definition. A sebaceous cyst is a small, mobile, superficial sac containing sebum or keratin. Sebaceous cysts are found frequently on the scalp, back, neck, or face. Other names commonly used to describe a sebaceous cyst are *wen* and *epidermal cyst.*

OVERVIEW

➤ Incidence unknown
➤ Areas of most frequent occurrence
  ➢ Hair follicles
  ➢ Back

OPTIONS

➤ *Method 1*
  ➢ Used when the cyst sac is identified and pulled easily through the incision
➤ *Method 2*
  ➢ Used when the cyst sac is not identified or pulled easily through the incision

RATIONALE

➤ To diminish pain
➤ To remove unsightly masses
➤ To prevent secondary infection

INDICATIONS

➤ Cosmetic
➤ Recurrent infection

CONTRAINDICATIONS

➤ Cyst on the face
➤ Client has bleeding disorder.
➤ Proceed cautiously with clients who are diabetic or immunocompromised.
➤ Cyst currently infected

✓ *Informed consent required*

PROCEDURE

Sebaceous Cyst Removal

Equipment

➤ Methods 1 and 2
  ➢ Antiseptic skin cleanser
  ➢ Gloves—sterile
  ➢ Drape—sterile
  ➢ 1% to 2% lidocaine
  ➢ 2 syringes—3 and 10 mL
  ➢ 27- to 30-gauge, $^1/_2$-inch needle—for anesthesia
  ➢ 18-gauge, $1^1/_2$-inch needle—for irrigation

> No. 11 scalpel
> Curved hemostats—sterile
> 0.9% sodium chloride—sterile
> **Iodoform gauze** $^1/_4$- to 1-inch
> Container with 10% **formalin**
> 4 × 4 gauze—sterile
> Scissors—sterile
> Tape

Procedure

METHOD 1—SEBACEOUS CYST REMOVAL

➤ Position the client with the cyst easily accessible.
➤ Cleanse the area and 3 inches surrounding with antiseptic skin cleanser.
➤ Drape the cyst with the sterile drape.
➤ Put on gloves.
➤ Perform a **field block** by anesthetizing the perimeter around the abscess with 1% or 2% lidocaine without epinephrine. Do not inject lidocaine into the abscess because it does not work well in an acidic medium.
➤ Using the No. 11 scalpel, incise the cyst lengthwise to allow easy extraction of the cyst material and sac (Fig. 12–1).
➤ With curved **hemostats,** pull sac out onto the surface of the skin (see Fig. 12–1).
➤ Using the No. 11 scalpel, cut the elastic tissue around the outer edges of the sac until released.
➤ Irrigate with 0.9% sodium chloride.

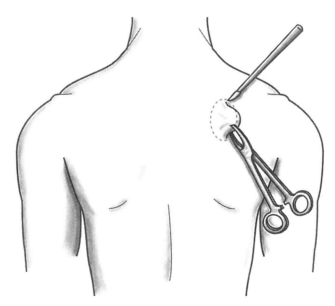

FIGURE 12 • 1 Cut the elastic tissue around the outer edges of the sac until released.

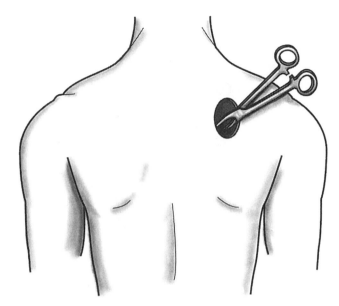

FIGURE 12 • 2 After expressing the contents of the cyst, explore the cavity with hemostats.

➤ Close wound with sutures.
➤ Apply a pressure dressing.

METHOD 2—SEBACEOUS CYST REMOVAL

➤ Position the client with the cyst easily accessible.
➤ Cleanse the area and 3 inches surrounding with antiseptic skin cleanser.
➤ Drape the cyst with the sterile drape.
➤ Put on gloves.
➤ Perform a field block by anesthetizing the perimeter around the abscess with 1% or 2% lidocaine without epinephrine. Do not inject lidocaine into the abscess because it does not work well in an acidic medium.
➤ Using the No. 11 scalpel, incise the cyst lengthwise to allow easy extraction of the cyst material and sac.
➤ Express cyst contents and put into a jar containing 10% formalin, and send to the pathology laboratory.
➤ Explore the cavity with curved hemostats (Fig. 12–2).
➤ Break down any sacs or septa using curved hemostats.
➤ After expressing all purulent material, pack the wound with iodoform gauze, leaving a small amount protruding from the wound. Advance the iodoform gauze daily for approximately 10 to 14 days until all is removed (Fig. 12–3).
➤ Cover with 4 × 4 gauze and tape.
  If the cyst is on the head, do not pack with iodoform gauze. Instead, roll 4 × 4 gauze into a gauze roll. Suture incision in two places, leaving room for drainage (Fig. 12–4). Leave ends of sutures 2 to 3 inches long. Place

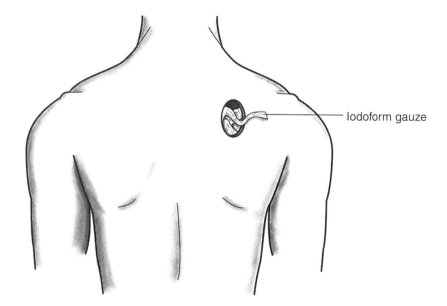

Iodoform gauze

FIGURE 12 • 3 Pack the wound with iodoform gauze, leaving a small amount protruding from the wound.

gauze roll on top of the incision, and tie tightly in place with the ends of the suture to form a pressure dressing. Remove the gauze roll in 7 days.

Client Instructions

➤ Observe for signs and symptoms of infection, such as
  ➤ Increase in pain after 24 hours
  ➤ Increase in temperature
  ➤ Redness or swelling
  ➤ Yellow or greenish drainage
  ➤ Foul odor
➤ If any signs and symptoms of infection are found, return to the office.
➤ *Pain and swelling*—Apply cool compresses to the area for 5 to 10 min/hr for the first 24 hours. After 24 hours, apply heat for 5 to 10 minutes four to six times per day for 2 to 3 days.
➤ Take Tylenol No. 3 one or two tablets every 4 to 6 hours for 24 hours for severe pain, then use plain or extra-strength acetaminophen.
➤ Return to the office in 48 hours for recheck.

B I B L I O G R A P H Y
Johnson, R.A. (1995). Cyst removal. Punch, push, pull. *Skin*, 1(1), 14–15.
Klin, B., and Ashkenazi, H. (1990). Sebaceous cyst excision with minimal surgery. *Am Fam Physician*, 41(6), 1746–1748.

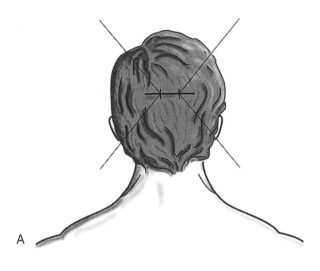

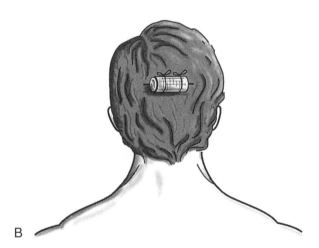

FIGURE 12 • 4 Head wounds. (A) Suture the incision in two places, leaving the ends of the suture long. (B) Place a gauze roll on top of the incision and tie tightly in place with the long ends of the suture.

Pfenninger, J.L., and Fowler, G.C. (1994). *Procedures for primary care physicians.* St. Louis: Mosby.

Swartz, G.R. (1992). *Emergency medicine.* Philadelphia: Saunders.

Tosti, A., et al (1992). Role of foods in the pathogenesis of chronic paronychia. *J Am Acad Dermatol,* 27(11), 706–710.

13

SKIN CLOSURE— DERMABOND APPLICATION

CYNTHIA R. EHRHARDT

CPT Code

12001-7 Simple repair of wounds

Skin closure using **Dermabond** (tissue adhesive) in combination with Steri strips is less invasive than, has a shorter time of application than, and results in similar outcome as suturing for smaller lacerations that do not have jagged edges and approximate well. Only about one third of wounds meet criteria for tissue adhesive closure.

OVERVIEW
- ➤ Incidence of use unknown
- ➤ Complicating factors of secondary infection similar to suturing

General Principles
- ➤ More efficient and less invasive method of wound repair
- ➤ Generally does not require anesthesia
- ➤ Lower incidence of irritation than with traditional suturing
- ➤ Equal to or better than cosmetic response with traditional suturing
- ➤ Within 2.5 minutes, bonding strength equivalent to 7 days of tissue healing by traditional suture closure
- ➤ Torso and extremity applications do better with subcutaneous suturing before application.
- ➤ High-tension locations and joints require splinting.

INDICATIONS
- ➤ Tissue adhesives such as Dermabond should be considered in place of 5-0 or smaller diameter sutures.
- ➤ Small wound repair
- ➤ Facial wounds

CONTRAINDICATIONS

➤ Adhesive sensitivity
➤ Jagged or irregular lacerations
➤ Mucosa or moist surface.
➤ Contaminated wounds
➤ Bites or punctured wounds
➤ Highly movable sites of hands and feet that cannot be splinted
➤ Crushed wounds
➤ Axillae and perineum areas
➤ Evidence of or potential for purulent exudate from the wound
➤ Wound greater than 5 cm

PROCEDURE

Skin Closure—Dermabond Application

Equipment

➤ Dermabond
➤ Povidone-iodine
➤ Alcohol prep pads
➤ Vaseline jelly
➤ Gloves—nonsterile
➤ Optional—topical anesthetic
➤ Optional—Steri strips

Procedure

➤ Assess the wound and irrigate with saline as needed.
➤ Apply povidone-iodine to the wound beginning at the wound edges and expanding out in a circular pattern.
  ➤ Allow to dry.
  ➤ Remove with alcohol prep pad before application of Dermabond.
➤ Put on gloves.
➤ If needed, apply topical anesthetic.
➤ Oppose the wound edges with good approximation.
➤ Crush the Dermabond vial and invert. You have only a few minutes to use this vial before polymerization results in the applicator orifice sealing. Excessive pressure to the vial results in dripping.
➤ When the adhesive is at the tip applicator, apply to the approximated wound edges with a gentle brushing motion to the edges. This method of application avoids tissue adhesive from oozing into the wound.
➤ Hold wound edges in place for 30 seconds.
➤ If edges are not approximated, you have 10 seconds to make any corrections before the wound is "glued." If an error is made, wipe as much of the adhesive off and apply liberal Vaseline jelly to the exterior site for 30 minutes to neutralize the adhesive.
➤ Apply a total of three layers of adhesive. The layer must be dry before the next can be applied. Blowing on or fanning the area does not accelerate drying time.

➤ *Optional*—Steri strips may be applied only if over high-tension areas.

Client Instructions

➤ No bandage is required for adults. In active children, a bandage may be used to prevent the child from picking at the wound.
➤ You may shower within 6 hours after the application.
  ➢ Avoid prolonged water exposure.
  ➢ Dry area immediately after showering.
➤ Do not use topical antibiotics. They weaken the glue.
➤ Adhesive spontaneously peels in 5 to 10 days.
➤ Observe for signs and symptoms of infection, such as
  ➢ Increase in pain after 24 hours
  ➢ Increase in temperature
  ➢ Redness or swelling
  ➢ Yellow or greenish drainage
  ➢ Foul odor
➤ If any signs and symptoms of infection are found, return to the office.
➤ Return to the office in 48 hours for wound recheck.

BIBLIOGRAPHY

Bruns, T., and Worthington, J. Using tissue adhesive for wound repair. A practical guide to Dermabond. *Am Fam Physician,* 61(5), 1382–1388.

King, M., and Kinney, A. (1999). Tissue adhesives. A new method of wound repair. *Nurse Practitioner,* 24(10), 66, 69–70, 73–74.

Quinn, J., et al (1997). A randomized trial comparing octylcyanoacrylate tissue adhesive and sutures in the management of lacerations. *JAMA,* 277(19), 1559–1560.

14 SKIN LESION REMOVAL
CAUTERY AND CRYOSURGERY

MARGARET R. COLYAR

CPT Code	
17000	Destruction, any method, including laser, with or without surgical curettement, all benign lesions/premalignant lesions any location or benign lesions other than cutaneous vascular proliferative lesions, including local anesthesia; one lesion

17003	Multiple lesions
17110	Destruction, any method, flat warts or molluscum contagiosum, milia; up to 14
17260	Destruction, malignant lesion, any method, trunk, arms, or legs; lesion diameter 0.5 cm or less
17261–66	Differing lesion diameters
17270	Destruction, malignant lesion, any method, scalp, neck, hands, feet, genitalia; 0.5 cm or less
17271–76	Differing lesion diameters

Two methods of removing skin lesions are **cautery** and **cryosurgery**. Another method, minor surgery (elliptical excision biopsy), is discussed in Chapter 2. Cautery is the destruction of tissue by the use of electricity, freezing, heat, or corrosive materials. Thermocautery is the process of tissue removal or destruction by the use of red-hot or white-hot heat.

Cryosurgery is a technique of exposing tissues to extreme cold to produce cell injury and destruction. This technique is safe and easy. Lesions heal with minimal or no scarring. No injections of local anesthetics or sutures are involved. Cryosurgery feels like an ice cube stuck to the skin. Temperatures that destroy tissues

➤ -10° C to -20° C
➤ To -50° C ensures malignant cells are completely destroyed

OVERVIEW

➤ Incidence is unknown.
➤ Freeze time guidelines for cryosurgery are recommended for different types of lesions (Table 14–1).

TABLE 14•1 Freeze Time Guidelines for Skin Lesions

TYPE OF SKIN LESION	FREEZE TIME, SEC
Full thickness (benign)	60–90
Plantar warts (after debridement)	30–40
Condylomata	45
Verrucae	60–90
Seborrheic keratoses (2 mm)	30
Actinic keratoses (c mm)	90
Molluscum contagiosum	30

OPTIONS

➤ *Method 1*—cautery
➤ *Method 2*—cryosurgery
  ➢ Superficial lesions—seborrheic keratoses
    • Freeze for 30 to 40 seconds or until a 2- to 3-mm ice ball forms beyond the lesion.
    • -89° C
  ➢ Benign or premalignant lesions—actinic keratoses
    • Freeze 1 to 1.5 minutes or until a greater-than-3-mm ice ball forms beyond the lesion (freeze, thaw, refreeze).
➤ -89° C
  ➢ Malignant lesions—basal cell carcinoma
    • Freeze for 1.5 minutes or until a greater-than-5- to 8-mm ice ball forms beyond the lesion (freeze, thaw, refreeze).
    • Activate rapid thaw.
  ➢ Large or irregular lesions
    • Same as malignant lesions except
      • Start on one side and progress to the opposite side.
        • Refreeze overlapping first freeze zone by 50% (Fig. 14–1).
  ➢ Keloids or hypertrophic scars
    • See Chapter 15.

RATIONALE

➤ To remove lesions for cosmetic reasons
➤ To remove cancerous lesions
➤ To prevent further tissue destruction caused by spread of malignant lesions

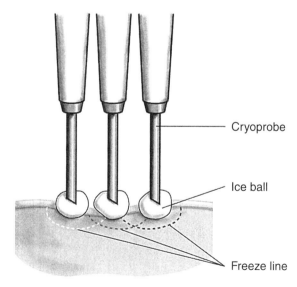

Cryoprobe

Ice ball

Freeze line

FIGURE 14 • 1 For large or irregular lesions—refreeze, overlapping first freeze zone by 50%.

INDICATIONS

- ➤ Skin tags
- ➤ Basal cell carcinoma
- ➤ **Condyloma acuminatum**
- ➤ Actinic keratoses
- ➤ Seborrheic keratoses
- ➤ **Lentigo** (freckles)
- ➤ Benign **nevi**—papular or acquired
- ➤ **Telangiectasias**—small
- ➤ Hypertrophic scars and keloids
- ➤ Warts—**verruca vulgaris** and plantaris

CONTRAINDICATIONS

- ➤ Face lesions
- ➤ Dark skin due to pigment changes
- ➤ Area that is hairy because freezing destroys hair follicles
- ➤ **Melanoma**
- ➤ Compromised circulation
- ➤ Areas in which biopsy is required
- ➤ Clients with high levels of cryoglobulins (abnormal proteins that precipitate when cooled and dissolve when reheated to body temperature)
  - ➤ Endocarditis
  - ➤ Syphilis
  - ➤ Epstein-Barr virus
  - ➤ Cytomegalovirus
  - ➤ Hepatitis B—chronic
  - ➤ On high-dose steroid treatment
- ➤ Collagen disease
- ➤ Active ulcerative colitis
- ➤ Glomerulonephritis
- ➤ Recurrent basal cell carcinoma

☑ *Informed consent required*

PROCEDURE
Skin Lesion Removal

Equipment

- ➤ Methods 1 and 2
  - ➤ Antiseptic skin cleanser
  - ➤ Gloves—nonsterile
  - ➤ Tape
  - ➤ Topical antibiotic (Bactroban, Neosporin, or Polysporin)
- ➤ Method 1 only

- ➤ Drape—sterile
- ➤ 3-mL syringe
- ➤ 27- to 30-gauge, $^1/_2$-inch needle
- ➤ 1% lidocaine
- ➤ 4 × 4 gauze—sterile
- ➤ Disposable cautery pen
➤ Method 2 only
- ➤ Verruca Freeze Kit or nitrous oxide cryosurgery unit (Fig. 14–2)
- ➤ Cotton-tipped applicators
- ➤ Water-soluble lubricant (K-Y jelly)
- ➤ 4 × 4 gauze soaked with water

Procedure

METHOD 1—CAUTERY

➤ Position the client so that the lesion is easily accessible.
➤ Cleanse the area and a 3-inch-diameter space around the lesion with anticeptic skin cleanser.
➤ Inject the tissue under the lesion with 1% lidocaine. If a large lesion (greater than 3 mm), perform a **field block**.
➤ Drape the lesion.
➤ Put on gloves.
➤ Cauterize the lesion with the disposable cautery pen.
➤ Wipe off the burned area.

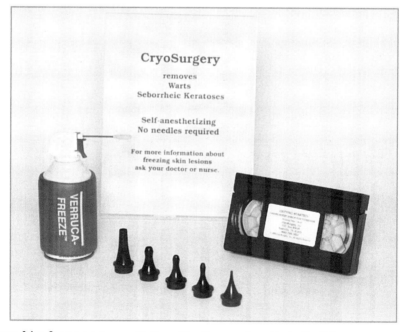

FIGURE 14 • 2 Veruca Freeze Kit (from CryoSurgery, Inc., Nashville, TN).

➤ Apply topical antibiotic.
➤ Cover with 4 × 4 gauze and tape.

METHOD 2—CRYOSURGERY

➤ Position the client so that the lesion is easily accessible.
➤ Cleanse the area and a 3-inch-diameter space around the lesion with antiseptic skin cleanser.
➤ Apply water-soaked gauze for 5 to 10 minutes.
➤ Drape the lesion.
➤ Put on gloves.
➤ Apply K-Y jelly with a cotton-tipped applicator to the lesion.
➤ Choose the tip desired (Fig. 14–3).
➤ Freeze the lesion for the appropriate amount of time (see Options).
➤ Apply topical antibiotic.
➤ Cover with 4 × 4 gauze and tape.

Client Instructions—Methods 1 and 2

➤ Although infection is unlikely, observe for signs and symptoms of infection, such as
  ➤ Increase in pain after 24 hours
  ➤ Increase in temperature
  ➤ Redness or swelling

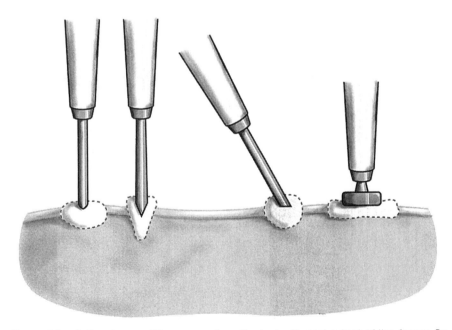

FIGURE 14 • 3 The shape of the cryoprobe affects depth and extent of the freeze. By applying pressure, a deeper freeze can be achieved.

- ➤ Yellow or greenish drainage
- ➤ Foul odor
- ➤ If any signs and symptoms of infection are found, return to the office.
- ➤ The following are considered normal reactions:
  - ➤ Redness—immediate response
  - ➤ Swelling and blisters form—within 24 to 48 hours—and decrease within 72 hours
  - ➤ Within 72 hours, crusts form and slowly wither over 1 week
  - ➤ Heals from outer margin toward the center
  - ➤ Skin may be lighter color and less hair may be present at the site
  - ➤ Not much scar formation
  - ➤ Wound weeping up to 8 weeks
  - ➤ Sensitive skin—wear sunscreen
- ➤ Return to the office in 1 week for recheck.

BIBLIOGRAPHY

American Medical Association (1996). *Physician's current procedural terminology.* Chicago: Author.

Brymill Corporation (1995). *Simplified cryosurgical techniques: Instruction manual.* Vernon, CT: Author.

Cryosurgery, Inc. (1995). *Verruca-Freeze instruction manual.* Nashville, TN: Author.

Habif, T. (1996) (3rd ed.). *Clinical dermatology: A color guide to diagnosis and therapy.* St. Louis: Mosby.

Hocutt, J. (1993). Skin cryosurgery for the family practice physician. *Am Fam Physician,* 48(3), 445–447.

Pfenninger, J.L., and Fowler, G.C. (1994). *Procedures for primary care physicians.* St. Louis: Mosby.

SKIN LESION REMOVAL

KELOIDS, MOLES, CORNS, CALLUSES

15

MARGARET R. COLYAR

CPT Code	
11050	Paring or curettement of benign hyperkeratotic skin lesion with or without chemical cauterization (verrucae, callus, corns), single lesion
11056	Two to four lesions

11057	Greater than four lesions
11300–33	Shaving of epidermal or dermal lesion, single lesion; trunk, arms, or legs
11305–38	Shaving of epidermal or dermal lesion, single lesion; scalp, neck, hands, feet, genitalia

Skin lesions such as **keloids,** moles, corns, and calluses are removed easily. Keloids are benign, hard, fibrous proliferations of collagen that expand beyond the original size and shape of the wound, sometimes 20 times normal size. They invade surrounding soft tissue in a clawlike fashion. Moles, or **nevi,** are discolorations of circumscribed areas of the skin resulting from pigmentation. They can be congenital or acquired. Acquired nevi usually appear first in childhood and in sun-exposed areas. These nevi extend into the dermis and epidermis (Fig. 15–1) by late adolescence and intradermis by late adulthood. Nevi always should be assessed for

➤ Asymmetry
➤ Border irregularities
➤ Color variation
➤ Diameter greater than 6 mm
➤ Elevation above the skin surface

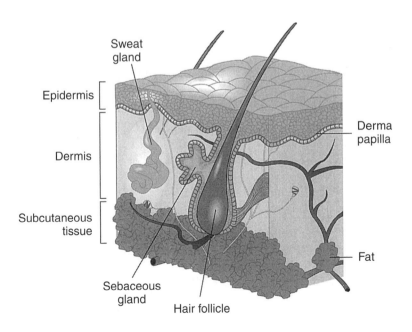

FIGURE 15 • 1 Anatomy and layers of skin.

Corns, or keratomas, are hyperkeratotic lesions or horny indurations with thickening and nucleation of the skin, usually on the toes. Hard corns are located on the dorsal aspect of the toes. Soft corns are located between the digits, usually the fourth interdigital space.

Calluses are hypertrophied hyperkeratotic thickenings of the stratum corneum usually located around the heel of the foot, great toe, metatarsal heel, and distal aspect of the first three digits of the dominant hand or palmar aspect of the metacarpal head. There is no underlying nucleus (core).

OVERVIEW

➤ Incidence—keloids
  ➢ 15 to 20 times greater in dark-skinned people. They develop more frequently in areas of motion or high skin tension, such as
    • Shoulders
    • Back
    • Presternum
    • Earlobe
    • Face
➤ Incidence—moles, corns, and calluses—unknown
➤ Causes
  ➢ Moles
    • Congenital
    • Acquired
  ➢ Corns
    • Pressure from poorly fitting shoes
  ➢ Calluses
    • Continuous friction
    • Pressure from poorly fitting shoes
    • Pencil and pen use
    • Physical labor using the unprotected hand

HEALTH PROMOTION/PREVENTION

Corns

➤ Wear properly fitting shoes.
➤ Use moleskin or felt spacer to relieve pressure of bony prominences.

OPTIONS

Keloids

➤ *Method 1*—**cryotherapy**—earlobe and all areas
➤ *Method 2*—corticosteroid injection—early, small, narrow, or softened lesions or to soften and/or flatten
➤ *Method 3*—surgical excision—any keloid

RATIONALE

➤ To remove unsightly skin lesions
➤ To relieve pain

INDICATIONS

➤ Cosmetic
➤ Pressure and pain
➤ Limitation of use
➤ Suspicion of malignancy

CONTRAINDICATIONS

➤ Poor circulation to the area
➤ Diabetic
➤ Immunocompromised

☑ *Informed consent required*

PROCEDURE

Keloid Removal

Equipment

➤ Methods 1, 2, and 3
  ➤ Antiseptic skin cleanser
  ➤ Gloves—nonsterile
➤ Methods 2 and 3
  ➤ 10-mL syringe
  ➤ 25- to 27-gauge, $1^1/_2$-inch needle (very small needles usually are unable to penetrate the lesions adequately)
  ➤ 1% lidocaine
  ➤ Corticosteroid of choice
➤ Method 1 only
  ➤ Water-soluble lubricant (K-Y jelly)
  ➤ Cotton-tipped applicators
  ➤ Liquid nitrogen (-89° C)
➤ Method 3 only
  ➤ 6-0 nylon suture
  ➤ Needle driver—sterile
  ➤ Scissors—sterile
  ➤ No. 15 scalpel

Procedure

METHOD 1—CRYOTHERAPY

➤ Position the client with the lesion easily accessible.
➤ Cleanse the area and a 3-inch-diameter space around the keloid with antiseptic skin cleanser.
➤ Apply water-soaked gauze for 5 to 10 minutes to soften the lesion.
➤ Apply K-Y jelly for 5 to 10 minutes.
➤ Using a cryotip narrower than the lesion

➤ Freeze for 10 to 15 seconds at −189° C, then
  ➤ Freeze for 30 to 45 seconds at −89° C.
➤ Wait 15 to 30 minutes for tissue edema to develop.
➤ Inject the keloid with corticosteroids (see Corticosteroid Injection following).

METHOD 2—Corticosteroid Injection

➤ Position the client with the keloid easily accessible.
➤ Cleanse the area and a 3-inch-diameter space around the keloid with antiseptic skin cleanser.
➤ Draw 2.5 mL of 1% lidocaine and 0.5 mL of corticosteroid into the syringe.
➤ Inject the medication into the lesion. The keloid will blanche. Do not inject the medication under or around the lesion.

METHOD 3—SURGICAL EXCISION

➤ See Chapter 2 (Method 3—Elliptical Excisional Biopsy).

Mole Removal

Equipment

➤ Antiseptic skin cleanser
➤ Gloves—sterile
➤ 10-mL syringe
➤ 25- to 27-gauge, $1^1/_2$-inch needle (very small needles usually are unable to penetrate the lesions adequately)
➤ 1% lidocaine
➤ Corticosteroid of choice
➤ 6-0 nylon suture
➤ Needle driver—sterile
➤ Scissors—sterile
➤ No. 15 scalpel

Procedure

Same as for cryosurgery, surgical excision, punch biopsy, and shave biopsy.

Corn Removal

Equipment

➤ Wash basin—nonsterile
➤ Warm water—tap
➤ Antiseptic skin cleanser
➤ Drape—nonsterile
➤ Gloves—nonsterile
➤ No. 15 scalpel
➤ 1% lidocaine

- 3-mL syringe
- 27- to 30-gauge needle
- Self-adherent web spacer
- Topical antibiotic (Bactroban, Neosporin, or Polysporin)
- 4 × 4 gauze—sterile
- Tape

Procedure

- Soak the foot for 15 to 20 minutes in warm water.
- Cleanse the skin around the corn with antiseptic skin cleanser.
- Anesthetize under the corn with 1% lidocaine.
- Drape the area.
- Put on gloves.
- Pare with No. 15 scalpel and remove core.
- Apply antibiotic, cover with 4 × 4 gauge, and tape.

Callus Removal

Equipment

- Pumice stone or file
- Wash basin—nonsterile
- Warm water
- Antiseptic skin cleanser
- Gloves—nonsterile
- No. 15 scalpel

Procedure

- Soak the foot for 15 to 20 minutes in warm water.
- Cleanse the foot with antiseptic skin cleanser.
- Put on gloves.
- Pare thick callous layers with No. 15 scalpel.
- File down with file or pumice stone.

Client Instructions

KELOIDS, MOLES, AND CORNS

- Apply antibiotic ointment, cover with 4 × 4 gauze, and tape or apply Band-Aid for 2 days; then leave open to air.
- Observe for signs of infections, such as
  - Green or yellow drainage
  - Red streaks
  - Increase in pain after 24 hours
  - Elevated temperature
  - Foul odor from wound
- If infection occurs, return to the office.
- Take acetaminophen or ibuprofen every 4 to 6 hours as needed for pain.
- Return to the office in 1 week for recheck.

CALLUSES

➤ Perform the following procedure weekly after bathing
  ➤ Pare thick callous layers.
➤ File down with file or pumice stone.
➤ Apply felt spacers or moleskin.
➤ Take acetaminophen or ibuprofen every 4 to 6 hours as needed for pain.
➤ Return to the office in 1 month, unless condition worsens.

B IBLIOGRAPHY
Berman, B., and Bieley, H.C. (1996). Adjunct therapies to surgical management of keloids. *Dermatol Surg, 22*(79), 126–130.
Pfenninger, J.L., and Fowler, G.C. (1994). *Procedures for primary care physicians.* St. Louis: Mosby.

16
SKIN TAG (ACROCHORDON) REMOVAL

CYNTHIA R. EHRHARDT

CPT Code	
11200	Removal of skin tags, multiple fibrocutaneous tags any area; up to and including 15 lesions
11201	Removal of skin tags, multiple fibrocutaneous tags any area; each additional 10 lesions

Skin tags, or **acrochordons,** are benign skin lesions that can be removed by scissoring, any sharp method, or chemical or electrocauterization of the wound. Local anesthesia may or may not be used. Removal usually is done because of irritation of the lesion or for cosmetic reasons.

OVERVIEW

➤ Incidence unknown

HEALTH PROMOTION/PREVENTION

➤ Avoid chronic irritation to the skin folds of the body.
➤ Examine the body regularly for changes in color and size of skin lesions.

OPTIONS

➤ *Method 1*—snips technique
  ➤ Use with small skin tags.
➤ *Method 2*—cryogenic technique
  ➤ Use with large skin tags.

RATIONALE

➤ To reduce the possibility of inflammation and infection caused by local irritation
➤ To promote cosmetic enhancement

INDICATIONS

➤ Unsightly skin tags
➤ Skin tags irritated by clothing

CONTRAINDICATIONS

➤ Any lesion that is suspect for malignancy
➤ High-dose steroid therapy
➤ Individuals with underlying medical diseases, such as
  ➤ Active severe collagen vascular diseases
  ➤ Acute poststreptococcal glomerulonephritis
  ➤ Acute severe subacute bacterial endocarditis
  ➤ Acute cytomegalovirus infection
  ➤ Acute Epstein-Barr virus infection
  ➤ Acute syphilis infection
  ➤ Chronic severe hepatitis B
  ➤ **Cryoglobulinemia**
  ➤ Diabetes with history of poor healing

☑ *Informed consent required*

PROCEDURE

Skin Tag Removal

Equipment

➤ Methods 1 and 2
  ➤ Antiseptic skin cleanser
  ➤ Water-soluble lubricant (K-Y jelly)
  ➤ Botton-tipped applicators—sterile

- ➤ Topical antibiotic (Bactroban, Neosporin, or Polysporin)—optional
- ➤ Band-Aids
- ➤ Drape—sterile
- ➤ Goggles—optional
- ➤ Tape—optional
➤ Method 1 only
  - ➤ Gloves—sterile
  - ➤ Sterile surgical kit that includes
    - 2 × 2 or 4 × 4 gauze
    - Forceps with teeth
    - Iris scissors
    - No. 11 or 15 scalpel
  - ➤ 1% lidocaine
  - ➤ 5-mL syringe
  - ➤ 27-gauge, $^1/_2$- to 1-inch needle
  - ➤ Hemostatic agent—aluminum chloride or ferrous subsulfate
  - ➤ Container with 10% **formalin**
➤ Method 2 only
  - ➤ Nitrous oxide cryosurgery unit or cryogun
  - ➤ Timer
  - ➤ Gloves—nonsterile

Procedure

METHOD 1—SNIPS TECHNIQUE

- ➤ Position the client for comfort.
- ➤ Put on gloves.
- ➤ Apply antiseptic skin cleanser to the skin tag and surrounding area.
- ➤ Infiltrate the base of the skin tag with 1% lidocaine (Fig. 16–1).
- ➤ Grasp the skin tag at the largest part (Fig. 16–2).
- ➤ Gently pull the skin tag until the stalk base is visible (Fig. 16–3).
- ➤ Using the iris scissors or scalpel, cut or slice the stalk as close to the base of the stalk as possible (Fig. 16–4).
- ➤ Apply a hemostatic agent (ferrous subsulfate or aluminum chloride) with cotton-tipped applicator. Hold to the area until the bleeding stops.
- ➤ Place the skin tags in the container with 10% formalin for laboratory pathology.
- ➤ Apply topical antibiotic—optional.
- ➤ Apply a Band-Aid.

METHOD 2—CRYOGENIC TECHNIQUE

See Chapter 14.
- ➤ Position the client so that the lesion is easily accessible.
- ➤ Cleanse the area and a 3-inch-diameter space surrounding with antiseptic skin cleanser.
- ➤ Drape the lesion.
- ➤ Put on gloves.

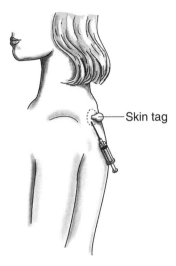

FIGURE 16 • 1 Infiltrate the base of the skin tag with lidocaine.

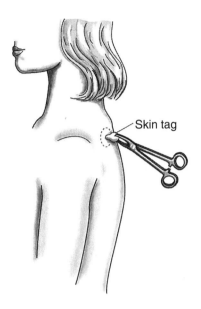

FIGURE 16 • 2 Grasp the skin tag at the largest part with hemostats.

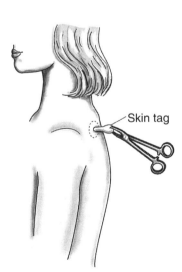

FIGURE 16 • 3 Pull the skin tag until the stalk base is visible.

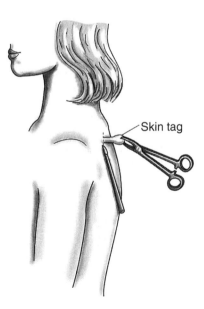

FIGURE 16 • 4 Cut the stalk of the skin tag as close as possible to the base of the stalk.

➤ Prepare equipment as manufacturer recommends.
➤ Select the appropriate-size device to match the size of the lesion.
➤ Anesthetize the site—optional.
➤ Use a cotton-tipped applicator to apply enough K-Y jelly to cover the skin tag but not beyond the tag.
➤ Apply the selected probe to the site and penetrate approximately halfway into the jelly.
➤ Squeeze the cryogun trigger to release the nitrogen oxide. The jelly is transformed into an ice ball.
➤ If area of skin is thin, when the jelly is frozen, pull up slightly on the skin to lessen depth of the tissue freezing.
➤ Application time is usually 30 seconds. Larger skin tags may require 45 seconds.
➤ Release the trigger.
➤ Allow the jelly to thaw before removing the probe from the site of the cryosurgery.
➤ Depending on the response of the lesion, a repeat freeze-thaw may be required for an additional 30 seconds.
➤ Do not apply any dressing until lesion becomes irritated and/or is bleeding.
➤ Topical antibiotic ointment is not recommended.
➤ Apply a Band-Aid to be removed when the client gets home.

Client Instructions

➤ On completion of treatment of the skin tag, the area appears erythematous and indurated (hard). A red ring may be visible around the site 2 weeks after removal. This is a normal response.
➤ Retreatment may be required if the entire lesion does not **slough** off.
➤ Keep the wound clean and dry.
➤ A Band-Aid is not required usually after 1 hour.
➤ Antibiotics are not required.
➤ Observe for signs and symptoms of infection, such as
  ➤ Increase in pain after 24 hours
  ➤ Increase in temperature
  ➤ Redness or swelling
  ➤ Yellow or greenish drainage
  ➤ Foul odor
➤ If any signs and symptoms of infection are found, return to the office.
➤ Pain—acetaminophen every 4 hours as needed for mild pain for the first 24 hours. After 24 hours ibuprofen or naproxen may be used.
  ➤ Acetaminophen with codeine rarely is used for severe pain because most skin lesions have few nerve endings. If discomfort continues and infection has been excluded, use Tylenol No. 3 every 4 to 6 hours as needed.
➤ Bathing is permitted 48 hours after the procedure.
➤ If the cryogenic technique was used
  ➤ First 24 to 48 hours, a blister may form; if it does, apply a small, non-stick Band-Aid until the weeping has stopped.

➤ Ideally, leave the wound exposed for more rapid healing.
➤ Redness to the site is common and lessens with time.
➤ The pain should lessen within 24 hours.
➤ A cotton swab with hydrogen peroxide may be used if the site becomes crusty.
➤ No topical antibiotic should be applied.
➤ Nonaspirin pain reliever is suggested.
➤ Rarely, painful and large blisters can occur. If they do, contact the practitioner to determine course of management. (Usually, these blisters are drained.)
➤ If infection is suspected, contact health-care provider.
➤ Within 7 to 10 days, a scab should form. Do not pick it. Let it fall off naturally.
  ➤ Most redness and decreased skin coloration resolve within 3 to 6 months.
  ➤ Some lesions may require retreatment.
➤ Remove the Band-Aid. Keep the area covered only if it is being irritated constantly. Continuous covering of the wound increases risk of infection.

BIBLIOGRAPHY

American Medical Association (1996). *Physicians' current procedural terminology.* Chicago: Author.

Habif, T. (1996) (3rd ed.). *Clinical dermatology: A color guide to diagnosis and therapy.* St. Louis: Mosby.

Matzen, R., and Lang, R. (1993). *Clinical preventive medicine.* St. Louis: Mosby.

Murtagh, J. (1995) (2nd ed.). *Practice tips.* New York: McGraw-Hill.

Pfenninger, J.L., and Fowler, G.C. (1994). *Procedures for primary care physicians.* St. Louis: Mosby.

17

SOFT TISSUE ASPIRATION

MARGARET R. COLYAR

CPT Code

20600	Arthrocentesis, aspiration, or injection: small joint, bursa, or ganglionic cyst (e.g., fingers or toes)

| 20605 | Arthrocentesis, aspiration, or injection: intermediate joint, bursa, or ganglionic cyst (e.g., temporomandibular; acromioclavicular; wrist, elbow, or ankle; olecranon bursa) |
| 20610 | Arthrocentesis, aspiration, or injection: major joint or bursa (e.g., shoulder, hip, knee joint, subacromial bursa) |

Soft tissue aspiration is the removal of fluid or exudate in an area of soft tissue for comfort and evaluation.

OVERVIEW

➤ Incidence unknown

RATIONALE

➤ To diagnose
  ➤ Infection
  ➤ Rheumatoid disease
  ➤ Crystals
  ➤ Bursitis
  ➤ Chondritis
➤ To provide symptomatic relief

INDICATIONS

➤ Pain and/or swelling in soft tissue
➤ Hematoma from trauma

CONTRAINDICATIONS

➤ Severe coagulation problems
➤ Swelling on the face
➤ Cellulitis or broken skin at the site
➤ Joint prosthesis

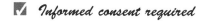 *Informed consent required*

PROCEDURE

Soft Tissue Aspiration

Equipment

➤ Antiseptic skin cleanser
➤ Drape—sterile
➤ Gloves—sterile

- **Hemostats**—sterile
- 6- to 10-mL syringe
- 18- to 20-gauge, 1-inch needle
- Container with 10% **formalin,** specimen tube, or microscope slide
- Ace wrap
- 4 × 4 gauze—sterile
- Tape

Procedure

- Position the client for comfort with the affected area easily accessible.
- Cleanse the area with antiseptic skin cleanser.
- Drape the area.
- Put on gloves.
- Insert 18- to 20-gauge needle into the area of soft tissue swelling and withdraw fluid.
- If the syringe becomes full (Fig. 17–1)

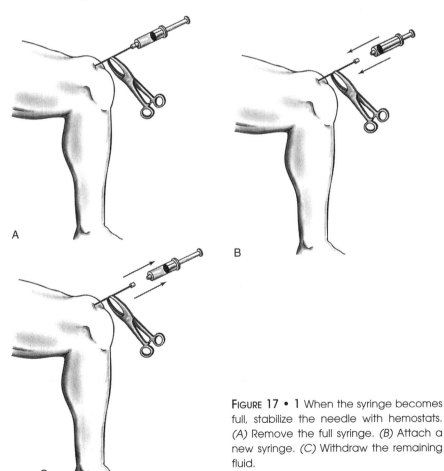

A

B

C

FIGURE 17 • 1 When the syringe becomes full, stabilize the needle with hemostats. *(A)* Remove the full syringe. *(B)* Attach a new syringe. *(C)* Withdraw the remaining fluid.

- ➤ Stabilize the needle with hemostats.
- ➤ Remove the full syringe.
- ➤ Attach a new syringe.
- ➤ Withdraw the remaining fluid.
- ➤ Inject the specimen into a tube or on a slide, and send to the laboratory for evaluation.
- ➤ Apply a pressure dressing and tape.
- ➤ Apply the Ace wrap.

Client Instructions

- ➤ Keep the pressure dressing in place for 24 hours, then remove.
- ➤ Observe for signs of infection, such as
  - ➤ Increase in pain and heat at the site
  - ➤ Red streaks
  - ➤ Yellow or green drainage
  - ➤ Chills and fever
  - ➤ Foul odor from wound
- ➤ Soft tissue swelling may recur. If this happens, return to the office.

BIBLIOGRAPHY

Dellacorte, M.P., Birrer, R.B., and Grisafi, P.J. (1994). Traumatic injuries. *Emerg Med*, 26(11), 46–64.
Pfenninger, J.L., and Fowler, G.C. (1995). *Procedures for primary care physicians*. St. Louis: Mosby.

18   STAPLE INSERTION

MARGARET R. COLYAR

CPT Code	
12001-7	Simple repair of superficial wounds of scalp, neck, axillae, external genitalia, trunk, or extremities (including hands and feet); based on length

Simple wound closure with the use of stapling devices can be done easily by the nurse practitioner.

OVERVIEW

- ➤ Incidence unknown
- ➤ Types of staple material available

> Ethicon
> 3M
> Deknatel

RATIONALE

> To prevent unsightly wound healing
> To promote accelerated wound healing

INDICATIONS

> Long, linear lacerations
> Scalp wounds
> Wounds in area of less cosmetic importance

CONTRAINDICATIONS

> Crush wounds
> Ischemic wounds
> Highly contaminated wounds

☑ *Informed consent required*

PROCEDURE

Staple Insertion

Equipment

> Antiseptic skin cleanser
> 0.9% sodium chloride—250 to 500 mL
> Drape—sterile
> Gloves—nonsterile
> Stapling device
> Staples
> 1% or 2% lidocaine with epinephrine if the area to be anesthetized is not on a digit, nose, ear, or penis
> 3-mL syringe
> 27- to 30-gauge, 1-inch needle
> 18-gauge, $1^1/_2$-inch needle
> Cotton-tipped applicator—sterile
> Topical antibiotic ointment (Bactroban, Neosporin, or Polysporin)
> Nonstick dressing such as Telfa
> 4 × 4 gauze—sterile
> Tape

Procedure

> Position the client for comfort with laceration easily accessible.
> Irrigate vigorously with 0.9% sodium chloride using 10-mL syringe and 18-gauge needle.

➤ Cleanse a 3-inch-diameter area around the laceration with antiseptic skin cleanser.
➤ Put on gloves.
➤ Infiltrate wound with 1% or 2% lidocaine. Epinephrine may be used if the wound is not on a digit, ear, nose, or penis.
➤ **Approximate** the skin edges.
➤ Place the stapling device perpendicular to the skin and depress the top handle.
➤ Insert staples perpendicular to the skin at $1/4$-inch intervals.
➤ Apply topical antibiotic ointment.
➤ Apply nonstick dressing.
➤ Cover with 4 × 4 gauze.
➤ Secure with tape.

Client Instructions

➤ You may remove the dressing in 48 hours.
➤ Keep the wound clean and dry.
➤ Observe for signs and symptoms of infection, such as
  ➤ Increase in pain after 24 hours
  ➤ Increase in temperature
  ➤ Redness or swelling
  ➤ Yellow or greenish drainage
  ➤ Foul odor
➤ If any of the signs and symptoms of infection are found, return to the office.
➤ Return to the office in _____ days for staple removal.

BIBLIOGRAPHY
Saunders, C.E., and Ho, M.T. (1994). *Current emergency diagnosis and treatment.* Norwalk, CT: Appleton & Lange.

19 STAPLE REMOVAL

MARGARET R. COLYAR

CPT Codes
None. Included as part of staple insertion.

Removal of staples after initial healing has occurred should be done within a specified time frame. The suggested times for removing staples are

- Face, neck—3 to 5 days
- Ear, scalp—5 to 7 days
- Arm, leg, hand, foot—7 to 10 or more days
- Chest, back, abdomen—7 to 10 or more days

OVERVIEW

- Incidence unknown

OPTIONS

- *Method 1*—staple removal (complete)
  - Used for wounds that are
    - Small
    - Well-approximated
    - Not oozing
- *Method 2*—staple removal (partial)
  - Used for wounds that are
    - Large
    - Healing poorly
    - Possibility of evisceration

RATIONALE

- To prevent scarring and infection from retained staples

INDICATIONS

- Staples in place for appropriate healing period
- Wound does not need extra stability of staples
- Allergic reaction to staples

CONTRAINDICATIONS

- Wound has not healed well

PROCEDURE

Method 1—Staple Removal (Complete)

Equipment

- Alcohol
- Staple remover—sterile
- Gloves—nonsterile
- Steri strips (method 2)
- Benzoin (method 2)
- Cotton-tipped applicators (method 2)
- Alcohol prep pads (method 2)

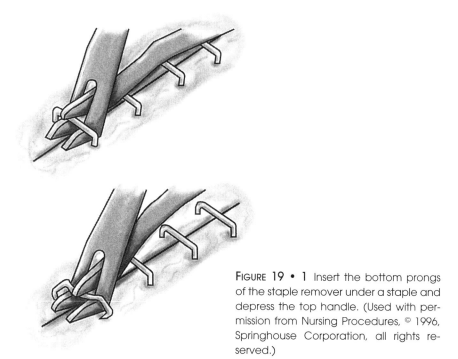

FIGURE 19 • 1 Insert the bottom prongs of the staple remover under a staple and depress the top handle. (Used with permission from Nursing Procedures, © 1996, Springhouse Corporation, all rights reserved.)

Procedure

- ➤ Position the client for comfort with laceration easily accessible.
- ➤ Put on gloves.
- ➤ Insert the bottom prongs of staple remover under a staple and depress the top handle.
  - ➤ Edges of the staple will rise (Fig. 19–1).
- ➤ Rock the staple gently side to side, if needed, to remove edges of the staple from the skin.
- ➤ Continue with each staple until all staples are removed.
- ➤ Cleanse incision with alcohol prep pads.

Method 2—Staple Removal (Partial)

Procedure

- ➤ Position the client for comfort with laceration easily accessible.
- ➤ Put on gloves.
- ➤ Insert the bottom prongs of staple remover under a staple and depress the top handle.
  - ➤ Edges of the staple will rise.
- ➤ Rock the staple gently side to side, if needed, to remove edges from skin.
- ➤ Continue with *alternate staples* until all staples are removed.

> Apply benzoin in spaces where staples have been removed. Start at wound edge and spread benzoin away from wound approximately $1^1/_2$ inches (see Chapter 20).
> When benzoin is tacky, apply Steri strips between every remaining staple.
> Cleanse the incision with alcohol prep pads.

Client Instructions

> Observe for signs and symptoms of infection, such as
> > Increase in pain after 24 hours
> > Increase in temperature
> > Redness or swelling
> > Yellow or greenish drainage
> > Foul odor
> > Wound separation
> If any signs and symptoms of infection are found, return to the office.

BIBLIOGRAPHY

Saunders, C.E., and Ho, M.T. (1994). *Current emergency diagnosis and treatment.* Norwalk, CT: Appleton & Lange.

20

STERI STRIP APPLICATION

MARGARET R. COLYAR

CPT Code

None. Included in evaluation and management charge (office visit charge).

Steri strips are noninvasive skin closure devices. They are used when sutures are not necessary but approximation of the wound is needed to promote healing.

OVERVIEW

> Incidence unknown

RATIONALE

> To provide wound stability while healing process takes place

INDICATIONS

➤ Small, superficial wounds
➤ Wounds under little tension
➤ Stapled or sutured wounds that need extra support

CONTRAINDICATIONS

➤ Large, deep wounds
➤ Wounds that are under tension

PROCEDURE

Steri Strip Application

Equipment

➤ Antiseptic skin cleanser
➤ Skin adhesive, such as **benzoin**
➤ Steri strips—1/8 to $^1/_2$ inch
➤ Cotton-tipped applicators—sterile
➤ 4 × 4 gauze—sterile
➤ Tape

Procedure

➤ Position the client with area to be Steri-stripped easily accessible.
➤ Cleanse skin 3 inches around the wound with antiseptic skin cleanser.
➤ Using cotton-tipped applicators, apply benzoin or other skin adhesive. Start next to the wound edges and extend outward approximately $1^1/_2$ inches (Fig. 20–1).
➤ Allow the skin adhesive to become tacky.
➤ Apply Steri strips toward the wound, pulling one skin edge to the other (Fig. 20–2).
➤ Apply a sufficient number of Steri strips to ensure wound closure.
➤ A nonocclusive dressing using 4 × 4 gauze may be applied to keep the wound clean and dry and to absorb drainage that oozes from the wound for the first 24 hours.

Client Instructions

➤ If you had a dressing applied over the Steri-stripped area, remove it in 24 hours and leave the area open to air.
➤ Keep Steri strips clean and dry.
➤ If Steri strips become dislodged and the wound separates, return to clinic for reapplication of Steri strips.
➤ A small amount of redness around the wound is normal.
➤ Observe for signs and symptoms of infection, such as
  ➤ Increase in pain after 24 hours
  ➤ Increase in temperature
  ➤ Redness or swelling

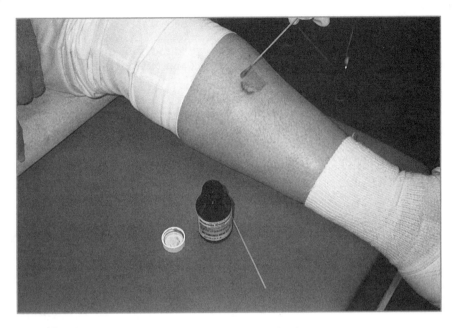

FIGURE 20 • 1 Apply skin adhesive next to the wound edges.

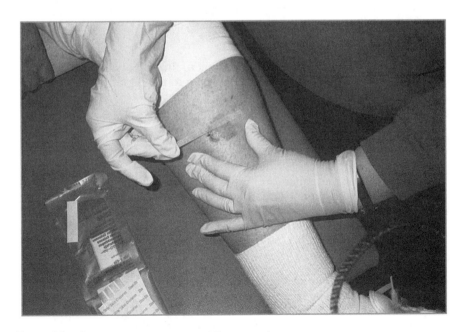

FIGURE 20 • 2 Apply Steri strips toward the wound.

- ➤ Yellow or greenish drainage
- ➤ Foul odor
- ➤ If any signs and symptoms of infection are found, return to the office.
- ➤ Return to the office in 1 week for recheck and removal of the Steri strips.

BIBLIOGRAPHY

Smeltzer, S., and Bare, B.G. (1996). *Brunner and Suddarth's textbook of medical-surgical nursing.* Philadelphia: Lippincott-Raven.

Sorensen, K.C., and Luckmann, J. (1986). *Basic nursing: A psychophysiologic approach.* Philadelphia: Saunders.

21

SUBUNGUAL HEMATOMA EXCISION

CYNTHIA R. EHRHARDT

CPT Code	
11740	Subungual hematoma evacuation

Subungual hematoma results from trauma to the nail plate in which bleeding occurs beneath the nail and results in pain to the digit.

OVERVIEW

- ➤ Incidence unknown
- ➤ Complicating factors
  - ➤ Temporary or permanent disfigurement to the nail
  - ➤ Temporary or permanent loss of the nail
  - ➤ Infection arising from the trauma or treatment
- ➤ Consider an x-ray if the subungual hematoma is greater than 25% of the nail.

General Principles

- ➤ Inspect the area for contraindications to the procedure.
- ➤ Palpate for tenderness beyond the nail bed.
- ➤ Determine the vascular and neurologic status of the digit.
- ➤ Perform active and passive range of motion of the distal joint.
- ➤ Test for instability of the digit's joint.

HEALTH PROMOTION/PREVENTION

➤ Follow safety measures around all machinery.
➤ Avoid placing digits in the path of closing doors.
➤ Use hammers carefully.
➤ Do not use unfamiliar machinery without proper instruction.

OPTIONS

➤ *Method 1*—cautery technique
➤ *Method 2*—paper clip technique

RATIONALE

➤ To relieve pain
➤ To prevent possible infection

INDICATIONS

➤ Complaint of digit pain following trauma with the presence of a subungual hematoma less than 4 hours old

CONTRAINDICATIONS

➤ Presence of hematoma greater than 50% of the nail surface
➤ Crushed or fractured nail
➤ Known history of poor healing (physician referral)
➤ Suspected distal phalanx fracture

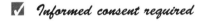 *Informed consent required*

PROCEDURES

Subungual Hematoma Excision

Equipment

➤ Method 1 only
  ➤ Battery-powered cautery device
  ➤ Basin—sterile
  ➤ Povidone-iodine soak or antibacterial soap
  ➤ Gloves—sterile
  ➤ 0.9% sodium chloride—sterile
  ➤ 4 × 4 gauze—sterile
➤ Method 2 only
  ➤ Alcohol lamp, Bunsen burner, or cigarette lighter
  ➤ Paper clip—medium or large
  ➤ **Hemostat**—sterile
  ➤ Safety goggles and mask—optional
  ➤ Magnifying lens—optional
  ➤ Finger protector—nonsterile

Procedure

METHOD 1—CAUTERY TECHNIQUE

➤ Soak the affected digit in lukewarm podivone-iodine or antibacterial soapy water for 5 to 10 minutes.
➤ Position the client for comfort.
➤ Drape the digit with the sterile 4 × 4 gauze to absorb the blood.
➤ If necessary, have someone hold the digit secure to prevent movement during the procedure.
➤ Put on gloves.
➤ Activate the cautery.
➤ When the cautery needle becomes red hot, apply the needle directly over the middle of the subungual hematoma at a 90-degree angle with firm, gentle pressure (Fig. 21–1).
➤ Be sure not to stand in the direct line of the hole because the release of the hematoma can result in the forceful splattering of blood.
➤ As the needle burns a hole (approximately 1 to 2 mm) through the nail, resistance can be felt.
➤ When resistance ceases, this indicates full penetration through the nail.
➤ Proceed to lift the cautery probe away from the nail, and allow blood to drain if clotting has not occurred (Fig. 21–2).
➤ Dab with the 4 × 4 gauze to facilitate drainage.
➤ Administer tetanus-diphtheria booster if immunization was more than 5 years ago.

METHOD 2—PAPER CLIP TECHNIQUE

➤ Soak the affected digit in lukewarm povidone-iodine or antibacterial soapy water for 5 to 10 minutes.
➤ Position the client for comfort.
➤ Drape the digit with the sterile 4 × 4 gauze to absorb the blood.
➤ If necessary, have someone hold the digit secure to prevent movement during the procedure.
➤ Straighten one end of a medium or large paper clip and clamp a hemostat to the opposite end.

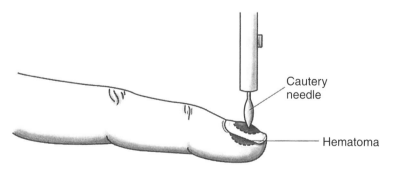

Cautery needle

Hematoma

FIGURE 21 • 1 Apply the heated cautery needle over the middle of the hematoma at a 90-degree angle.

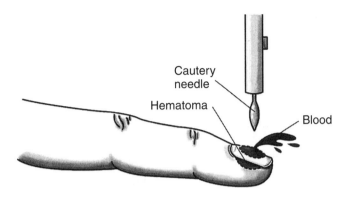

FIGURE 21 • 2 Remove the cautery probe and allow the blood to drain.

➤ Light the alcohol lamp, Bunsen burner, or cigarette lighter.
➤ Put on gloves.
➤ Place the tip of the paper clip into the hottest part of the flame and heat until red hot.
➤ Using firm, gentle pressure, apply the paper clip to the nail surface at a 90-degree angle (Fig. 21–3).
➤ As the nail burns a hole (approximately 1 to 2 mm) through the nail, resistance can be felt.
➤ Resistance ceases with full penetration through the nail.
➤ Lift the paper clip away from the nail, and allow blood to drain if clotting has not occurred.
➤ Dab with the 4 × 4 gauze to facilitate drainage.
➤ Administer tetanus-diphtheria booster if immunization was more than 5 years ago.

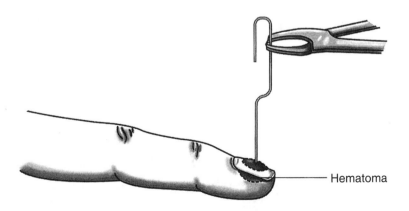

FIGURE 21 • 3 Apply the heated paper clip to the nail surface at a 90-degree angle.

Client Instructions

➤ Keep wound clean and dry.
➤ To lessen pain, apply cool compresses and elevate the hand above the heart.
➤ Antibiotics are not required.
➤ Observe for signs and symptoms of infection, such as
  ➤ Increase in pain after 24 hours
  ➤ Increase in temperature
  ➤ Redness or swelling
  ➤ Yellow or greenish drainage
  ➤ Foul odor
➤ If any signs and symptoms of infection are found, return to the office.
➤ To relieve pain
  ➤ Take acetaminophen every 4 to 6 hours as needed for mild pain for first 24 hours.
  ➤ Ibuprofen, naproxen, and other nonsteroidals should be avoided for the first 24 hours to lessen the risk of increased bleeding.
  ➤ After 24 hours, alternating nonsteroidals with acetaminophen may be beneficial.
  ➤ Tylenol No. 3 is used rarely for severe pain.
  ➤ Return to the office if the nail appears to need removal.

BIBLIOGRAPHY

American Medical Association (1996). *Physicians' current procedural terminology.* Chicago: Author.
Habif, T. (1996) (3rd ed.). *Clinical dermatology: A color guide to diagnosis and therapy.* St. Louis: Mosby.
Hoffman, D., and Schaffer, T. (1991). Management of common finger injuries. *Am Fam Physician,* 43(5), 850–862.
Pfenninger, J.L., and Fowler, G.C. (1994). *Procedures for primary care physicians.* St. Louis: Mosby.
Trott, A. (1991). *Wounds and lacerations: Emergency care and closure.* St. Louis: Mosby.

22 SUTURE INSERTION

CYNTHIA R. EHRHARDT

CPT Code	
12001–7	Simple repair, superficial wounds; scalp, neck, axillae, external genitalia, trunk, or extremities
12011–18	Simple repair, superficial wounds; face, ears, eyelids, nose, lips, or mucous membranes

12020	Superficial dehiscence, simple
12031–37	Intermediate repair with layer closure; scalp, axillae, trunk, or extremities (not hands and feet)
12041–47	Intermediate repair with layer closure; neck, hands, feet, or external genitalia
12051–57	Intermediate repair with layer closure; face, ears, eyelids, nose, lips, or mucous membranes

Suturing is a procedure used to repair lacerations of the skin. The length of time sutures are left in depends on location. Leaving sutures in too long or removing them too soon increases the risk of unnecessary scarring (Table 22–1).

OVERVIEW

➤ Incidence unknown
➤ Complicating factors of secondary infection are usually due to
　➤ Gram-positive bacteria
　　• *Staphylococcus aureus* (3% resistance)
　　• Streptococci
　➤ Gram-negative bacteria
　　• *Proteus*
　　• *Klebsiella*
　　• Pseudomonas

General Principles

➤ Minimize the amount of pain to the site with anesthesia.
➤ Irrigate all wounds with sterile 0.9% sodium chloride (60 to 120 mL) to ensure removal of foreign matter and to improve clean closure.
➤ Avoid infection and poor wound healing, minimize scarring, and obtain good cosmetic results by

TABLE 22•1 SUGGESTED LENGTH OF TIME SUTURES SHOULD BE LEFT IN PLACE

BODY PART	LENGTH OF TIME (DAYS)
Face	3–4
Neck	5
Scalp	6–7
Arms and back of hands	7
Chest and abdomen	7–10
Legs and top of feet	10
Back	10–12
Palms of hands, soles of feet	14

- Maintaining uniform tensile strength
- Precise approximation of skin edges
- Closure of all dead space in wound
- Avoiding excessive suturing
➤ If laceration is located over a joint, it is recommended after suturing that the joint be splinted for the length the sutures are in place to prevent rupture of the suture line. It is permitted to remove the splint a minimum of four times a day for gentle active range of motion to prevent loss of joint mobility.
➤ If sutures are needed in a hairy area of the body, use a different color of suture material (e.g., blue filament in a person with black hair).
➤ Prophylactic antibiotic therapy no longer is recommended.
➤ Oral antibiotic therapy should be considered when the risk for infection is greater than side effects of medication.
  - Guidelines include
    • Wounds more than 6 hours old
    • Wounds caused by crushing mechanism with tissue compromise
    • Contaminated or soiled wounds that require extensive cleansing and/or debridement
    • Extensive lacerations to the hand
    • Immunocompromised and diabetic clients

Selection of Suture Needles

➤ The ideal suture needle should be
  - Inexpensive
  - Appropriate to the type of wound repair
  - Maximum sharpness and strength to complete the task with the least amount of tissue injury
➤ For most superficial and intermediate suture repair use a P-1 to P-3 (Ethicon) 3/8- to $1/2$-inch cutting circle. Deep suturing or buried sutures may require PS-1 or PS-2 (Ethicon) needle.

Selection of Suture Material

➤ The advantages and disadvantages of each suture material should be taken into consideration (Table 22–2). The ideal suture material should
  - Be inexpensive
  - Be strong
  - Form secure knots
  - Handle easily
  - Stretch and recoil easily during wound healing
  - Minimize tissue inflammation
  - Retard tissue infections

General Recommendations for Suture Use

➤ The larger the number of the suture (e.g., 3-0), the smaller the filament thickness.
  - *Extremities*—4-0 or 5-0 polypropolyene (Prolene) nonabsorbable, 3-0 or 4-0 mild chromic gut (Vicryl) for buried sutures

TABLE 22•2 SUTURE MATERIAL

SUTURE MATERIAL	ADVANTAGES	DISADVANTAGES
Silk (nonabsorbable)	Natural product; easiest-handling of suture material; least amount of wound irritation	Lowest in tensile strength and breaks easily; high absorption capacity increases wound infections
Nylon (nonabsorbable) (Ethilon, Dermalon)	Synthetic product; hydrolyzes slowly; high elasticity and tensile strength; minimal tissue reaction; inexpensive	Stiff; difficult to knot
Polypropylene (nonabsorbable) (Prolene, Surgilene)	Synthetic; low tissue adherence; stretches	Knots poorly; loose after tissue edema resolves; expensive
Braided polyester (nonabsorbable) (Ethibond, Dacron)	Synthetic; handles easily; good knot control	Uncoated— leads to increased tissue friction and drag; increases incidence of wound infection; expensive
Polybutester (nonabsorbable) (Novafil)	Elastic; accommodates change in wound edema; less stiffness and tissue drag	Moderately expensive
Treated catgut (absorbable) (Mild chromic gut)	Natural product; inexpensive; good tensile strength for 4–5 days	Poor knot handling; moderate tissue inflammation
Polyglycolic (absorbable) (Dexon)	Synthetic; less tissue reactivity; prolonged tensile strength	Poor knot tying; stiff
Polyglactic acid (absorbable) (Vicryl)	Synthetic; easy to handle; prolonged tensile strength; decreased tissue reactivity	Dyed for visibility
Polyglyconate (absorbable) (Maxon)	Extended duration of tensile strength– 80% after 2 weeks; easy to handle	Expensive; recent market introduction

➤ *Trunk*—4-0 or 5-0 polypropolyene nonabsorbable; 3-0 or 4-0 mild chromic gut for buried sutures
➤ *Face*—5-0 to 6-0 nylon (Ethilon); 4-0 or 5-0 absorbable for buried sutures

HEALTH PROMOTION/PREVENTION

➤ Use basic safety techniques around machinery and tools.

OPTIONS
Suturing Techniques

➤ Each technique has advantages and disadvantages (Table 22–3 and Fig. 22–1).

TABLE 22 •3   SUTURING TECHNIQUES (SEE FIG. 22-1 A TO H)

TECHNIQUE	ADVANTAGES	DISADVANTAGES
Buried suture (Fig. 22–1A)	Allows good approximation	Minimal eversion occurs
Buried vertical mattress suture (Fig. 22–1B)	Has prolonged eversion; allows early removal of top layer sutures	If too superficial, more likely to split
Running continuous suture (Fig. 22–1C)	Quick; good for children; even tension	Entire suture must be removed
Interrupted suture (Fig. 22–1D)	Permits precise adjustments between sutures; allows selection of sutures	Increased risk of uneven tension over the suture line; higher incidence of "rail-road track" scarring
Vertical mattress suture (Fig. 22–1E)	Good dead space wound closure; increased wound eversion; increases wound strength	Time consuming; increased risk of suture marking; difficult to approximate wound edges
Corner (half-buried) suture (Fig. 22–1F)	Used in skin flap suturing; decreases risk of obstruction of blood supply to sutured skin flap	Edge approximation more difficult; risk of trauma to skin flap; increased risk of dead space
Subcuticular suture (Fig. 22–1G)	Lower incidence of scarring; best for edge approximation	Poor tensile strength; time consuming; poor wound eversion
Horizontal mattress suture (Fig. 22–1H)	Good dead space closure; good wound eversion; some hemostasis occurs	Increased risk of scarring; increased risk of epidermal necrosis
Wound closure tapes (Steri strips)	Minimal wound trauma; more resistant to wound infections	Poor wound eversion; more difficult wound edge approximation

Note: Application of a technique to the laceration depends on size, shape, location, and depth of the injury. The number of sutures depends on the size of the laceration, location of the laceration, and amount of tension that would be placed on the sutured wound. Generally the rule of thumb for sutures on nonfacial areas is that spacing should be no closer than 0.25 cm from the next or adjacent suture.

Commonly Used Anesthetic Agents

➤ Lidocaine (Xylocaine) 1% to 2.5%—1 to 2 hours of relief
➤ Bupivacaine (Marcaine) 0.25% to 1.5%—6 to 8 hours of relief

RATIONALE

➤ To avoid infection
➤ To promote good wound healing
➤ To minimize scarring
➤ To obtain good cosmetic results
➤ To repair the loss of tissue integrity because of trauma

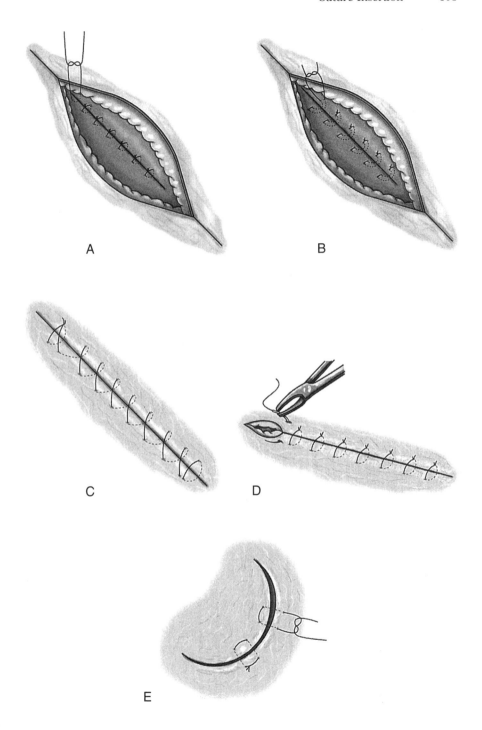

A

B

C

D

E

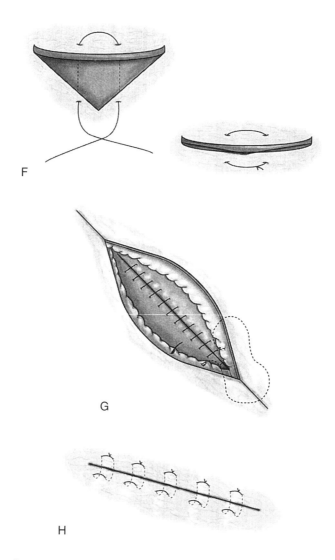

F

G

H

FIGURE 22 • 1 Suturing techniques. *(A)* Buried suture (interrupted); *(B)* buried vertical mattress suture; *(C)* running continuous suture; *(D)* interrupted suture; *(E)* vertical mattress suture; *(F)* corner (half-buried suture); *(G)* subcuticular suture; and *(H)* horizontal mattress suture.

INDICATIONS

➤ Superficial or intermediate laceration to the skin without artery, bone, ligament, nerve, or tendon involvement

CONTRAINDICATIONS

➤ Complex laceration, REFER to a physician.
➤ Involvement of artery, bone, ligament, nerve, or tendon, REFER to a physician.
➤ More than 6 hours after the occurrence. *(Consultation with collaborative physician is strongly advised with delayed treatment of lacerations.)*

☑ *Informed consent required*

PROCEDURE

Suture Insertion

Equipment

➤ Povidone-iodine solution or swabs
➤ 1% lidocaine with or without epinephrine
  ➤ Lidocaine with epinephrine generally is reserved for wounds that have considerable bleeding characteristics, such as wounds in the scalp and eyebrow areas.
  ➤ *Lidocaine with epinephrine should never be used in digits and appendages of the body because of vasoconstriction.*
➤ Two syringes—5 mL and 30 mL
➤ Angiocath—16- or 18-gauge
➤ 25- to 27-gauge, 1- to $1^1/_2$-inch needle
➤ Appropriately selected suturing material for the laceration
➤ Gloves—sterile
➤ 0.9% sodium chloride—sterile
➤ Sterile towels (fenestrated and nonfenestrated)
➤ Sterile suture kit (prepackaged or self-made) should include
  ➤ Curved and straight **hemostats**
  ➤ Needle holders ($4^1/_2$- and 6-inch)
  ➤ Skin hooks
  ➤ Forceps with teeth
  ➤ Iris scissors
  ➤ Knife handle and blades (usually No. 11 blade)
  ➤ Cup to hold povidone-iodine and sterile normal saline solution
  ➤ 4 × 4 sterile gauze

Procedure

➤ Position client comfortably with area of laceration easily accessible.
➤ Apply povidone-iodine to the wound beginning at the wound edges and expanding out in a circular pattern.
➤ Put on gloves.
➤ Infiltrate wound with 1% lidocaine (5-mL syringe with 25- to 27-gauge needle).
➤ Insert the needle parallel along each side of the edge of the laceration to the farthest point, and begin to infiltrate the wound while slowly

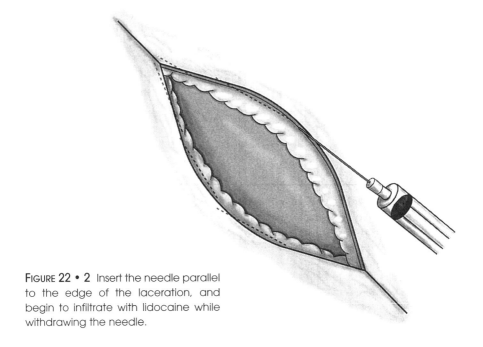

FIGURE 22 • 2 Insert the needle parallel to the edge of the laceration, and begin to infiltrate with lidocaine while withdrawing the needle.

withdrawing the needle (Fig. 22–2). This procedure results in a more uniform anesthesia with fewer injections.

➤ Carefully explore the wound for foreign bodies and involvement of the joint capsule, tendons, and other related anatomic structures.

➤ If there are no anatomic contraindications to suturing, irrigate the wound with 60 to 100 mL of sterile normal saline. (Be sure to document this in your procedure note.)

➤ If wound edges are ragged, trim with iris scissors. Minimize the amount of debridement of epidermis (Fig. 22–3). Occasionally, undermining may be required to give good approximation of the edges (Fig. 22–4).

➤ Place suture needle in needle holder, using proper hand position.

➤ With the opposite hand, use forceps with teeth to grasp wound edge and evert the edges. Penetrate the wound edge with the suture needle (Fig. 22–5), ensuring the suture is far enough from the wound edge to prevent tearing (generally 0.5 cm, but no greater than 1 cm from wound edge).

➤ Tie suture off as determined by chosen technique.

➤ Trim leftover suture to a length suitable for grasping with forceps for easy removal.

➤ When wound is completely sutured, cleanse area with 0.9% sodium chloride.

➤ Pat dry.

➤ Apply dressing. (If highly vascular, consider a pressure dressing for several hours.)

➤ Be precise and descriptive when documenting the procedure performed in the medical record. Include

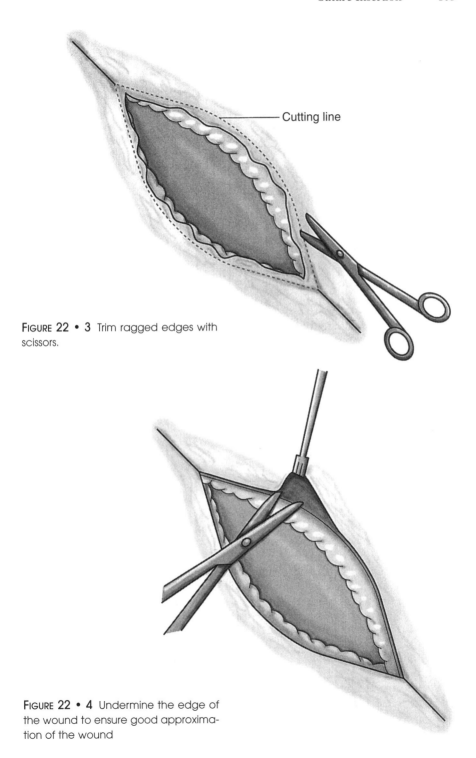

Cutting line

FIGURE 22 • 3 Trim ragged edges with scissors.

FIGURE 22 • 4 Undermine the edge of the wound to ensure good approximation of the wound

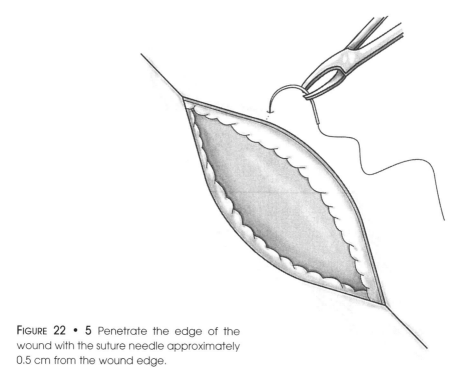

FIGURE 22 • 5 Penetrate the edge of the
wound with the suture needle approximately
0.5 cm from the wound edge.

- ➤ Anesthetic used
- ➤ Cleansing preparation performed
- ➤ Whether irrigation occurred (amount of irrigation)
- ➤ Type of suture material
- ➤ Number of sutures
- ➤ Outcome of the suturing
- ➤ How the procedure was tolerated

Client Instructions

- ➤ Keep wound clean and dry.
- ➤ Do not wash area for 24 hours after the procedure. After 24 hours, dressing may be removed, and site may be left open to air.
  - ➤ Continuous covering of wound increases risk of infection.
- ➤ Bathing 48 hours after the procedure is permitted.
- ➤ If crust develops over the sutured site
  - ➤ Cleanse with a cotton-tipped swab saturated with hydrogen peroxide.
  - ➤ Take the swab and gently roll over the wound site.
  - ➤ Gently rinse the area with warm water.
  - ➤ Blot dry with clean towel or cotton gauze.
- ➤ To decrease pain
  - ➤ Use Tylenol No. 3 for severe pain every 4 to 6 hours as needed for the first 24 hours.

➤ Then use acetaminophen, ibuprofen, or naproxen every 4 hours for mild pain.
➤ Observe for signs and symptoms of infection, such as
  ➤ Increase in pain after 24 hours
  ➤ Increase in temperature
  ➤ Redness or swelling
  ➤ Yellow or greenish drainage
  ➤ Foul odor
➤ If any of the signs and symptoms of infection are found, return to the office.
➤ Apply antibiotic ointment to the wound to lessen the development of scab formation.
➤ Return to the office in 48 hours for wound recheck.

BIBLIOGRAPHY

American Medical Association (1996). *Physicians' current procedural terminology.* Chicago: Author.
Edlich, R., et al (1990) (4th ed.). *A manual for wound closure.* St. Paul, MN: 3-M Medical-Surgical Division.
Moy, R., et al (1991). Commonly used suturing techniques in skin surgery. *Am Fam Physician,* 44(5), 1625–1634.
Moy, R., et al (1991). Commonly used suturing materials in skin surgery. *Am Fam Physician,* 44(6), 2121–2129.
Pfenninger, J., and Fowler, G. (1994). *Procedures for primary care physicians.* St. Louis: Mosby.
Trott, A. (1991). *Wound and lacerations: Emergency care and closure.* St. Louis: Mosby.
Weitekamp, M., and Caputo, G. (1995). Antibiotic prophylaxis. *Am Fam Physician,* 48(4).

23 SUTURE REMOVAL

CYNTHIA EHRHARDT

CPT Code
V 058.3   Simple removal

Suture removal is the withdrawal of artificially inserted polyfilament thread used to repair a laceration. Leaving foreign material in the body after healing increases inflammation and scarring to the site.

OVERVIEW

➤ Incidence is unknown.
➤ Sutures should be removed in a timely manner to prevent scarring and inflammation (see Table 22–1).

OPTIONS

➤ *Method 1*—Standard suture removal technique
➤ *Method 2*—Running suture line technique
➤ *Method 3*—Small loop sutures, closed sutures, and difficult anatomic position sutures technique

RATIONALE

➤ To diminish the occurrence of inflammation and scarring

INDICATIONS

➤ Presence of suture material in superficial layers of the skin

CONTRAINDICATIONS

➤ Removal before recommended length of time for healing of the laceration

PROCEDURE

Suture Removal

Equipment

➤ Methods 1 and 2 only
  ➤ Scissors—sterile
  ➤ **Forceps** without teeth—sterile
➤ Methods 1, 2, and 3
  ➤ Gloves—sterile
  ➤ Hydrogen peroxide
  ➤ Cotton-tipped applicators—clean or sterile
  ➤ 4 × 4 gauze—clean or sterile
  ➤ Steri strips or butterfly Band-Aids—optional
➤ Method 3 only
  ➤ No. 11 scalpel

Procedure

Method 1—Standard Suture Removal Technique

➤ Position the client comfortably with sutured area easily accessible.
➤ Examine sutures to determine the type of suture technique that was used.
➤ Locate the end tie knot(s).
➤ If crust is present over suture site
  ➤ Gently roll a cotton-tipped applicator saturated with hydrogen peroxide over the site to remove crust.
  ➤ Rinse with cotton-tipped applicator saturated with 0.9% sodium chloride.
  ➤ Blot the site dry.
  ➤ Grasp the tip of the suture (tail) with forceps and gently lift upward on the suture.
  ➤ Slide scissors under the suture (Fig. 23–1).

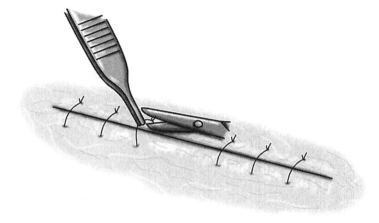

FIGURE 23 • 1 Pull the suture tail upward with forceps, slide the scissors under the suture, and cut.

- ➤ Cut the suture.
- ➤ Gently remove the suture.
- ➤ Repeat this procedure until all sutures are removed.
- ➤ Blot the area dry as needed with 4 × 4 gauze.
- ➤ If the suture line appears slightly unstable, a Steri strip or butterfly Band-Aid may be used (see Chapter 20).

METHOD 2—RUNNING SUTURE LINE TECHNIQUE

- ➤ Position the client comfortably with sutured area easily accessible.
- ➤ Examine sutures to determine the type of suture technique that was used.
- ➤ Locate the end tie knot(s).
- ➤ If crust is present over suture site
  - ➤ Gently roll a cotton-tipped applicator saturated with hydrogen peroxide over the site to remove crust.
  - ➤ Rinse with cotton-tipped applicator saturated with 0.9% sodium chloride.
  - ➤ Blot the site dry.
  - ➤ Cut the knot at the distal end of the suture line (Fig. 23–2).
  - ➤ Grasp the opposite knot with forceps.
  - ➤ Pull gently with a continuous steady motion until suture is removed.
  - ➤ Blot the area dry as needed with 4 × 4 gauze.
  - ➤ If the suture line appears slightly unstable, a Steri strip or butterfly Band-Aid may be used (see Chapter 20).

METHOD 3—SMALL LOOP SUTURES, CLOSED SUTURES, AND DIFFICULT ANATOMIC POSITION SUTURES TECHNIQUE

- ➤ Position the client comfortably with sutured area easily accessible.
- ➤ Examine sutures to determine the type of suture technique that was used.
- ➤ Locate the end tie knot(s).

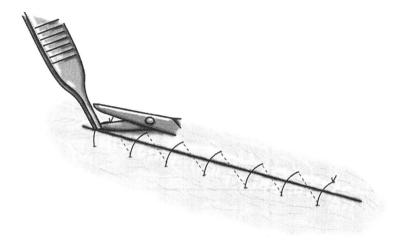

FIGURE 23 • 2 Cut the knot at the distal end of the running suture line, grasp the knot at the opposite end with forceps, and gently pull.

➤ If crust is present over suture site
  ➤ Gently roll a cotton-tipped applicator saturated with hydrogen peroxide over the site to remove crust.
  ➤ Rinse with cotton-tipped applicator saturated with 0.9% sodium chloride.
  ➤ Blot the site dry.
➤ Take No. 11 scalpel and place flat on skin (Fig. 23–3).
➤ Slide the scalpel under the suture, and exert the sharp edge against suture.
➤ Use forceps to remove the suture.
➤ Blot the area dry as needed with 4 × 4 gauze.

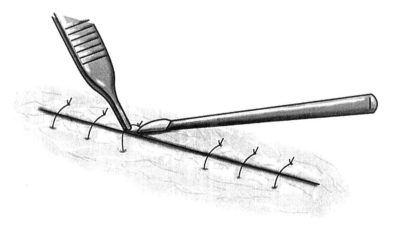

FIGURE 23 • 3 Pull the suture tail upward with forceps, slide the No. 11 scalpel under the suture, and cut.

➤ If the suture line appears slightly unstable, a Steri strip or butterfly Band-Aid may be used (see Chapter 20).

Client Instructions

➤ If Steri strip sutures are used, they may be removed in 24 to 48 hours.

BIBLIOGRAPHY

American Medical Association (1996). *Physicians' current procedural terminology.* Chicago: Author.

Edlich, R., et al (1980) (2nd ed.). *A manual for wound closure.* St. Paul, MN: 3-M Medical-Surgical Division.

Trott, A. (1991). *Wound and lacerations: Emergency care and closure.* St. Louis: Mosby.

Walt, A., and Wilson, R. (1975). *Management of trauma: Pitfalls and practice.* Philadelphia: Lea & Febiger.

24

TICK REMOVAL

CYNTHIA R. EHRHARDT

CPT Code

10120   Removal of superficial foreign body, skin
10121   Removal of foreign body, complex

Ticks are small, blood-sucking ectoparasites. Ticks burrow into the skin and may become buried, resulting in pain and infection.

OVERVIEW

➤ Incidence unknown
➤ Demographic characteristics of tick infestation victims
  ➤ Average age 31 to 42 years
  ➤ 75% affect males
  ➤ 80% participate in outdoor activities
  ➤ 75% are rural residents
➤ Ascertain the following
  ➤ Length of time the tick has been embedded
  ➤ What attempts have been made to remove it
  ➤ Locale (camping, woods, contact with animals) where the tick may have been picked up
  ➤ Presence or absence of **erythema migrans**
  ➤ If the tick has been removed, did the individual bring the tick to the office

> ➤ Is the tick intact (no missing parts)
> ➤ Knowledge of ticks indigenous to the geographic location where the individual had spent time
> ➤ Allergies to medication
> ➤ History of immunosuppressive disorders or poor wound healing

General Principles

- ➤ Avoid use of finger to "pull tick out."
- ➤ Use gloves to protect self from contamination.
- ➤ If possible, attempt to identify the tick (dog tick versus deer tick).
- ➤ Avoid manipulating the tick because this increases the release of more irritant juices into the tissue.
- ➤ Avoid crushing the tick.
- ➤ Avoid tearing tissue on removal of the tick.
- ➤ Prevent residual parts of the tick from being left in tissue.
- ➤ Alcohol, nail polish, and burning tick off no longer are considered appropriate intervention therapies because these techniques increase the chance of the tick releasing juices and leaving body parts embedded in the skin.

Different types of ticks cause different diseases that are endemic to different areas (Table 24–1). Ticks are known vectors of the following diseases

TABLE 24•1 TYPES OF TICKS

TYPE AND SUBTYPE	DISEASE CAUSES	ENDEMIC AREA
Hard-shelled tick (ixodidae)		
	Highest frequency in causing localized reaction; highest percentage vector of disease	
Spirochete	Lyme disease (*Borrellia burgdorferi*)	Northeast United States, Wisconsin, Minnesota, California
Soft-shelled ticks (ornithodoros, dermacentor, amblyomma)		
Spirochete	Relapsing fever (*Borrelia* spp.)	Western United States
Rickettsia	Q fever	Southeastern United States
	Rocky mountain spotted fever (*Rickettsia rickettsii*); Ehrlichiosis (*Ehrlichia chaffeensis*)	Western United States, South-central United States
	Typhus (*Rickettsia* spp.)	South-central and southern Atlantic United States
Bacteria	Tularemia (*Francisella tularensis*)	Arkansas, Missouri, Oklahoma
Protozoa	Babesiosis (*Babesia* spp.)	Northeastern United States
Virus	Colorado tick fever (*Coltivirus* spp.)	Western United States
Toxin	Neurotoxin	Northwestern and southern United States

- Babesiosis
- Colorado tick fever
- Ehrlichiosis
- Lyme disease
- Q fever
- Relapsing fever
- Rocky Mountain spotted fever
- Tick fever
- Tularemia
- Typhus

Antibiotic therapy for tick infestations (especially Lyme disease) should not be initiated unless the clinical presentation includes erythema migrans and/or bacterial **cellulitis.**

HEALTH PROMOTION/PREVENTION

Environmental

- Avoid areas that support tick populations.
- Avoid direct contact with mammals with a high population of ticks (especially deer and rodents).
- Avoid wooded areas and activities such as
  - Camping
  - Hunting

Physical

- When out in the woods, wear the following
  - Light-colored clothing, which allows ticks to be spotted before they become embedded in the skin
  - Tight-fitting clothes around the wrists, neck, and ankles
  - Closed-toe shoes
- Inspect for tick infestations
  - All sleeping bags
  - Tents
  - Body, especially crevices during and after outdoor exposure
- Prompt and proper technique in removal of the tick lessens the risk of transmission of the disease. *Most disease transmission (including Lyme disease) requires 24 to 48 hours of contact for vector transmission.*

Chemical

- Wear insect repellents such as
  - Natural repellents, including oil of citronella (Treo and Avon's Skin-So-Soft)
  - DEET (N,N-diethyl-meta-toluamide) on body and clothing to retard tick infestations
  - Permethrins in aerosols for clothing to retard tick infestations

Tetanus

- Give prophylactic injection if not received within the last 5 years.

OPTIONS

➤ *Method 1*—forceps/tweezers technique
➤ *Method 2*—thread technique
➤ *Method 3*—punch biopsy technique
  ➤ Use if the other two methods are unsuccessful.

RATIONALE

➤ Prompt and proper removal of an embedded tick reduces the incidence of disease transmission to the individual.

INDICATIONS

➤ Presence of embedded tick

CONTRAINDICATIONS

➤ Near eye
➤ Near artery

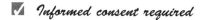 *Informed consent required*

PROCEDURE

Tick Removal

Equipment

➤ Methods 1, 2, and 3
  ➤ Antiseptic skin cleanser
  ➤ Gloves—nonsterile
  ➤ 1% lidocaine
  ➤ 3-mL syringe
  ➤ 25- to 27-gauge, $^1/_2$- to 1-inch needle
  ➤ Magnifying lens—optional
  ➤ Blunted curve forceps or tweezers—sterile
  ➤ 4 × 4 gauze—sterile
  ➤ Band-Aids
  ➤ 0.9% sodium chloride—sterile
➤ Method 2 only
  ➤ Suture material (nylon), 4-0 or 5-0
➤ Method 3 only
  ➤ Iris scissors—sterile
  ➤ Punch biopsy

Procedure

Method 1—Forceps/Tweezers Technique

➤ Position client comfortably with tick site easily accessible. Cleanse area with topical antiseptic cleanser.

➤ Determine which technique to use for removal. Each technique depends on the individual's preference and success with the chosen technique.
➤ Put on gloves.
➤ Inject 1 mL of 1% lidocaine at the base of the embedded tick until a small wheal has formed, being careful not to inject the tick until the wheal has formed (Fig. 24–1).
➤ Grasp tick as close to the skin as possible (Fig. 24–2).
  ➤ Use extra caution if the tick is buried in areas where there is hair.
➤ Pull on the tick using gentle and steady upward pressure for 2 to 4 minutes. This should permit the tick to back out of the site.
  ➤ Do not twist or jerk the tick out because this may result in incomplete removal of the tick and tearing of the skin.
➤ Dispose of tick in a container to prevent reinfestation.
➤ Wash area gently with topical antiseptic cleanser.
➤ Rinse with 0.9% sodium chloride.
➤ Topical antibiotic ointment is not recommended.
➤ Apply a Band-Aid. Instruct the client to remove the Band-Aid as soon as he or she arrives home. Exposure to air lessens risk of secondary infection.

METHOD 2—THREAD TECHNIQUE

➤ Position client comfortably with tick site easily accessible. Cleanse area with topical antiseptic cleanser.

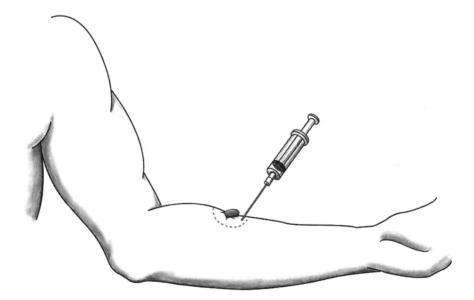

FIGURE 24 • 1 Inject lidocaine at the base of the embedded tick, but do not inject the tick.

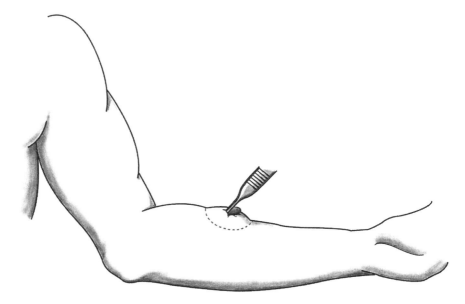

Figure 24 • 2 Method 1—Grasp the tick as close to the skin as possible, and pull gently, allowing the tick to back out of the site.

➤ Determine which technique is to be used for removal. Each technique depends on the individual's preference and success with the chosen technique.
➤ Put on gloves.
➤ Inject 1 mL of 1% lidocaine at the base of the embedded tick until a small wheal has formed, being careful not to inject the tick until the wheal has formed.
➤ Cut a 6-inch length of 4-0 or 5-0 polyfilament suture.
➤ Make a loop knot.
➤ Slide it over the embedded tick.
➤ Gently draw it tight over the smallest part of the tick as close to the skin as possible.
➤ Pull both ends of the suture firmly upward until the skin is lifted (Fig. 24–3).
➤ Hold tension on the tick for 3 to 4 minutes to allow the tick to back out.
➤ Dispose of the tick in a container to prevent reinfestation.
➤ Wash the area gently with antiseptic skin cleanser.
➤ Rinse with 0.9% sodium chloride.
➤ Topical antibiotic ointment is not recommended.
➤ Apply Band-Aid. Instruct the client to remove the Band-Aid as soon as he or she gets home. Exposure to air lessens risk of secondary infection.

METHOD 3—PUNCH BIOPSY TECHNIQUE

Used in situations where other techniques have not been successful or body parts of the tick have been retained in the skin.

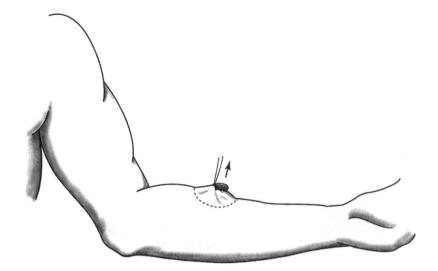

FIGURE 24 • 3 Method 2—Slide a loop of suture over the tick, and pull gently, allowing the tick to back out of the site.

➤ Position client comfortably with tick site easily accessible. Cleanse area with topical antiseptic cleanser.
➤ Determine which technique is to be used for removal. Each technique depends on the individual's preference and success with the chosen technique.
➤ Put on gloves.
➤ Inject 1 mL of 1% lidocaine at the base of the embedded tick until a small wheal has formed, being careful not to inject the tick until the wheal has formed.
➤ Follow the steps for punch biopsy technique in Chapter 1.
➤ Dispose of the tissue in a container to prevent reinfestation.
➤ Consider sending tissue for pathology to ensure all tick body parts have been removed.
➤ Irrigate wound with 0.9% sodium chloride (approximately 30 to 60 mL).
➤ Apply pressure to the site for 2 minutes.
➤ If persistent bleeding occurs despite pressure to site, use of coagulant agent (aluminum chloride, Gelfoam) or suture may be required.
➤ Apply 4 × 4 gauze dressing and tape in place.

Client Instructions

METHODS 1 AND 2

➤ Keep the wound clean and dry.
➤ After 24 hours, the dressing may be removed, and the site may be left open to air. Continuous covering of wounds increases the risk of infection.

- If crust develops over the bite site
  - Cleanse by gently rolling a cotton-tipped swab saturated with hydrogen peroxide over the wound site.
  - Gently rinse the area with warm water.
  - Blot dry with clean towel or cotton gauze.
- Observe for signs and symptoms of infection, such as
  - Increase in pain after 24 hours
  - Increase in temperature
  - Redness or swelling
  - Yellow or greenish drainage
  - Foul odor
- If any signs and symptoms of infection are found, return to the office.
- To decrease pain, use Tylenol No. 3 for severe pain every 4 to 6 hours as needed. After 24 hours, use acetaminophen, ibuprofen, or naproxen every 4 to 6 hours as needed for mild pain.

METHOD 3 ONLY

- Keep dressing clean, dry, and in place for 48 hours to decrease the chance of bleeding and oozing.
- Avoid touching or contaminating the area biopsied.
- To prevent the chance of infection, take cephalexin 500 mg three times per day or cefadroxil 500 mg twice per day for 5 days.
- Some redness, swelling, and heat are normal.
- Return to the office if symptoms of infection occur, such as
  - Yellow or greenish drainage
  - Red streaks
  - Pain
  - Elevated temperature
- Take acetaminophen or ibuprofen every 4 to 6 hours as needed for pain.
- Return to the office in 48 hours for wound recheck.

BIBLIOGRAPHY

American Medical Association (1996). *Physicians' current procedural terminology.* Chicago: Author.

Goldman, D., et al (1993). Human ehrlichiosis. A newly recognized tick borne disease. *Am Fam Physician,* 46(1), 128–132.

Habif, T. (1996) (3rd ed.). *Clinical dermatology: A color guide to diagnosis and therapy.* St. Louis: Mosby.

Murtagh, J. (1995) (2nd ed.). *Practice tips.* New York: McGraw-Hill.

Pfenninger, J.L., and Fowler, G.C. (1994). *Procedures for primary care physicians.* St. Louis: Mosby.

25

TOPICAL HEMOSTATIC AGENT APPLICATION

CYNTHIA R. EHRHARDT

CPT Code

None

Application of a chemical agent ensures rapid hemostasis of capillaries and small blood vessels and is used frequently as an initial agent in situations where rapid hemostasis or vasoconstriction to small areas of tissue is required and/or where there is the lack of available electrocautery. It also commonly is used in dermatologic situations.

OVERVIEW

- ➤ Incidence unknown
- ➤ Complications
  - ➤ Rare hypopigmentation or hyperpigmentation of skin
  - ➤ Rare localized inflammation and scarring of skin
- ➤ Obtain the following information
  - ➤ Sensitivity to the agent being used
  - ➤ Medical contraindications to use of epinephrine (if used)
  - ➤ History of poor healing characteristics
  - ➤ History of exaggerated hypopigmentation or hyperpigmentation of the skin caused by chemical agents

RATIONALE

- ➤ To promote hemostasis without the use of electrocautery

INDICATIONS

- ➤ Skin lesions

CONTRAINDICATIONS

- ➤ With a distal digit or skin appendage, may cause ischemia and necrosis
- ➤ Cardiovascular diseases

PROCEDURE

Topical Hemostatic Agent Application

Equipment

➤ Gloves—nonsterile
➤ Cotton-tipped applicators—sterile
➤ Fenestrated drape—sterile
➤ 4 × 4 gauze—sterile
➤ Topical **hemostatic agent** of choice (Table 25–1)

Procedure

➤ Position the client with the area easily accessible.
➤ Put on gloves.
➤ Establish a clean field around lesion using fenestrated drape.
➤ Choose topical hemostatic agent.
➤ Prepare the topical applicator.
  ➤ If solution, dip the cotton-tipped applicator to impregnate it with the solution. Caution should be taken not to spill or splash the solution.
➤ Using two digits, apply tension to the skin surrounding the lesion.
➤ Wipe excess blood off with sterile gauze.
➤ Apply the chemically impregnated cotton-tipped applicator to the desired site for approximately 15 seconds.
➤ Remove the cotton-tipped applicator and release the skin.

TABLE 25 • 1 TYPES OF COMMON TOPICAL HEMOSTATIC AGENTS

Monsel's Solution (Ferric Subsulfate)
➤ Allows rapid hemolysis
➤ Good agent with **seborrheic keratoses** and **basal cell carcinoma**
➤ Disadvantage: Can cause pigment changes and staining

Aluminum Chloride 30% (Drysol)
➤ Fast hemolysis, but not as fast as Monsel's solution
➤ Not as irritating to the skin
➤ Liquid application or cotton applicator
➤ Less incidence of pigment changes and staining

Silver Nitrate
➤ Fast hemolysis, equal to aluminum chloride
➤ Least expensive of topical hemostatic agents
➤ Usually in the form of impregnated cotton applicators
➤ Disadvantage: Sensitive to moisture exposure
  ➤ High incidence of pigment changes and staining

Epinephrine (Topical or Injectable Application). *Never use in digit applications.*
➤ Extremely potent vasoconstriction agent
➤ May be applied topically, intradermally, or subcutaneously
➤ Disadvantage: Use of large amount can result in tissue necrosis and sloughing

➤ Observe to determine if successful hemolysis has occurred.
  ➤ May need to repeat the procedure twice for successful hemolysis

Client Instructions

➤ Infection rarely is associated with this procedure. Observe for signs and symptoms of infection, such as
  ➤ Increased redness and warmth at the site
  ➤ Red streaks
  ➤ Swelling with drainage
  ➤ Pus from site
➤ Skin may appear inflamed and reddened for 24 to 48 hours from normal chemical irritation of the hemostatic agent.
➤ Hyperpigmentation and hypopigmentation changes can occur and usually do not resolve.
➤ Pain is usually minimal and may be relieved with acetaminophen taken every 4 hours as needed.
➤ Tetanus injection is not indicated if the wound was surgically induced.
➤ Return to the office if rebleeding occurs.

BIBLIOGRAPHY

American Medical Association (1996). *Physicians' current procedural terminology.* Chicago: Author.

Habif, T. (1996) (3rd ed.). *Clinical dermatology: A color guide to diagnosis and therapy.* St. Louis: Mosby.

Pfenninger, J.L., and Fowler, G.C. (1994). *Procedures for primary care physicians.* St. Louis: Mosby.

Trott, A. (1991). *Wounds and lacerations: Emergency care and closure.* St. Louis: Mosby.

Musculoskeletal Procedures

26

BONE MARROW ASPIRATION AND BIOPSY

CYNTHIA R. EHRHARDT

> **CPT Code**
> 85095 Bone marrow aspiration
> 85102 Bone marrow biopsy, needle or trocar

Bone marrow aspiration is one of the diagnostic tools used to assess the status of the hematopoietic system. It involves extracting small amounts of myeloid tissue from a bony cavity (e.g., the sternum or iliac crest). Bone marrow aspiration provides accurate information on the relative number of stem cells and their development and morphologic structure. A follow-up technique, bone marrow **biopsy,** provides a more specific morphology of the bone.

OVERVIEW

- Incidence unknown
- Used as second-line diagnostic tool
- Complications
  - Potentially painful
  - Potential hemorrhage at the site
  - Risk of introducing infection to the bone, which can lead to **osteomyelitis**
  - Retroperitoneal hemorrhage caused by penetration into the bowel cavity by too deep a penetration of the iliac crest
  - Unsuccessful biopsy (known as *dry tap*)

General Principles

- There are two sites for bone marrow aspiration.
  - Sternum
  - Iliac crest
- The posterior-superior spine portion of the iliac crest is considered the first-choice site because there is a higher percentage of success in obtaining quantities of bone marrow sufficient for diagnostic testing.
- Sterile technique must be used for the procedure.
- Universal precautions should be used in handling of the specimen.

➤ All specimen containers and slides should be labeled properly and transported in the appropriate containers.
➤ Further diagnostic testing is possible when initial evaluation by patient history, drug history, physical examination, and initial hematopoietic evaluation (complete blood count and antinuclear antibody tests) has not yielded a diagnosis.

OPTIONS

➤ Bone marrow aspiration
➤ Bone marrow biopsy

RATIONALE

➤ To assess the hematopoietic system
➤ To evaluate hematopoietic abnormalities

INDICATIONS

➤ Unexplained anemia
➤ Unresolved neutropenia after withdrawal from antibiotic therapy
➤ Suspected metastatic disease
➤ Abnormal hematopoietic disorder (leukemia, idiopathic thrombocytopenia, pancytopenia)
➤ Lymphoproliferative disorders, including lymphoma
➤ Immunodeficiency disorders, including human immunodeficiency virus (HIV)
➤ Fever of unknown etiology
➤ Suspected unusual presentation of an infectious disorder (fungal, tuberculosis)
➤ Chromosomal analysis
➤ Bone marrow transplantation

CONTRAINDICATIONS

➤ Severe osteoporosis
➤ Hemophilia
➤ Known radiation to bone site

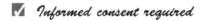 *Informed consent required*

PROCEDURE

Bone Marrow Aspiration and Biopsy

Equipment

Prepackaged disposable kits are available.
➤ Gloves—sterile
➤ Povidone-iodine (Betadine)

➤ Fenestrated drape—sterile
➤ 3-mL syringe
➤ 2 needles—21-gauge and 25-gauge, $1\frac{1}{2}$ inch
➤ 1% or 2% lidocaine without epinephrine
➤ 10-mL syringe prepared with ethylenediamine tetra-acetic acid (EDTA) solution rinse
➤ Complete blood count purple-top (EDTA) laboratory test tube
➤ No. 11 scalpel
➤ Bone marrow aspiration needle
➤ Jamshidi bone marrow biopsy needles (optional)
➤ Microscope glass slides
➤ Fixative specimen container
➤ 4 × 4 gauze—sterile
➤ Tape

Procedure

BONE MARROW ASPIRATION

➤ Position the client comfortably on abdomen. A pillow under the area of the procedure may relax the individual.
➤ Identify the posterior-superior landmarks.
➤ Cleanse the area of the aspiration and 3 inches surrounding with povidone-iodine.
➤ Open the bone marrow kit.
➤ Put on sterile gloves.
➤ Draw up lidocaine in the 3-mL syringe with the 25-gauge needle.
➤ Insert the needle intradermally at the site, and inject a small amount of lidocaine until a wheal has formed.
➤ Replace the 25-gauge needle with the 21-gauge needle, and penetrate deeper into the tissue until the periosteum of the site is felt. Inject approximately 1 mL into the area, then slowly withdraw while infiltrating the needle tract with the remaining solution.
➤ While waiting for local anesthetic to work (5 to 10 minutes), confirm that the obdurator of the biopsy needle is locked in place and the cap is secured.
➤ When the skin is anesthetized, use the No. 11 scalpel and make a small (0.25 cm or less) stab wound.
➤ Insert the biopsy needle at a 90-degree angle into the incision with the capped end in the palm of hand and the shaft between two fingers (usually index and middle finger) until resistance of the periosteum is felt.
➤ Instruct the client that the next part of the procedure may cause a pressure sensation.
➤ Simultaneously begin to apply downward pressure and alternate clockwise and counterclockwise motion to penetrate the cortex of the bone.
➤ Continue this until penetration for approximately 1 cm until the "give" of the cortex is felt. Halt downward pressure, and advance approximately 1 to 2 mm farther to ensure placement in the marrow. The biopsy needle should be held in place by the skin and bone.

➤ Unlock the cap of the syringe, withdraw the obdurator, and attach the EDTA-prepared 10-mL syringe.
➤ Counsel client that pain may be felt at this time and to remain as still as possible.
➤ Pull up on the plunger of syringe. This creates a vacuum, allowing bone marrow contents to be aspirated. If no material is withdrawn, advance the needle an additional 1 to 2 mm, and repeat aspiration.
➤ If still no response, withdraw the needle from that periosteum site, and try another site within the incision.
➤ Withdraw a minimum of 5 mL of marrow. A good specimen shows grossly visible bone **spicules**.
➤ Prepare the smears (may be performed by nonsterile assistant) in the following manner
  ➢ Thinly spread the bone marrow aspiration material over one glass specimen slide and cover with second slide.
  ➢ Gently squeeze the two slides together, and allow any excess blood to drain off the slides.
  ➢ After excess blood is removed, roll the slides apart lengthwise.
    • This allows thinning of any layering of the specimen.
➤ On successful aspiration, remove the needle, and apply pressure over the area using a quarter-folded 4 × 4 gauze and tape as a pressure dressing.
➤ Have the client remain supine for 1 hour with pressure dressing in place.
➤ After 1 hour, the pressure dressing may be removed and a standard dressing applied to area.

BONE MARROW BIOPSY

Usually performed on the iliac crest.
➤ Position the client comfortably on abdomen. A pillow under the area of the procedure may relax the individual.
➤ Identify the posterior-superior landmarks.
➤ Cleanse the area of the aspiration and 3 inches surrounding with povidone-iodine.
➤ Open the bone marrow kit.
➤ Put on sterile gloves.
➤ Draw up lidocaine in the 3-mL syringe with the 25-gauge needle.
➤ Insert the needle intradermally at the site and inject a small amount of lidocaine until a wheal has formed.
➤ Replace the 25-gauge needle with the 21-gauge needle, and penetrate deeper into the tissue until the periosteum of the site is felt. Inject approximately 1 mL into the area, then slowly withdraw while infiltrating the needle tract with the remaining solution.
➤ While waiting for local anesthesia to work (5 to 10 minutes), confirm that the obdurator of the biopsy needle is locked in place and cap is secured.
➤ When the skin is anesthetized, use the No. 11 scalpel and make a small (0.25 cm or less) stab wound.
➤ Insert the biopsy needle at a 90-degree angle into the incision with the capped end in the palm of hand and the shaft between two fingers (usually index and middle finger) until resistance of the periosteum is felt.

➤ Simultaneously begin to apply downward pressure and alternate clockwise and counterclockwise motion to penetrate the cortex of the bone.
➤ Continue this until penetration for approximately 1 cm until the "give" of the cortex is felt. Halt downward pressure, and advance approximately 1 to 2 mm farther to ensure placement in the marrow. The biopsy needle should be held in place by the skin and bone.
➤ When the biopsy syringe has been placed in the marrow, withdraw the needle 3 mm to have it placed in the cortex.
➤ Redirect the angle of the needle toward the anterior iliac spine, and advance it into the cortex until resistance decreases.
➤ Remove the obdurator and perform an alternate clockwise and counter-clockwise motion for a distance of 2 cm.
➤ Proceed to rock the needle clockwise five times then counterclockwise five times, to ensure a good specimen.
➤ Change the angle approximately 15 degrees, and repeat previous step. This allows the specimen to be severed from the marrow.
➤ Cover the opening of bone marrow needle with your thumb and withdraw.
➤ Insert the obdurator and allow the specimen to be pushed out onto sterile 4 × 4 gauze.
➤ Prepare the smears (may be performed by nonsterile assistant) in the following manner
   ➤ Using a light touch, gently touch four glass slides to the specimen on the gauze.
   ➤ Place the specimen in a container with the fixative agent.
➤ On completion, remove needle, and apply pressure over the area using a quarter-folded sterile 4 × 4 gauze and tape as a pressure dressing.
➤ Have the client remain supine for 1 hour with pressure dressing in place.
➤ After 1 hour, client may get up and leave.

Client Instructions

➤ Infection rarely is associated with this procedure. Observe for signs and symptoms of infection, however, such as
   ➤ Increased redness and warmth at the site
   ➤ Red streaks
   ➤ Swelling with drainage
   ➤ Pus from site
➤ Contact your health-care provider if any of the following symptoms occur within 48 hours
   ➤ Fever
   ➤ Abdominal pain
   ➤ Unrelieved site pain
➤ Leave the pressure dressing on for 12 hours. After that time, the dressing may be removed and a standard dressing applied.
➤ Keep the site clean and dry for 24 hours.
➤ Avoid strenuous exercise for 48 hours.
➤ Pain is usually minimal and may be relieved with acetaminophen (Tylenol) or acetaminophen with codeine (Tylenol No. 3).
➤ Return to the office in 48 hours for recheck.

BIBLIOGRAPHY

American Medical Association (1996). *Physicians' current procedural terminology.* Chicago: Author.

American Society of Hematology (1996). Diagnosis and treatment of idiopathic thrombocytopenia purpura. *Am Fam Physician,* 54(8), 2437–2445.

Davenport, J. (1995). Macrocytic anemia. *Am Fam Physician,* 53(1), 155–160.

McCance, K., and Huether, S. (1996). *Pathophysiology: The biological basis for disease in adults and children.* St. Louis: Mosby.

Paulman, P. (1989). Bone marrow sampling. *Am Fam Physician,* 40(6), 85–87.

Pfenninger, J.L., and Fowler, G.C. (1994). *Procedures for primary care physicians.* St. Louis: Mosby.

27 LUMBAR PUNCTURE

MARGARET R. COLYAR

CPT Code

62270   Spinal puncture, lumbar, diagnostic

Lumbar puncture is the introduction of a hollow needle into the subarachnoid space of the lumbar portion of the spinal column to diagnose suspected infection and remove blood or pus. Cerebrospinal fluid (CSF) is completely replaced about three times a day. Although about 500 mL of CSF is formed every day, much of it is reabsorbed into the blood. There are about 120 to 150 mL of CSF in the system at any one time.

RATIONALE

➤ To determine or to rule out central nervous system infection
➤ To determine the level of pressure in spinal column

INDICATIONS

➤ Symptoms of fever, malaise, and central nervous system irritability

CONTRAINDICATIONS

➤ Lumbar skin infection
➤ Platelet count less than 50,000/µL
➤ Degenerative joint disease
➤ Increased intracranial pressure

COMPLICATIONS

➤ Severe headache
➤ Meningitis from introducing bacteria into CSF
➤ Back or leg pain/paresthesia
➤ Accidental puncture of spinal cord
➤ Accidental puncture of aorta or vena cava
➤ Herniation of brain due to sudden decrease in pressure

☑ *Informed consent required*

PROCEDURE

Lumbar Puncture

Equipment

➤ Spinal tap tray
  ➤ Mask
  ➤ 22- to 23-gauge needle
  ➤ Syringe
  ➤ Manometer
  ➤ CSF specimen collection bottles
  ➤ Skin spray
  ➤ 1% lidocaine
  ➤ Povidine-iodine
  ➤ 22-gauge spinal needle
➤ Sterile gloves
➤ Fenestrated drape
➤ 2 × 2 gauze
➤ Tape

Procedure

➤ Position client in tripod (fetal) or lateral recumbent (fetal/child/adult) position.
➤ Have client clasp hands on the knees.
➤ Draw a line across the back between the top of the iliac crests. Locate the interspace between either L4-5 or L5-S1 (preferred) (Fig. 27–1). Mark with barrel of syringe.

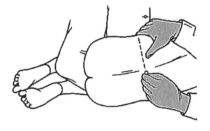

FIGURE 27 • 1 Draw a line across back between top of iliac crests. (From Colyar MR: *Well-child assessment for primary care providers*. Philadelphia, F.A. Davis, 2003.)

- ➤ Open the spinal tray.
- ➤ Apply mask.
- ➤ Apply sterile gloves.
- ➤ Cleanse the skin 6 inches around the interspace with povidone-iodine in a circular motion.
- ➤ Cleanse the same area with 70% alcohol.
- ➤ Draw up 3 mL of 1% lidocaine.
- ➤ Assemble the manometer with the three-way stopcock.
- ➤ Inject the lidocaine at the site, raising a wheal in the skin. Inject 0.5 mL of lidocaine into the posterior spinous region.
- ➤ Insert the spinal needle with stylet in place through the skin just below the palpated spinous process. Angle about 15 degrees cephalad.
- ➤ If you hit bone or the needle meets with resistance, withdraw the needle slightly and redirect.
- ➤ Advance the needle slowly.
- ➤ After the needle is inserted a few millimeters, withdraw the stylet to see if CSF is present. You may hear a popping sound when the needle penetrates the dura.
- ➤ Advance the needle 1 to 2 mm further.
- ➤ Remove the stylet.
- ➤ Attach the manometer to the hub of the inserted needle. Note the level of pressure on the manometer.
- ➤ Open the stopcock to allow the CSF to flow into the test tubes. CSF collection usually takes 5 to 10 seconds. **Do *not* attempt to aspirate CSF with a syringe**.
- ➤ If blood returns, remove needle and discard.
- ➤ Repeat procedure with fresh needle.
- ➤ Remeasure level of pressure. Do *not* withdraw CSF if pressure is significantly different.
- ➤ Label the tubes (Table 27–1).

TABLE 27•1 LABELING TUBES

TUBE NO	PURPOSE OF TEST
1— Biochemistry	Glucose, protein
2— Bacteriology	Gram stain, culture (bacterial)
	Indicate if the following are needed
	Fungal culture
	TB culture
	Viral culture
3— Hematology	Cell count, differential
4— Optional	VDRL
	India Ink (fungal)
	Cytology
	Myelin basic protein
	Oligoilonal bands

TB, tuberculosis; VDRL, Venereal Disease Research Laboratory.

TABLE 27•2 NORMAL CEREBROSPINAL FLUID

TEST	NORMAL VALUE	INDICATION
Opening pressure	50–200 mm H_2O	No intracranial pressure No obstruction
WBC	$<5/mm^3$	No infection
Glucose	50–80% of serum glucose	No hypoglycemia or hyperglycemia
Protein	15–45 mg/dL	No hemorrhage No tumors Nontraumatic tap
Color	Clear and colorless	No bacteria, WBCs, or bleeding
RBC	<20	Nontraumatic tap

WBC, white blood cell; RBC, red blood cell.

➤ When enough CSF has been obtained, replace the stylet and remove the needle.
➤ Spray the skin.
➤ Cover the insertion site with a 2 × 2 pressure dressing and leave in place for 2 hours.
➤ Send tubes to laboratory within 2 hours for analysis (Tables 27–2 and 27–3). Do *not* refrigerate the tubes.

Client Instructions

➤ To prevent a headache
  ➤ Have the client lie still for 4 to 8 hours after the procedure.

TABLE 27•3 ABNORMAL CEREBROSPINAL FLUID VALUES

TEST	NORMAL	ABNORMAL	INDICATION
Appearance	Clear	Cloudy	Infection
		Bloody	Hemorrhage, obstruction, or traumatic tap
		Brown, yellow, orange	Elevated protein, RBC hemolysis present for ≥3 days
Protein	15–45 mg/dL	Increase	Tumors, trauma, hemorrhage, diabetes mellitus, polyneuritis, blood in CSF
		Decrease	Rapid CSF production
Gamma globulin	3–12%	Increase	Multiple sclerosis, neurosyphilis, Guillain-Barré syndrome

(*Continued on following page*)

TABLE 27•3 ABNORMAL CEREBROSPINAL FLUID VALUES   *(Continued)*

TEST	NORMAL	ABNORMAL	INDICATION
Glucose	50–80%	Increase	Systemic hyperglycemia
		Decrease	Systemic hypoglycemia, bacterial or fungal infection, meningitis, mumps
Cell count	0–5 WBCs	Increase	Active disease, meningitis, tumor, abscess, infarction, multiple sclerosis
	No RBCs	RBCs present	Hemorrhage, traumatic tap
VDRL	Nonreactive	Positive	Neurosyphilis
Chloride	118–130 mEq	Decrease	Meningitis, TB
Gram stain	Negative	Gram positive or negative organisms	Bacterial meningitis

RBC, red blood cell; CSF, cerebrospinal fluid; WBC, white blood cell; VDRL, Venereal Disease Research Laboratory; TB, tuberculosis.

> ➤ Encourage fluids by offering at least one to two 8-oz. glasses. Popsicles are often a great substitute.
> ➤ Ask the caregiver to assist the client with activities and have the client rest while lying down over the following 4 to 8 hours.
> ➤ Have the client avoid strenuous activity for first 24 hours after procedure.

B IBLIOGRAPHY
American Thoracic Society (2000). *Lumbar puncture.* Available at: Http://www.thoracic.org.
Ewald, G.A., and McKenzie, C.R. (eds.) (1999) (32nd ed.). Manual of medical therapeutics. Boston: Little, Brown.
Fischbach, F. (2001) (6th ed.). *A manual of laboratory and diagnostic tests.* Philadelphia: Lippincott.
Intermed Communications, Inc. (2000). *Diagnostics: an A-Z guide to laboratory tests.* Springhouse, PA: Author.
Neurology (2002). *Protocol for lumbar puncture.* Available at: http://www.neuro.nwu.edu.
Siberry, G.K., and Iannone, R. (2000) (15th ed.). *The Harriet Lane handbook.* St. Louis: Mosby.
Wellington School of Medicine (1999). *Lumbar puncture.* Available at: http://medmico2.wnmeds.ac.nz.

28

X-RAY INTERPRETATION— BONES

MARGARET R. COLYAR

CPT Code

Multiple listings based on area of body being x-rayed.

X-rays of the musculoskeletal system are taken to determine the presence of disease, including arthritis, spondylitis, bone lesions, and fractures.

OVERVIEW

➤ Incidence unknown

Basic Principles

➤ Approach must be systematic.
➤ The health-care provider must know normal body structures.
➤ In children or adolescents, the contralateral side always should be x-rayed for comparison purposes.
➤ Long bones should not be x-rayed without the joint.
➤ When putting x-rays on the view box, remember the following
  ➤ Place them so that you seem to be facing the client.
  ➤ X-rays usually are marked by the technician to indicate which side was the client's right side or, in the case of films of the extremities, whether it was the client's right or left leg or arm.
  ➤ Always view a chest x-ray as if you are facing the client. The client's right will be on your left.
➤ Food and drinks are *not* restricted before musculoskeletal x-rays.
➤ Clothing, jewelry, hairpins, and dentures should be removed, depending on the area of the body being x-rayed.
➤ The genital area should be shielded unless the area to be x-rayed is the pelvis.

OPTIONS

➤ Various positions are assumed, based on the area to be x-rayed.

RATIONALE

➤ To determine the presence of

- Fractures
- Dislocations
- Soft tissue injury
- Disease processes

INDICATIONS

- Clinical suspicion of disease, injury, or deformity
- Pain of unknown origin

CONTRAINDICATIONS

- Pregnancy

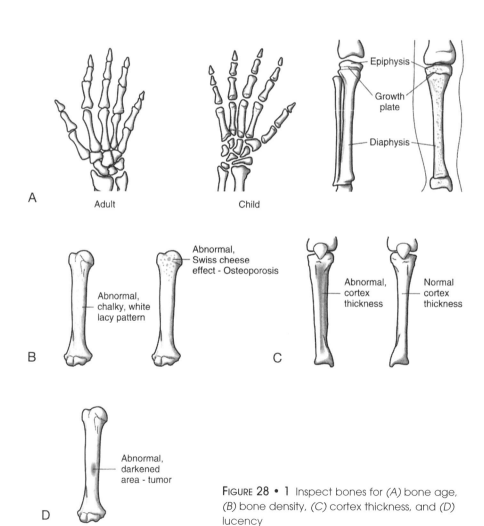

FIGURE 28 • 1 Inspect bones for (A) bone age, (B) bone density, (C) cortex thickness, and (D) lucency

PROCEDURE

Interpretation of Musculoskeletal X-Rays

Equipment

➤ View box

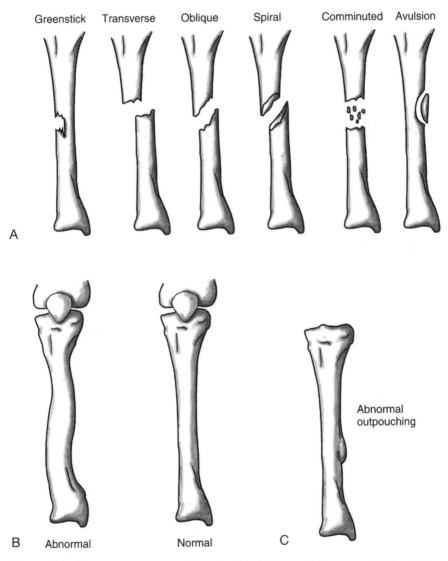

FIGURE 28 • 2 Inspect bones for (A) continuity, (B) size and shape, and (C) soft tissue inflammation.

Procedure

Systematic approach to bone x-ray interpretation includes (Fig. 28–1)

➤ *Anatomic alignment and position*
  ➤ *Bone age*—Check epiphyseal growth plates. Epiphyses begin to appear at birth and are completed at puberty. Ossification usually is completed by age 20 in females and age 23 in males.
  ➤ *Bone density*—Density should be consistent over the entire bone. Changes in density indicate fractures, tumors, and sclerosis.
  ➤ *Continuity*—Check for fractures in bones and joint capsules (Fig. 28–2).
  ➤ *Cortex thickness*—As an adult ages, the cortex thins. If greater than 50% of the cortex is gone, REFER to an orthopedic surgeon.
➤ *Lucency*—Spotted lucency and dense sclerosis indicate
  ➤ Bone metastases—spine and skull usually involved
  ➤ Congenital diseases
  ➤ Infectious diseases
  ➤ Neoplastic diseases
  ➤ Metabolic diseases—hyperparathyroidism or nutritional deficits—osteoporosis, malformation, and others
➤ *Periosteum*—Thickening indicates stress fractures or inflammation.
➤ *Size and shape of the bone*—Check for abnormalities in contour or excess calcification.
➤ *Soft tissue inflammation*—Inflammation indicates **osteomyelitis**.

BIBLIOGRAPHY

Edmunds, M.W., and Mayhew, M.S. (1996). *Procedures for primary care practice.* St. Louis: Mosby.

Kee, J.L. (1995). *Laboratory and diagnostic tests with nursing implications.* Norwalk, CT: Appleton & Lange.

Merier, L.R. (1991). *Practical orthopedics.* St. Louis: Mosby.

Pierro, J.A., et al (1989). *Manual of diagnostic radiology.* Philadelphia: Lea & Febiger.

29 ARTHROCENTESIS

MARGARET R. COLYAR

CPT Code	
20600	Arthrocentesis, aspiration, or injection; small joint, bursa
20605	Arthrocentesis, intermediate joint or bursa
20610	Arthrocentesis, major joint or bursa

Arthrocentesis is the aspiration of fluid from a joint space. It is performed to decrease inflammation or differentiate the diagnosis between intra-articular and extra-articular origin. Knowledge of the injection site anatomy is crucial.

OVERVIEW

➤ Incidence unknown
➤ Sites for arthrocentesis (see Chapter 34)

OPTIONS

➤ *Method 1*—arthrocentesis only
  ➤ Used to remove fluid for diagnostic purposes
➤ *Method 2*—arthrocentesis with intra-articular corticosteroid injection
  ➤ Used to remove fluid and inject corticosteroid to decrease inflammation and pain

RATIONALE

➤ To diminish inflammation of the joint
➤ To differentiate the diagnosis between intra-articular and extra-articular origin

INDICATIONS

➤ Remove joint fluid
➤ Decrease pain in a joint
➤ Diagnose the cause of joint inflammation

CONTRAINDICATIONS

➤ Anticoagulation therapy
➤ Presence of joint prosthesis
➤ Recent joint injury

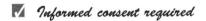 *Informed consent required*

PROCEDURE

Arthrocentesis

Equipment

➤ Methods 1 and 2
  ➤ Alcohol prep pads
  ➤ Povidone-iodine prep pads
  ➤ Gloves—nonsterile
  ➤ 1 or 2 syringes—10 to 20 mL
  ➤ 18- to 20-gauge, 1½-inch needle

- ➤ 4 × 4 gauze—sterile
- ➤ Tape
- ➤ Elastic bandage—3 or 4 inches
- ➤ Culture tubes
- ➤ **Hemostats**—sterile
- ➤ Method 2 only
  - ➤ 1% lidocaine (single-dose vial)
  - ➤ Corticosteroid of choice

Procedure

METHOD 1—ARTHROCENTESIS ONLY

- ➤ Position the client with the affected joint slightly flexed.
- ➤ Mark the injection site with your thumbnail.
- ➤ Cleanse the injection site with alcohol first, then with povidone-iodine.
- ➤ Let povidone-iodine air dry.
- ➤ Put on gloves.
- ➤ Insert the syringe with the 18-gauge needle at a 90-degree angle, and aspirate the fluid.
- ➤ If blood is aspirated and a hematoma is not suspected, withdraw the needle.
- ➤ If more fluid needs to be removed (Fig. 29–1)
  - ➤ Stabilize the needle with the hemostats.
  - ➤ Remove the filled syringe and replace with an empty syringe.
  - ➤ Reaspirate.
  - ➤ Withdraw the fluid, and inject into the culture tubes.
  - ➤ Apply a pressure dressing with the 4 × 4 gauze and tape securely.
  - ➤ Apply an elastic bandage.

METHOD 2—ARTHROCENTESIS WITH INTRA-ATRICULAR CORTICOSTEROID INJECTION

- ➤ Position the client with the affected joint slightly flexed.
- ➤ Mark the injection site with your thumbnail.
- ➤ Cleanse the injection site with alcohol first, then with povidone-iodine.
- ➤ Let povidone-iodine air dry.
- ➤ Put on gloves.
- ➤ Insert the syringe with the 18-gauge needle at a 90-degree angle, and aspirate the fluid.
- ➤ If blood is aspirated and a hematoma is not suspected, withdraw the needle.
- ➤ If more fluid needs to be removed
  - ➤ Stabilize the needle with the hemostats.
  - ➤ Remove the filled syringe and replace with an empty syringe.
  - ➤ Reaspirate.
- ➤ Withdraw the fluid, and inject into the culture tubes.
- ➤ If you are planning to inject the joint with a steroid and lidocaine mixture after the aspiration
  - ➤ Stabilize the needle with the hemostat.

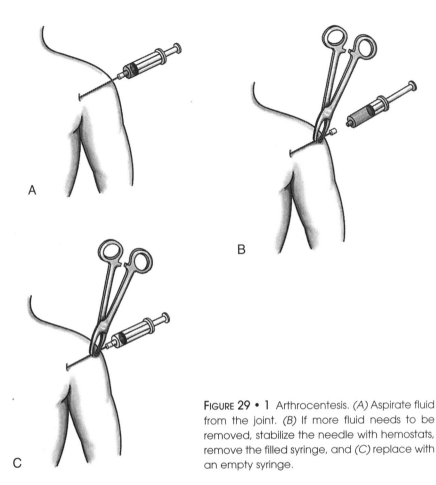

A

B

C

FIGURE 29 • 1 Arthrocentesis. *(A)* Aspirate fluid from the joint. *(B)* If more fluid needs to be removed, stabilize the needle with hemostats, remove the filled syringe, and *(C)* replace with an empty syringe.

- Remove the filled syringe and inject fluid into the culture tubes.
- Replace the first syringe with the second syringe, holding the lidocaine and steroid mixture.
- Inject the mixture steadily into the joint.
- Remove the syringe from the joint.
- Apply a pressure dressing with 4 × 4 gauze and tape securely.
- Apply an elastic bandage.

Client Instructions

- Rest the joint for the next 24 hours.
- Remove the dressing and elastic bandage in 24 hours.
- Observe for signs of infection, such as
  - Increase in pain
  - Fever
  - Yellow or greenish discharge
  - Red streaks

➤ Sometimes fluid recollects in the joint. If this occurs, return to the office.
➤ Your culture should be back by _____. We will call you with the results.

BIBLIOGRAPHY

Clark, C.R., and Bonfiglio, M. (eds.) (1994). *Orthopaedics: essentials of diagnosis and treatment.* New York: Churchill Livingstone.
Pfenninger, J.L., and Fowler, G.C. (1994). *Procedures for primary care physicians.* St. Louis: Mosby.
Stitik, T.P. (1995) Practical pointers. *Consultant,* December.

CLAVICLE IMMOBILIZATION TECHNIQUES
CLAVICLE STRAP, FIGURE EIGHT, SLING AND SWATH

30

MARGARET R. COLYAR

CPT Code	
23500	Closed treatment without manipulation
23505	Closed treatment with manipulation

Clavicle fractures usually result from a fall on the extended arm or a direct blow to the shoulder. Fractures of the clavicle require immobilization for proper healing to occur. Three types of immobilization are clavicle strap, figure eight, and sling and swath. The clavicle strap technique holds the shoulder upward, outward, and away from the thorax, as does the figure eight technique. The sling and swath technique restricts the use of the arm on the side of the clavicle fracture.

OVERVIEW

➤ Clavicle fractures—80% occur in the middle or inner two thirds of the clavicle

OPTIONS

- ➤ Method 1—clavicle strap technique
  - ➤ For fracture at the middle or inner two thirds of the clavicle
  - ➤ Used to pull the shoulder back and hold the clavicle in **alignment**
- ➤ Method 2—figure eight technique
  - ➤ For fracture at the middle or inner two thirds of the clavicle
  - ➤ Used to pull the shoulder back and hold the clavicle in alignment
- ➤ Method 3—sling and swath technique
  - ➤ For fracture at the distal third without displacement or ligament disruptions
  - ➤ Used to restrict use of the arm

RATIONALE

- ➤ To provide proper alignment
- ➤ To immobilize
- ➤ To promote proper healing

INDICATIONS

- ➤ Fracture of middle clavicle
- ➤ Fracture of inner two thirds of clavicle

CONTRAINDICATIONS

- ➤ Fracture of distal third of the clavicle with disruption and displacement—REFER

PROCEDURE

Clavicle Immobilization Techniques

Equipment

- ➤ Method 1
  - ➤ Clavicle strap
- ➤ Methods 2 and 3
  - ➤ Long (approximately 4 to 6 feet), 6-inch-wide bandage
  - ➤ 2 to 4 safety pins—nonsterile

Procedure

METHOD 1—CLAVICLE STRAP TECHNIQUE

See Figure 30–1.

- ➤ Place the straps over the client's shoulders, one strap over each shoulder.
- ➤ Pull straps gently toward the middle of the back and fasten.
- ➤ Palpate the fractured clavicle, checking that the displaced clavicle is pulled into alignment.
- ➤ Obtain an x-ray of the chest after placement of the clavicle strap to check for alignment. Tighten strap if needed.

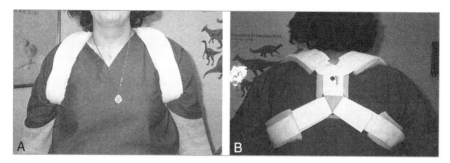

FIGURE 30 • 1 Clavicle strap. *(A)* Front. *(B)* Back.

METHOD 2—FIGURE EIGHT TECHNIQUE

See Figure 30–2.

➤ Starting at midback, go over, around, and under the right shoulder.
➤ Pull the end of the bandage across the back diagonally.
➤ Place the bandage over, around, and under the left shoulder.
➤ Pull across the back.
➤ Tie or pin in place.

METHOD 3—SLING AND SWATH TECHNIQUE

See Figure 30–3.

➤ Apply the sling.
➤ Wrap the 6-inch bandage around the torso and upper arm on the affected side.

Client Instructions

➤ Do *not* raise the arm above the shoulder for 6 weeks.
➤ Flex wrist, elbow, and fingers daily.

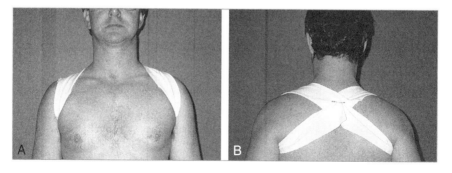

FIGURE 30 • 2 Figure eight clavicle strap. *(A)* Front. *(B)* Back.

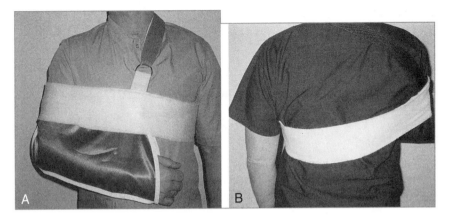

FIGURE 30 • 3 Sling and swath. *(A)* Front. *(B)* Back.

➤ Perform the following shoulder exercises after 6 weeks
   ➤ Pendulum—bend over and gently swing arm to and fro.
   ➤ External rotation—lying down and using unaffected arm, push affected arm to lateral side.
   ➤ Elevation—pull affected arm up in front of chest.
   ➤ Internal rotation—lying down and using unaffected arm, pull affected arm across chest.
   ➤ Wall climbing—walk fingers up a wall as far as possible.
➤ Heavy activity usually may be initiated after 3 months.

BIBLIOGRAPHY
Eiff, M.P. (1997). Management of clavicle fractures. *Am Fam Physician,* 55(1), 121–128.
Smeltzer, S., and Bard, B.G. (1996). *Brunner and Suddarth's textbook of medical-surgical nursing.* Philadelphia: Lippincott-Raven.

31 CRUTCH WALKING

MARGARET R. COLYAR

CPT Code
None

Crutch walking is a method of support and balance for transferring or walking employed by a person who is lame, weak, or injured. Instruction in proper crutch-walking technique is essential in many orthopedic disorders.

OVERVIEW

➤ Incidence unknown

RATIONALE

➤ To ensure proper support and balance
➤ To prevent injury

INDICATIONS

➤ Fractured leg, knee, ankle, or foot
➤ Ankle sprain
➤ Postsurgical procedures of lower extremities

CONTRAINDICATIONS

➤ Client unable to balance well
➤ Elderly

PROCEDURE

Crutch Walking

Equipment

➤ Crutches—adjustable with rubber suction tips
➤ Measuring tape

Procedure

Measure the client for crutches using the following technique.

MEASUREMENTS—CRUTCH LENGTH

➤ Have client stand if possible.
➤ Measure from anterior axillary fold to sole of foot, then add 2 inches, or measure from 2 inches below the axilla to 6 inches in front of the client.
➤ Adjust crutches based on measurements.

MEASUREMENTS—HAND PIECE

➤ Have client position crutch under axilla and grasp hand piece. Arm rest should be 1 to 2 inches below the axilla. Elbow should be flexed 20 to 30 degrees.
➤ Axilla should not rest on the crutch arm rest because of the possibility of damage to the brachial plexus.
➤ Adjust crutches to fit the client's measurements.
➤ Demonstrate the following
  ➤ Tripod stance

- Crutches 10 to 12 inches in front and to the side of the client. Weight is supported on hands, *not* axilla (Fig. 31–1).
- Crutch gaits
  - •Weight bearing on both legs—use four-point gait (Fig. 31–2).
    - Advance in the following sequence: right crutch, left foot, left crutch, right foot.
  - Weight bearing on one leg only—use three-point gait (Fig. 31–3).
    - Advance both crutches and swing the non–weight-bearing leg through while standing on the weight-bearing leg.
    - When the crutches are securely in place, put weight on the hand pieces and advance the weight-bearing leg.
- To sit down (Fig. 31–4)
  - Grasp both crutch hand pieces in one hand on the side of the weaker leg.
  - Grasp the hand rail of the chair.
  - Lower self into chair by bending the knee of the weight-bearing leg while lifting the weaker leg out in front.

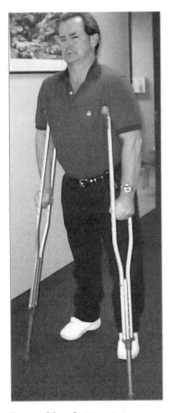

FIGURE 31 • 1 Tripod stance.

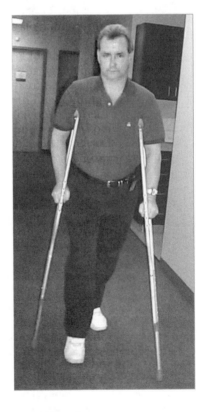

FIGURE 31 • 2 Four-point gait.

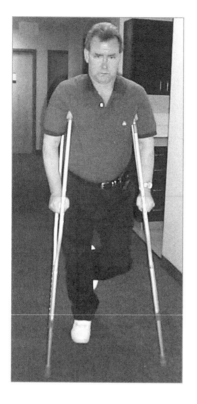

FIGURE 31 • 3 Three-point gait.

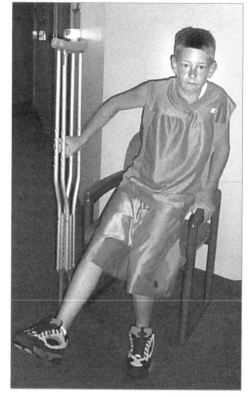

FIGURE 31 • 4 Sitting down with crutches.

> To stand up (Fig. 31–5)
  • Move forward to edge of the chair.
  • Grasp the hand pieces of both crutches in one hand on the side of the weaker leg.
  • Grasp the hand rail of the chair.
  • Use the weight-bearing leg to lift while pushing down on the hand pieces of crutches.
> To go down stairs (down with the weaker leg) (Fig. 31–6)
  • Stand on the weight-bearing leg.
  • Advance both crutches to the next step and advance the weaker leg.
  • Advance weight-bearing leg.
> To go up stairs (up with the weight-bearing leg) (Fig. 31–7)
  • While stabilizing self with hands on the hand pieces, advance the weight-bearing leg up to the next step.
  • Next, advance crutches and weaker leg up to the step.
> Have the client give a repeat demonstration.

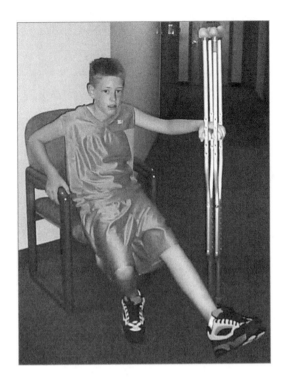

FIGURE 31 • 5 Standing up with crutches.

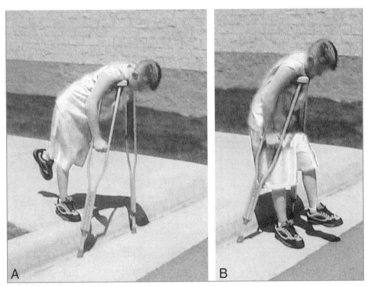

A   B

FIGURE 31 • 6 Going down stairs with crutches. (A) Stand on weight-bearing leg. (B) Advance both crutches to next step, then advance weaker leg, followed by weight-bearing leg.

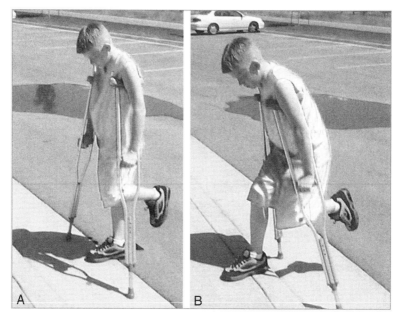

FIGURE 31 • 7 Going up stairs with crutches. (A) Stabilize self with hands on hand pieces. (B) Advance weight-bearing leg up to next step.

BIBLIOGRAPHY
Smeltzer, S.C., and Bare, B.G. (1996). *Brunner and Suddarth's textbook of medical-surgical nursing.* Philadelphia: Lippincott-Raven.

32

DISLOCATION REDUCTION

MARGARET R. COLYAR

CPT Code	
21480	Closed treatment of temporomandibular joint (TMJ) dislocation
23650–55	Closed treatment of shoulder dislocation, with manipulation

24600–5	Treatment of closed elbow dislocation
26700–5	Closed treatment of metacarpophalangeal (MCP) dislocation, single, with manipulation
26770–75	Closed treatment of interphalangeal joint dislocation, single, with manipulation

Dislocation indicates the partial or complete displacement of one bone from another bone. Displacement can occur spontaneously as a result of a structural defect, traumatic injury, or joint disease. A dislocated joint is reduced when it is restored to normal position. Reduction of a joint facilitates proper healing.

OVERVIEW

➤ Incidence
  ➤ TMJ dislocations
    • 5% to 6% of the population. Dislocation is usually anterior but can be posterior, lateral, and superior.
  ➤ Shoulder dislocation
    • 90% to 95% anterior
    • 2% posterior
    • 2% to 3% acromioclavicular (AC)
  ➤ Recurrence of shoulder dislocations
    • Younger than 20 years of age—90% to 95%
    • Older than 40 years of age—10% to 15%
  ➤ Elbow dislocations
    • Greater incidence than shoulder dislocations
  ➤ Hand dislocations
    • Proximal interphalangeal (PIP) joint—most common dislocation in the body
    • MCP joint—index finger most common dislocation, then thumb and fifth digit
➤ Causes
  ➤ TMJ dislocations
    • Spontaneous—eating, talking, yawning, or rinsing mouth
    • Traumatic—blow to mandible
  ➤ Shoulder dislocations
    • Anterior shoulder dislocation—trauma with arm abducted, extended, and externally rotated
    • Posterior shoulder dislocation—direct force to the shoulder while flexed, adducted, and internally rotated
    • AC shoulder dislocation—persistent upward displacement of lateral end of the clavicle

➤ Elbow dislocations
  • Posterior dislocations—direct trauma on outstretched forearm held in extension; also may have wrist injury
➤ Hand dislocations
  • MCP joint dislocations—hyperextension of finger at the MCP joint
  • PIP joint dislocations—hyperextension or "jamming" injury

OPTIONS

➤ TMJ dislocation reduction
  ➤ Method 1—passive reduction
    • Requires no anesthesia and can be done easily without force
  ➤ Method 2—manual reduction
    • Use if method 1 fails
➤ Shoulder dislocation reduction
  ➤ Anterior shoulder dislocation
    • Method 1—passive reduction
      • Requires no anesthesia and can be done easily without force
    • Method 2—manual reduction
      • Use if method 1 fails
  ➤ Posterior shoulder dislocation reduction
  ➤ AC shoulder dislocation reduction
➤ Elbow dislocation reduction
➤ Hand dislocation reduction
  ➤ MCP joint dislocation reduction
  ➤ Dorsal PIP joint dislocation reduction
  ➤ Volar PIP joint dislocation reduction
  ➤ Thumb dislocation reduction

RATIONALE

➤ To diminish pain
➤ To prevent loss or decreased use of a joint
➤ To prevent structural defects

INDICATIONS

➤ Dislocation of mandible, shoulder, elbow, or finger

CONTRAINDICATIONS

➤ Dislocation with fracture of the mandible, shoulder, elbow, or finger
➤ Separation of the AC joint
➤ Fracture of the joint capsule
➤ Abnormal neurovascular status of the extremity
➤ Dislocation of the hip or knee

☑ *Informed consent required*

PROCEDURE

Dislocation Reduction

Equipment

TMJ DISLOCATION REDUCTION

➤ Methods 1 and 2
  ➤ Gloves—nonsterile
  ➤ Gauze—nonsterile
  ➤ Tongue blade—nonsterile

Procedure

METHOD 1—PASSIVE REDUCTION—TMJ

➤ Examine the client. Your examination should show
  ➤ Malocclusion
  ➤ Mandibular fossa empty
  ➤ Moderate pain
  ➤ Mouth held open
➤ X-ray the TMJ if traumatic injury or if diagnosis of dislocation is in doubt.
  ➤ Lateral view—check for fracture
  ➤ Towne's view—shows medial or lateral offset (dislocation)
➤ Induce the gag reflex by probing the soft palate with tongue blade (Fig. 32–1).

METHOD 2—MANUAL REDUCTION—TMJ

➤ Position the client sitting on the floor with head stabilized by an assistant.
➤ Put on gloves.
➤ Stand above and in front of the client.

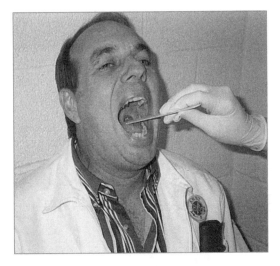

FIGURE 32 • 1 Passive reduction of TMJ. Probe the soft palate with a tongue blade to induce the gag reflex.

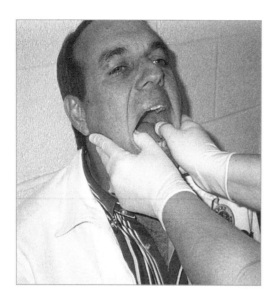

FIGURE 32 • 2 Manual reduction of TMJ. Place your thumbs on the bottom molars and fingers submentally. Ask the client to yawn.

➤ Place your thumbs in the client's mouth on the bottom molars (Fig. 32–2). Place digits 3, 4, and 5 of each hand submentally.
➤ Place second digits of each hand at the mandibular angle.
➤ Ask the client to yawn.
➤ Apply your body weight downward on the mandible.
➤ Elevate the chin.
➤ Slide the mandible backward into position.
➤ Obtain an x-ray to determine if the mandible is in correct position.

Client Instructions

TMJ DISLOCATION REDUCTION

➤ Eat soft food for several days.
➤ Avoid opening the mouth wide for 3 to 4 weeks.
➤ Place your hand under your chin when yawning.
➤ Take acetaminophen every 4 hours as needed for pain.
➤ Perform jaw muscle–strengthening exercises.

Shoulder Dislocation Reduction

Equipment

➤ Method 1 only
  ➢ Weights—5- to 10-lb free weights or sandbag
  ➢ Towel—nonsterile
  ➢ Roll of gauze
➤ Methods 1 and 2
  ➢ 1% lidocaine, 20 mL, or muscle relaxer
  ➢ Syringe—20 mL
  ➢ 25-gauge, 1½-inch needle

Procedure

ANTERIOR SHOULDER DISLOCATION REDUCTION

➤ Method 1—passive reduction (Fig. 32–3)
   ➤ Examine the client. You should find
      • Fullness in the anterior capsule
      • Sulcus sign (space under the acromion)
      • Severe pain
      • Limited range of motion
      • Arm held slightly abducted and externally rotated
      • Shoulder contour flattened with protruding acromion
   ➤ Examine the client's neurovascular status and document.
   ➤ Give a muscle relaxer or inject 20 mL of 1% lidocaine inferiorly off the
      tip of the acromion (Fig. 32–4)
   ➤ X-ray the shoulder (three views) to determine dislocation and whether
      a fracture is present. X-ray should show anterior and slight inferior
      displacement of the humerus out of the glenoid fossa. If a fracture is
      present, REFER.
      • Anteroposterior view—shows internal and external rotation of the
         shoulder, upper humerus, AC joint, and clavicle

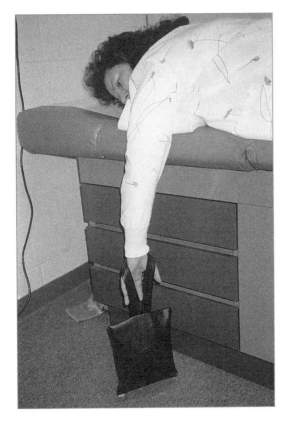

FIGURE 32 • 3 Passive reduction
of anterior shoulder dislocation.

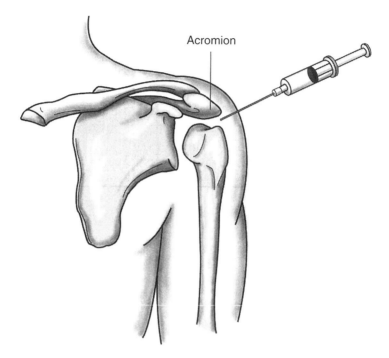

FIGURE 32 • 4 Passive reduction of anterior shoulder dislocation. Inject lidocaine inferiorly off the tip of the acromion.

- • Y view—needed to verify a dislocation
- • Load-bearing view—to differentiate an AC joint separation from a dislocation
- ➤ Position the client prone on an examination table with the affected arm hanging downward.
- ➤ Place a folded towel under the shoulder.
- ➤ Wrap gauze snugly around the wrist of the affected arm.
- ➤ Hook weights into the gauze.
  - • If weights are not available, a sandbag may be used.
- ➤ Allow weights to pull on arm for 15 to 20 minutes.
- ➤ If no progress after 15 to 20 minutes, apply a sling and REFER to an orthopedic surgeon.
- ➤ If successful, immobilize the affected arm in a sling and swath to immobilize the shoulder.
- ➤ Method 2—manual reduction (Fig. 32–5)
  - ➤ Position the client in a sitting position.
  - ➤ Grasp the wrist and elbow of the affected arm.
  - ➤ With the arm against the body
    - • Flex the elbow 90 degrees.
    - • Externally rotate the arm to approximately 70 to 85 degrees or until resistance is felt.

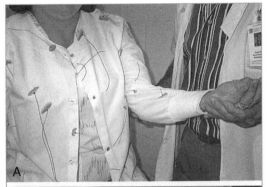

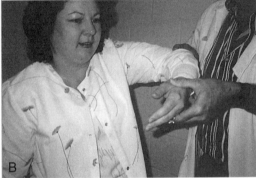

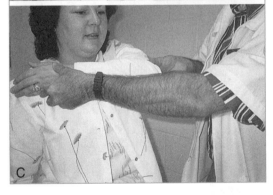

FIGURE 32 • 5 Manual reduction of anterior shoulder dislocation. (A) Flex the elbow 90 degrees, externally rotating the arm 70 to 85 degrees until resistance is felt; (B) lift the elbow in the sagittal plane while (C) internally rotating the arm.

- Lift the elbow in the sagittal plane as far as possible.
- Internally rotate the arm. The head of the joint should slip into place; the pain immediately decreases.
➤ Obtain an x-ray of the shoulder to determine if reduction was successful.
➤ Check neurovascular status and document.

POSTERIOR SHOULDER DISLOCATION REDUCTION

➤ Examine the client. You should find
  ➤ Minimal posterior swelling

➤ Severe pain with any motion
➤ Do not attempt to reduce; REFER to an orthopedic surgeon.

AC SHOULDER DISLOCATION REDUCTION

➤ Examine the client. You should find
  ➤ Slight pain—worse on elevation of the arm
  ➤ Lateral end of the clavicle prominent
  ➤ Distinct step palpable between the clavicle and the acromion
➤ No active reduction is needed.
➤ Apply sling for 1 week or until the pain subsides.
➤ Instruct the client to avoid overhead work.

Client Instructions

SHOULDER DISLOCATION REDUCTION

➤ Apply an ice pack for the first 24 hours.
➤ Give acetaminophen every 4 hours as needed for pain.
➤ Start deltoid isometric exercises immediately.
➤ In 3 weeks, start the following exercises (Fig. 32–6):

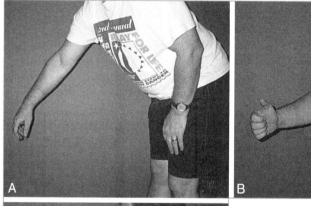
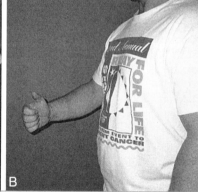
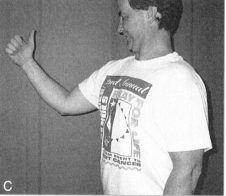

FIGURE 32 • 6 Shoulder exercises. *(A)* While leaning over, make hanging circles (clockwise/counterclockwise). *(B)* Flex the arm 90 degrees at the elbow, make a fist with the thumb up, and move the forearm and hand rotating at the elbow. *(C)* Flex the arm 90 degrees at the elbow, make a fist with the thumb up, and raise the arm at the shoulder in abduction.

➤ Lean over with affected arm hanging, and make increasingly larger circles clockwise and counterclockwise.
➤ Standing upright with affected arm flexed 90 degrees at the elbow, make a fist with the thumb up. Move the forearm and hand rotating at the elbow to and away from the body.
➤ Standing upright with affected arm flexed 90 degrees at the elbow, make a fist with the thumb up; raise the arm at the shoulder in abduction.
➤ Return to the office in _____ for recheck.

Elbow Dislocation Reduction

Equipment

➤ Metal splint with foam on one side
➤ Gauze—nonsterile
➤ Tape

Procedure

➤ Examine the client. You should find
  ➤ Pain
  ➤ Limited range of motion
➤ Assess and document neurovascular status.
  ➤ Radial and brachial pulses
  ➤ Capillary refill of the fingers
  ➤ Nerve function of the median, ulnar, and radial nerves (Fig. 32–7)
  ➤ Muscle function (Fig. 32–8)
➤ X-ray both arms for comparison—check for fat pad sign.
  ➤ Anteroposterior, lateral, and oblique views
  ➤ If fracture is present, REFER.
➤ Assistant applies countertraction on the distal humeral shaft.
➤ Nurse practitioner applies continuous gentle downward traction to proximal portion of the forearm and brings the elbow into flexion (Fig. 32–9).
➤ X-ray the dislocated elbow to ensure that it is reduced.
➤ Repeat the neurovascular assessment and document.
➤ Apply a posterior splint (see Chapter 36) with the elbow at 100 to 110 degrees of flexion.

Client Instructions

ELBOW DISLOCATION REDUCTION

➤ Take acetaminophen every 4 hours as needed for pain.
➤ Return to the office in 1 week.
➤ Start range-of-motion exercises in 1 week if the elbow is stable. Gradually increase range-of-motion exercises (Fig. 32–10) after 10 to 14 days.
➤ Keep the splint in place until full extension is achieved.
➤ A follow-up x-ray must be taken in 2 to 3 weeks to determine stability of the elbow.

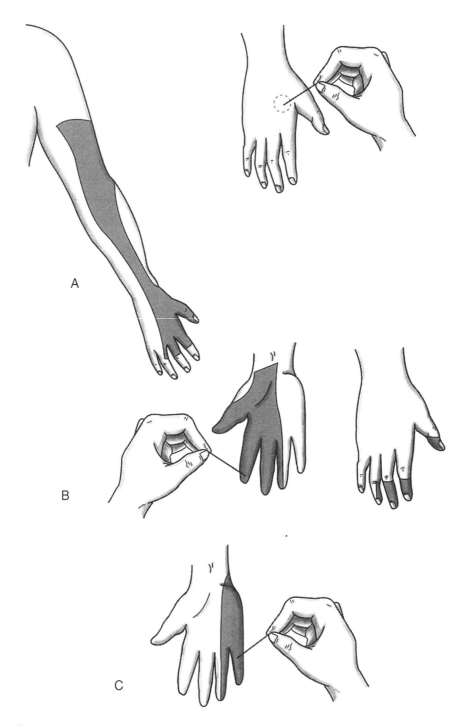

FIGURE 32 • 7 *(A)* Median, *(B)* ulnar, and *(C)* radial nerves.

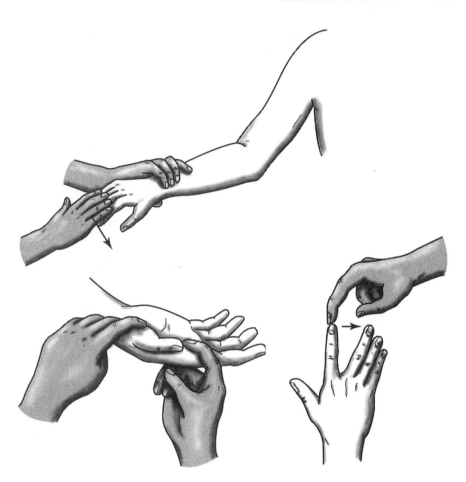

FIGURE 32 • 8 Muscle function.

Hand Dislocation Reduction

Equipment

- ➤ Splint
- ➤ Syringe—5 mL
- ➤ 25-gauge, 1½-inch needle
- ➤ 1% lidocaine—5 mL
- ➤ Gauze—nonsterile
- ➤ Tape

Procedure

MCP JOINT DISLOCATION REDUCTION

- ➤ Examine the client. You should find
  - ➤ Digit held in extension or hyperextension

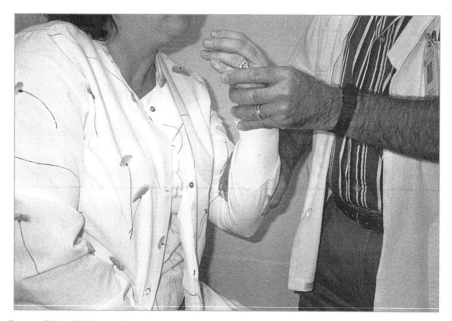

FIGURE 32 • 9 Elbow dislocation reduction. Pull down on the proximal portion of the forearm and bring the elbow into flexion.

- ➤ Dimpling of the palmar skin over the protruding metacarpal head
➤ Assess neurovascular status and document.
➤ X-ray the affected hand.
  - ➤ Anteroposterior view shows obliteration of normal joint space.
  - ➤ Lateral view shows proximal phalanx is dorsal to the metacarpal head.

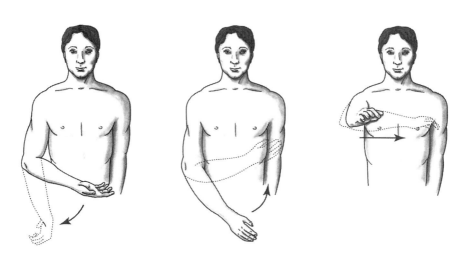

FIGURE 32 • 10 Elbow exercises.

➤ If a fracture is found, immobilize the joint and REFER to an orthopedic surgeon.
➤ Hyperextend the finger at the MCP joint.
➤ Apply traction by pulling the finger in an outward and upward direction.
➤ Apply pressure of the dorsal aspect of the base of the proximal phalanx (Fig. 32–11).
➤ Remove traction.
➤ Flex the finger.
➤ Obtain another x-ray of the hand to determine successful reduction.
➤ Assess neurovascular status and range of motion.
➤ Apply a posterior splint (see Chapter 36) with MCP flexed 70 degrees. Keep the posterior splint in place for 3 to 4 weeks.

DORSAL PIP JOINT DISLOCATION REDUCTION

➤ Examine the client. You should find
    ➤ Finger swollen and malformed
    ➤ Limited range of motion
➤ Assess neurovascular status and document.

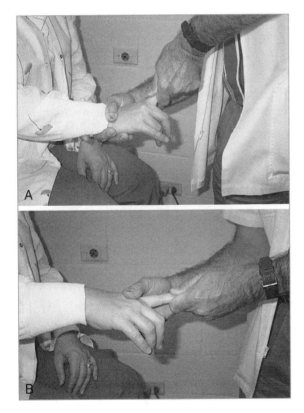

FIGURE 32 • 11 MCP joint dislocation reduction. (A) Hyperextend the MCP joint while pulling the finger outward and upward. (B) apply pressure on the dorsal aspect the proximal phalanx.

- ➤ X-ray the hand.
  - ➤ Anteroposterior view shows obliteration of joint space.
  - ➤ Lateral view shows dorsal dislocation of middle phalanx.
- ➤ If a fracture is present, immobilize, and REFER to an orthopedic surgeon.
- ➤ Perform a digital nerve block (see Chapter 8).
- ➤ Apply direct longitudinal traction.
- ➤ Obtain another x-ray of the hand to determine if the PIP joint has been reduced.
- ➤ Reassess neurovascular status and document.
- ➤ Apply a dorsal extension block splint (see Chapter 36), blocking the last 15 degrees of extension. Keep splint in place for 3 to 4 weeks.

VOLAR PIP JOINT DISLOCATION REDUCTION

- ➤ Examine the client. You should find
  - ➤ Finger swollen and malformed
  - ➤ Limited range of motion
- ➤ Assess neurovascular status and document.
- ➤ X-ray the hand.
  - ➤ Lateral view shows base of middle phalanx is palmar to head of proximal phalanx.
  - ➤ If a fracture is present, immobilize, and REFER to an orthopedic surgeon.
  - ➤ No active reduction is required.
  - ➤ Splint in full extension of PIP joint on the volar side. Keep splint in place for 4 to 6 weeks.

THUMB DISLOCATION REDUCTION

- ➤ Usually a ligament tear is involved. REFER to an orthopedic surgeon.

Client Instructions

HAND DISLOCATION—MCP AND PIP—DORSAL

- ➤ Take acetaminophen every 4 hours as needed for pain.
- ➤ Return to the office in 1 week.
- ➤ Start flexion and extension exercises in 1 week.
- ➤ The splint can be removed in 3 to 4 weeks.

HAND DISLOCATION—PIP—VOLAR

- ➤ Take acetaminophen every 4 hours as needed for pain.
- ➤ Return to the office in 1 week.
- ➤ Keep the splint in place for 4 to 6 weeks.
- ➤ After 4 to 6 weeks, start flexion and extension exercises.

BIBLIOGRAPHY

Diamond, S. (1996). The mechanism and management of shoulder pain. *Adv Nurse Practitioners*, March, 16, 18, 20–21, 50.

Gates, S.J., and Mooar, P.A. (eds.) (1989). *Orthopaedics and sports medicine for nurses.* Baltimore: Williams & Wilkins.

Hansen, S.T., and Swiotkowski, J.F. (eds.) (1993). *Orthopaedic trauma protocols.* New York: Raven Press.

Pfenninger, J.L., and Fowler, G.C. (1995). *Procedures for primary care physicians.* St. Louis: Mosby.

Small, A.J., and DelGross, C. (1995). Spontaneous temporomandibular joint dislocation in an 80 year old. *J Fam Pract,* 40(4), 395–398.

Thakur, A.J., and Narayan, R. (1990). Painless reduction of shoulder dislocation by Kocher's method. *J Bone Joint Surg Am,* 72(3), 524.

GANGLION CYST ASPIRATION AND INJECTION

33

MARGARET R. COLYAR

CPT Code

20600	Arthrocentesis, aspiration, or injection; small joint, bursa, or ganglion cyst (leg, fingers, toes)
20605	Arthrocentesis, aspiration, or injection; intermediate joint, bursa, or ganglion cyst (e.g., TMJ, acromioclavicular, wrist, elbow, ankle, olecranon bursa)
25111	Excision of ganglion, wrist; primary
25112	Excision of ganglion, wrist; recurrent
26160	Excision of lesion of tendon sheath or capsule (e.g., cyst, mucous cyst, or ganglion); hand or finger

A simple **ganglion cyst** is a cystic tumor that develops on or in a tendon sheath containing a thick, gel-like material. This gel-like material leaks from the joint into the weakened tendon sheath and forms a cyst sac (Fig. 33–1). The ganglion cyst usually is caused by frequent strains and contusions.

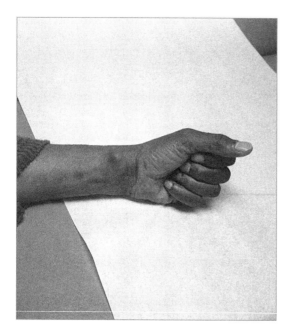

FIGURE 33 • 1 Ganglion cyst.

OVERVIEW

➤ Incidence unknown
➤ Cause—joint inflammation
➤ Usual location—back of the wrist

RATIONALE

➤ To diminish pain
➤ To promote joint mobility

INDICATIONS

➤ Pain over a joint
➤ Limitation of joint movement

CONTRAINDICATIONS

➤ On anticoagulant therapy
➤ Problems with clotting
➤ Lack of response to previous injections
➤ Sepsis
➤ Recent joint fractures
➤ Inform the client of the following
  ➤ Chance of infection and recurrence
  ➤ Chance of steroid flare 24 to 36 hours after injury
  ➤ Chance of subcutaneous atrophy

☑   *Informed consent required*

PROCEDURE

Ganglion Cyst Aspiration and Injection

Equipment

- ➤ Antiseptic skin cleanser
- ➤ Gloves—sterile
- ➤ Drape—sterile
- ➤ 2 syringes—10 mL and 3 mL
- ➤ 18-gauge, 1½-inch needle
- ➤ 22- to 25-gauge, 1½-inch needle
- ➤ 1% lidocaine
  - ➤ Use single-dose vials because they do not contain preservatives that are likely to cause allergic reactions.
- ➤ Culture tubes
- ➤ Corticosteroid (Table 33–1)
- ➤ 4 × 4 gauze—sterile
- ➤ Tape

Procedure

- ➤ Position the client with the ganglion cyst easily accessible.
- ➤ Cleanse the skin in a 3-inch-diameter area around the ganglion cyst with antiseptic skin cleanser.
- ➤ Drape the ganglion cyst.

TABLE 33•1 COMMONLY USED CORTICOSTEROIDS

TYPE	USE	DOSE (MG)
Short-Acting	Quick relief in self-limiting	20
Hydrocortisone	disorders, such as bursitis	
Intermediate-Acting	Longer relief to decrease inflammation	
Methylprednisolone		4
Prednisolone (Depo-Medrol) 20 mg/ml		5–10
Triamcinolone acetonide (Kenalog) 10 mg/mL		5–10
Triamcinolone diacetate (Aristocort) 25 mg/mL		12.5–25
Long-Acting	Chronic conditions such as tendinitis	
Dexamethasone (Decadron) 4 mg/ml or 10 mg/mL		0.6
Betamethasone (Celestone) 6 mg/mL		0.6

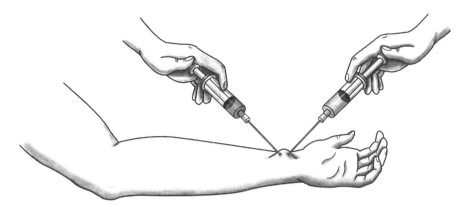

FIGURE 33 • 2 Aspirate the ganglion cyst with an 18-gauge needle. Then inject the medication into the cyst with the second needle.

➤ Put on gloves.
➤ Using the 22- to 25-gauge needle on 3-mL syringe, draw up 2.5 mL of 1% lidocaine and 0.5 mL of corticosteroid. Mix well by gently rotating syringe back and forth.
➤ Insert the 10-mL syringe with the 18-gauge needle into the ganglion cyst (for aspiration) (Fig. 33–2).
➤ Insert the syringe with the medication into the ganglion cyst, and aspirate for blood.
➤ If no blood, aspirate the fluid from cyst. If the aspirate is cloudy, send it to the pathology laboratory for culture and sensitivity.
    ➤ If blood is aspirated, remove the needle and dress the wound.
➤ Inject the medication.
➤ Remove both needles.
➤ Apply a pressure dressing.

Client Instructions

➤ Keep the wound covered for 8 to 12 hours.
➤ Some redness, swelling, and heat are normal. If you notice yellow or green drainage from wound or red streaks, return to the office.
➤ Take acetaminophen or ibuprofen every 4 to 6 hours as needed for pain.
➤ Rest the joint for 24 hours.
➤ Elevate the joint above the heart as much as possible for 24 hours.
➤ Return to the office in 1 week for recheck.
➤ If the cyst recurs, removal may be indicated.

BIBLIOGRAPHY

Hashimoto, B.E., et al (1994). Sonographic diagnosis and treatment of ganglion cysts causing suprascapular nerve entrapment. *J Ultrasound Med,* 13(9), 671–674.
Pfenninger, J.L., and Fowler, G.C. (1994). *Procedures for primary care physicians.* St. Louis: Mosby.

34

INTRA-ARTICULAR AND BURSA CORTICOSTEROID INJECTION

MARGARET R. COLYAR

CPT Code	
20550	Injection; tendon sheath, ligaments, trigger points
20600	Arthrocentesis, aspiration, or injection; small joint, bursa
20605	Arthrocentesis, aspiration, or injection; intermediate joint, bursa
20610	Arthrocentesis, aspiration, or injection; major joint or bursa

Injection of corticosteroids into a joint space or bursa is done to decrease pain in overuse injury and to improve function. Injection of corticosteroids may be done immediately after joint aspiration. Anesthetic agents are used in conjunction with corticosteroid injection to decrease injection pain. For overuse injuries, a general rule of thumb is that two injections can be done over 2 weeks and then in 3 to 4 months, if necessary. No more than three injections within a 12-month period are recommended.

OVERVIEW
➤ Incidence is unknown.
➤ Familiarity with the anatomy of the injection site is crucial to effective intra-articular injection. Common conditions for which intra-articular injection is indicated are
  ➤ Tendinitis
    • de Quervain's disease
    • Tennis elbow
    • Plantar fasciitis
    • Trigger finger

> Bursitis
> Neuritis
  • Carpal or tarsal tunnel syndrome
  • Costochondritis
  • Tietze's syndrome
  • Postherpetic neuralgia
> Myofascial pain syndrome
> Arthritis
  • Osteoarthritis (degenerative)
  • Rheumatoid arthritis

Complications

➤ Tendon rupture
➤ Joint injection
➤ Postinjection flare (pain)
➤ Injection into a blood vessel
➤ Tissue atrophy

Commonly Used Corticosteroids

See Table 33–1.

Commonly Used Anesthetic Agents

➤ Lidocaine (Xylocaine) 1%—1 to 2 hours of relief
➤ Bupivacaine (Marcaine) 0.25%—6 to 8 hours of relief

RATIONALE

➤ To diminish pain
➤ To promote joint function

INDICATIONS

➤ Painful joint
➤ Inflamed joint

CONTRAINDICATIONS

➤ Infected joint
➤ Cellulitis over the joint
➤ More than three injections in a 12-month period
➤ Joint instability
➤ Joint surgery or prosthesis
➤ Fracture
➤ Sickle cell anemia
➤ Coagulation disorders

➤ Diabetes
➤ Children or adolescents

☑ *Informed consent required*

PROCEDURE

Intra-Articular and Bursa Corticosteroid Injection

Equipment

➤ Alcohol prep pads
➤ Povidone-iodine prep pads
➤ Gloves—nonsterile
➤ Syringe—3 to 10 mL
➤ 22-gauge, $1\frac{1}{2}$-inch needle
➤ 1% lidocaine—single-dose vial (5 to 10 times the amount of steroid to be used—e.g., 2.5 mL of lidocaine to 0.5 mL of steroid)
➤ Corticosteroid of choice (see Table 33–1)
➤ Adhesive bandage (Band-Aid)

Procedure

➤ Draw lidocaine and corticosteroid into the syringe.
➤ Mix by rolling or gently rocking the syringe back and forth.
➤ Mark the injection site with your thumbnail.
➤ Position the client with the joint slightly flexed to open the joint space (Fig. 34–1).
➤ Don gloves.
➤ Cleanse the site with alcohol and then povidone-iodine.
    ➤ Allow the povidone-iodine to air dry.
➤ Insert the needle at the thumbnail mark at 45- to 90-degree angle, depending on the site of injection.
➤ Aspirate.
    ➤ If blood is obtained, remove the needle.
    ➤ If using injection for a bursa, aspirate for cloudy bursal fluid. This indicates the appropriate site.
➤ Inject the corticosteroid mixture steadily and gently into the area.
➤ Remove the needle.
➤ Apply pressure for 1 minute.
➤ Cover with Band-Aid.

Client Instructions

➤ Rest the joint for the next 24 hours.
➤ You may remove the dressing and bandage in 24 hours.
➤ Observe for signs and symptoms of infection, such as
    ➤ Increase in pain after 24 hours

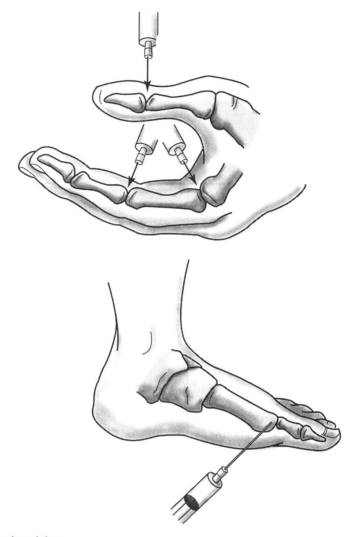

Finger and toe joints —
- Flex the finger or toes to open the joint.
- Inject corticosteroid medial or lateral to the extensor tendon.

FIGURE 34 • 1 Sites for injections.

    ➤ Increase in temperature
    ➤ Redness or swelling
    ➤ Yellow or greenish drainage
    ➤ Foul odor
➤ If any signs or symptoms of infection are found, return to the office.
➤ Steroid flare or postinjection pain lasting 36 hours may occur. If this does occur, do the following

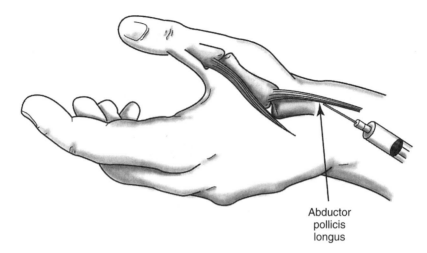

Abductor
pollicis
longus

de Quervains Disease —
* Abduct the thumb.
* Inject parallel to the tendon at the point of tenderness.

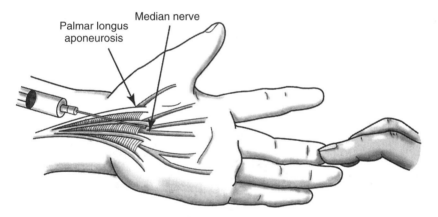

Median nerve

Palmar longus
aponeurosis

Carpal Tunnel Syndrome —
* Dorsiflex the wrist.
* Insert the needle at the distal crease of the wrist lateral to the tendon toward the middle finger.
* 45-degree angle.
* 1–2 cm in depth.

FIGURE 34 • 1 *(Continued)*

> ➤ Apply an ice pack.
> ➤ Take ibuprofen (Motrin) every 6 hours as needed.
> ➤ Call the office if the pain does not subside within 36 hours.
➤ Sometimes fluid recollects in the joint. If this occurs, return to the office.
➤ Your culture should be back by _____. We will call you with the results.

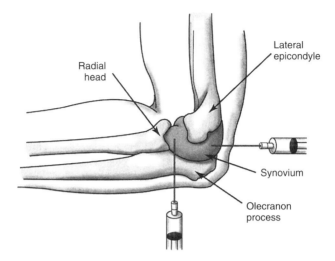

Tennis Elbow —
- Flex the elbow 45 degrees.
- Inject the corticosteroid in the joint space inferior to the lateral epicondoyle.
- Inject superior to the olecranon process.

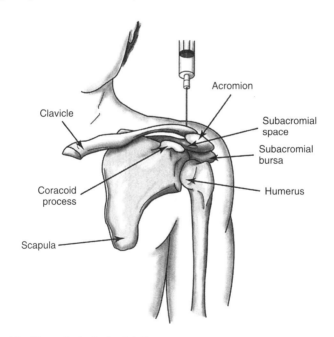

Shoulder (Acromioclavicular Joint) —
- Palpate distal clavicle until a moveable prominence is felt.
- Insert the needle anteriorly at a 90-degree angle.
- Inject the corticosteroid into the joint.

FIGURE 34 • 1 *(Continued)*

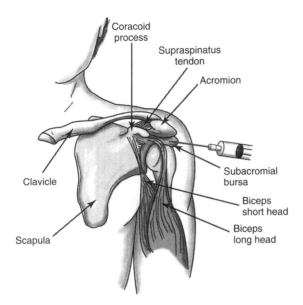

Shoulder (Subacromial Bursa) —
- Palpate the lateral edge of the acromion.
- The soft spot just below the acromion is the subacromial bursa.
- Insert the needle at 90-degree angle into the bursa which should feel soft.
- Be careful not to inject in the supraspinatus tendon or the deltoid.

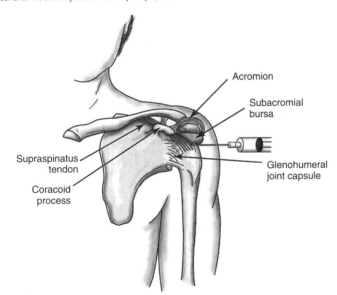

Shoulder (Rotator Cuff — supraspinatus tendonitis) —
- Use the same technique as for the subacromial bursa.
- Insert the needle farther into the area to the point of tenderness.
- Withdraw the needle slightly and inject the corticosteroid.

FIGURE 34 • 1 *(Continued)*

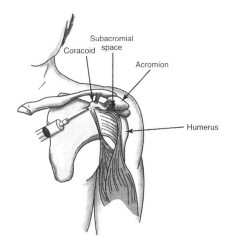

Shoulder (Short head of the biceps) —
- Identify the anterior coracoid bony process.
  - Inferior to the clavicle.
  - Medial to the humerus.
- Insert needle at the point of tenderness at a 90-degree angle until the bone is reached.
- Withdraw the needle 1–2 mm.
- Inject the corticosteroid.

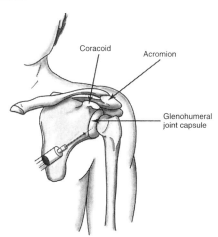

Shoulder (Glenohumeral or Scapulohumeral Joint) —
- **_Anterior (Glenohumeral)_** —
  - Rotate the shoulder joint toward the back and identify the joint space.
  - Insert the needle at a 90-degree angle into the glenohumeral joint.
  - No bone should be encountered.
  - Inject the corticosteroid.
- **_Posterior (Scapulohumeral)_** —
  - Rotate the shoulder anteriorly and identify the joint space.
  - Insert the needle at a 90-degree angle into the scapulohumeral joint.
  - No bone should be encountered.
  - Inject the corticosteroid.

FIGURE 34 • 1 *(Continued)*

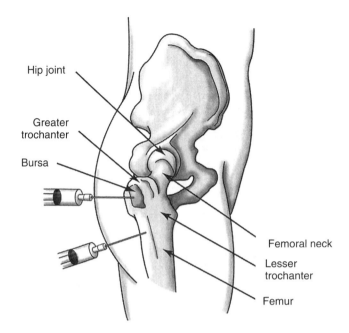

Hip Bursa —
- Identify the hip joint by having the client flex the joint.
- Insert the needle until you hit the bone.
- Withdraw 2–3 mm and inject the corticosteroid.

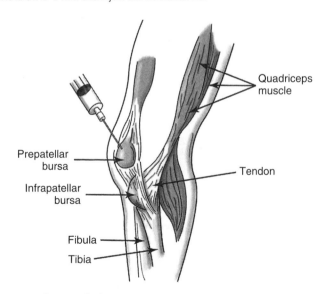

Knee Bursa (Prepatellar) —
- Inject above the patella.
- 90-degree angle.

FIGURE 34 • 1 *(Continued)*

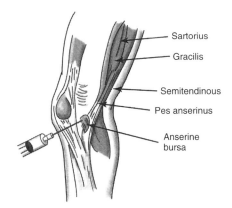

Knee-Anserine Bursa —
- Below patella find the lateral concavity.
- Inject the needle at 90-degree angle.
- Inject until you hit bone, then withdraw 2–3 mm.
- Inject the corticosteroid.
- Redirect the needle several times and inject in several areas.

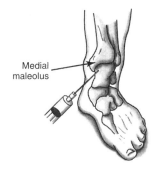

Ankle —
- Dorsiflex the ankle.
- Inject at the medial malleolous and tibia.

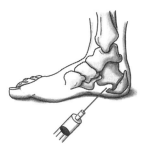

Heel Spur (Calcaneal) —
- Insert the needle on the lateral side of the foot at the heel at the point of maximal tenderness.
- Inject the corticosteroid.

FIGURE 34 • 1 (Continued)

BIBLIOGRAPHY

Larson, H.M., et al (1996). Shoulder pain: The role of diagnostic injections. *Am Fam Physician,*
53(5), 1637–1643.

Nelson, R.H., et al (1995). Corticosteroid injection therapy for overuse injuries. *Am Fam
Physician,* 52(6), 1811–1816.

Tibone, J.E., and Shaffer, B. (1995). A functional approach to managing shoulder impinge-
ment. *J Medical Surgical Med,* 12(7), 37–41.

35 SLING APPLICATION

MARGARET R. COLYAR

CPT Code
None

Slings are devices used to immobilize, support, and elevate the shoulder, arm,
and hand. A sling can be used by itself or in combination with other immobilization devices.

OVERVIEW

➤ Incidence is unknown.
➤ Before sling application, always assess the extremity for and document
  ➤ Pulse
  ➤ Paresthesias
  ➤ Paralysis
  ➤ Pallor
  ➤ Pain
  ➤ Edema

OPTIONS

Sling Application

➤ *Method 1*—manufactured sling application
➤ *Method 2*—triangular sling application

RATIONALE

➤ To immobilize a joint
➤ To support and elevate the shoulder, arm, and hand

INDICATIONS

➤ Strain or sprain of the shoulder, elbow, or arm

CONTRAINDICATIONS

➤ Unstable fracture
➤ Loss of pulse
➤ Signs or symptoms of compartment syndrome

PROCEDURE

Sling Application

Equipment

➤ Method 1
  ➢ Sling
➤ Method 2
  ➢ Triangular piece of cloth 16 to 20 inches on each side—optional
  ➢ Two large safety pins—nonsterile

Procedure

METHOD 1—MANUFACTURED SLING APPLICATION

➤ Position the client sitting or supine with
  ➢ Injured arm across the chest in 90-degree angle
  ➢ Forearm slightly above the level of the elbow
  ➢ Thumb pointed upward and toward the body
  ➢ With the sling outside the clothing
➤ Using manufactured sling
  ➢ Secure the elbow snugly in the sling.
  ➢ Extend the sling to include the hand to the MCP joints.
    • This prevents ulnar deviation and supports the wrist.
  ➢ Cross the strap over the unaffected shoulder and around the back of the neck (Fig. 35–1).
  ➢ Buckle or tie the strap. Do not allow the buckle or knot to rest on a bony prominence or put pressure on the neck.
  ➢ Tighten the strap so that the arm is supported.

METHOD 2—TRIANGULAR SLING APPLICATION

➤ Fasten corner of cloth at elbow with safety pins (Fig. 35–2).

METHODS 1 AND 2

➤ After application of the sling, assess the extremity for and document
  ➢ Pulse
  ➢ Grasp strength
  ➢ Paresthesias
  ➢ Warmth of hand

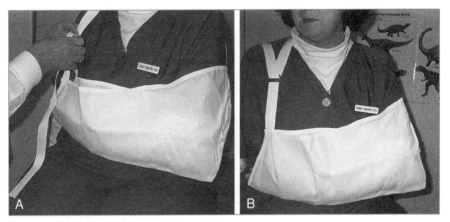

FIGURE 35 • 1 Manufactured sling application.

- Color of hand
- Presence of edema

Client Instructions

- You must keep the sling in place for _____.
- If the hand becomes cold, pale in color, numb, or tingly, contact the nurse practitioner.
- Observe for signs of skin irritation around the neck. If skin irritation occurs, pad the strap with a soft cloth.

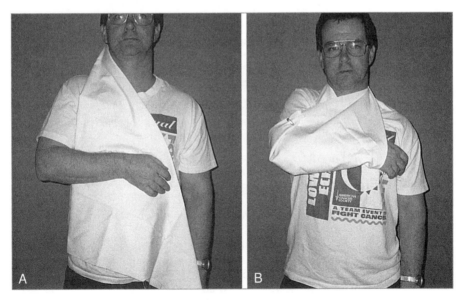

FIGURE 35 • 2 Triangular sling application.

- ➤ Do the following exercises while the sling is in place
  - ➤ Isometrics of the deltoid—flex and relax.
  - ➤ Wiggle the fingers.
  - ➤ Return to the office for recheck on _____.

B IBLIOGRAPHY

Kenney, D.E., and Klima, R.R. (1993). Modified armsling for soft-tissue injuries of the shoulder and glenohumeral subluxation. *J Hand Ther,* 6(3), 215–216.

McConnell, E.A. (1991). Correctly positioning an arm sling. *Nursing 91,* 21(7), 70.

Potter, P.A., and Perry, A.G. (1995). *Basic nursing: theory and practice.* St. Louis: Mosby.

36

SPLINTING AND TAPING

CYNTHIA R. EHRHARDT

CPT Code	
29260–80	Strapping; elbow or wrist, hand or finger
29530–50	Strapping; ankle, knee, toes
99070	Splinting

Splinting and taping provide effective temporary methods of immobilizing a joint after a mild-to-moderate musculoskeletal joint inflammation or injury. Splinting frequently is used in place of casting.

OVERVIEW

- ➤ Incidence is unknown.
- ➤ The most common musculoskeletal injuries (85%) involve the ankle joint following the mechanism of inversion and plantar flexion stretching of the lateral ligaments.
- ➤ The second most common musculoskeletal injury involves overuse syndrome of the wrist and thumb.
- ➤ General principles include the following
  - ➤ During application, frequently reassess neurovascular status.
  - ➤ Apply material firmly but not tightly.
  - ➤ Avoid skin irritation wherever possible.
  - ➤ Instruct on precautions of skin irritation if stockinette is not used.

➤ Remove splint at least four times a day for gentle range-of-motion exercises to reduce the incidence of "frozen joint syndrome."

➤ Do not discharge client until 30 minutes after completion of the procedure, to ensure satisfactory application without compromise of neurovascular system.

➤ Determination of the appropriate appliance to use (taping versus splinting) depends on
  ➤ Joint injured
  ➤ Nature of joint injury and ligaments involved
  ➤ Mechanism of joint injury
  ➤ Time of injury
    • Immediate
    • Acute (within 24 hours without onset of swelling)
    • Intermediate acute (within 24 hours with onset of swelling)
    • Delayed acute (beyond 48 hours)
  ➤ Previous history of injury to the joint
  ➤ Severity of injury
    • Most grade II and III ligamental and musculoskeletal injuries respond well with splinting or immobilization.
  ➤ Physical examination findings
  ➤ Requirement to return to activity

HEALTH PROMOTION/PREVENTION

➤ Use of
  ➤ Properly fitting athletic equipment
  ➤ Appropriate footwear for participation in the sport
  ➤ Proper stretching and warm-up exercises before sports participation
  ➤ Proper conditioning to play the sport
  ➤ Prophylactic use of taping of chronic joint injuries before sports participation

OPTIONS

See Table 36–1.

Splinting

➤ Ankle splinting
  ➤ *Method 1*—posterior splint
  ➤ *Method 2*—Aircast technique
➤ Knee immobilization
  ➤ Use with grade II and III knee strains
➤ Wrist splinting
  ➤ *Method 1*—premade wrist splint
  ➤ *Method 2*—volar splinting
➤ Thumb splinting
  ➤ Use for adductor pollicis tendinitis
    • *Method 1*—premade wrist splint with thumb support

TABLE 36•1 PROCEDURE OPTIONS

Splinting
  Advantages
  ➤ Restricts movement 100%
  ➤ Allows stabilization of suspected joint fractures
  ➤ Prevents further trauma to the joint and skeletal structure
  ➤ Allows adjustment of the orthopedic device in the presence of soft tissue edema
    and its resolution
  ➤ Can replace bulky casting
  Disadvantages
  ➤ Bulky prosthetic device
  ➤ Cannot be used as a prophylactic measure
  ➤ Can be overused and misused by the client
  ➤ Can cause skin irritation
  ➤ More expensive than taping

Taping
  Advantages
  ➤ Facilitates to limit movement
  ➤ Does not restrict movement 100%
  ➤ May immediately return to activity without an obtrusive prosthetic device
  ➤ Not as bulky as a prosthetic device
  ➤ Prophylactic use prevents further aggravation of a chronic injury
  Disadvantages
  ➤ 50% of taping loosens within 10 min of application
  ➤ Requires some skill in application
  ➤ Can cause skin irritation
  ➤ Not as effective as splinting if joint immobilization is required

---

  • *Method 2*—aluminum thumb splint
  • *Method 3*—thumb spica

Taping

➤ Ankle taping
  ➤ *Method 1*—Louisiana ankle wrap technique
  ➤ *Method 2*—open Gibney technique with heel lock
  ➤ *Method 3*—open Gibney technique without heel lock
  ➤ *Method 4*—basket-weave technique with heel lock
➤ Knee taping
➤ Wrist taping
➤ Elbow taping
  ➤ Lateral epicondylar taping
➤ Foot taping
  ➤ For plantar fasciitis, overuse, and blunt injury
    • *Method 1*—figure eight technique
    • *Method 2*—full plantar taping technique

RATIONALE

➤ To protect ligaments from abnormal stress
➤ To diminish muscle spasms
➤ To maintain range of motion

INDICATIONS

➤ Splinting and taping
  ➤ Mild grade II or III ankle strains (Table 36–2)
  ➤ Tenosynovitis from overuse syndrome, such as
    • Carpal tunnel syndrome
    • Abductor pollicis tendon inflammation (computer game syndrome)
    • Extensor retinaculum inflammation
  ➤ Suspected peroneal tendon dislocation
  ➤ Suspected fracture
  ➤ Suspected unstable joint structure
➤ Taping only
  ➤ Grade I and II strains (see Table 36–2)

TABLE 36•2 GRADING OF INJURED LIGAMENTS

Grade I
➤ Injury history
  ➤ Short-lived or minimal experience of pain. Joint was forced beyond normal range of motion
➤ Pain
  ➤ Momentary
  ➤ May proceed with activity but without significant interference of activity
➤ Physical examination
  ➤ Abnormal laxity of ligament present
  ➤ Localized tenderness at the insertion points of the ligament
  ➤ Minimal soft tissue edema

Grade II
➤ Injury history
  ➤ Sharp initial sensation with or without a "popping" or "snapping" sensation
  ➤ Joint was forced beyond normal range of motion
➤ Pain
  ➤ Generally progressive with continued stress to the joint
  ➤ Eventually, activity must be halted
➤ Pathology
  ➤ Incomplete disruption of the musculotendinous unit
  ➤ Lengthening or partial tearing of the ligament
➤ Physical examination
  ➤ Laxity of the joint
  ➤ Soft tissue edema with obliteration of landmarks
  ➤ Possible ecchymosis

(Continued on following page)

TABLE 36•2 GRADING OF INJURED LIGAMENTS *(Continued)*

Grade III
- Injury history
  - Sharp initial sensation with or without a "popping" or "snapping" sensation
  - Joint was forced beyond normal range of motion
- Pain
  - Short-lived and disappears within a few minutes
- Pathology
  - Complete tearing of the ligament
  - Complete disruption of the musculotendinous unit
- Physical examination
  - Marked laxity
  - Presence of drawer sign

  - Tenosynovitis from overuse syndromes, such as
    - Epicondylitis
    - Chondromalacia patellae
    - Iliotibial band tendinitis, also known as runner's knee
    - Osgood-Schlatter syndrome—occasionally beneficial
  - Plantar **fasciitis**

CONTRAINDICATIONS

- Sprains accompanied by soft tissue compression or open injury
- Neurovascular compromise
- Emergency department or orthopedic referral should be considered if
  - Injury is suspicious for fracture.
  - Joint is unstable.
  - Injury represents potential loss of limb or function.
  - Internal derangement of ligamental structure is suspected.
  - Pain persists.
  - Injury is not resolved.
  - Joint instability persists.

PROCEDURE

Splinting

Equipment

- Tube stockinettes in various diameters
- Precast casting material or casting material of various widths (4 and 6 inches are used most often)
- Elastic wrap tape (2-, 4-, or 6-inch widths)
- Adhesive tape in various widths (1- or 2-inch widths)
- Bucket with water
- Soft padding material—optional
- Lubricated foam padding—optional

> Scissors—nonsterile
> Sling—for upper extremity injuries
> Aluminum splits (1- or 2-inch widths)
> Wrist splints
> Knee immobilizer
> Arm sling

Procedure

ANKLE SPLINTING

> *Method 1*—posterior splint (Fig. 36–1)
> > Position the client onto the abdomen with knee flexed at 90 degrees.
> > Have the ankle in a neutral position ensuring adequate stretching of the Achilles tendon.
> > Apply stockinette distal to proximal approximately 2 to 3 inches above and below the projected splint area.
> > Optional—Apply cotton web padding from distal to proximal until a 2-inch thickness is obtained.
> > • Extra cushion and thickness may be necessary around the bony prominences of the ankle.
> > Select appropriate width of casting material (usually 6-inch width).
> > Cut casting material to the length needed.
> > • If not precast with preset thickness, fold in 10 to 12 overlapping layers equaling the length plus 4 cm of the projected splint.

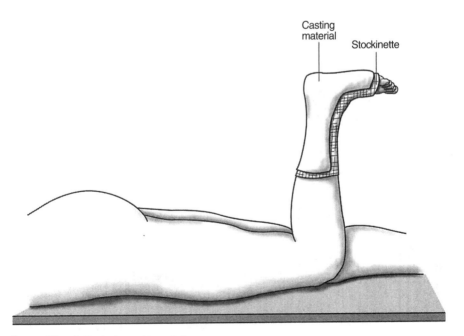

FIGURE 36 • 1 Posterior ankle splint.

- ➤ Moisten plaster (fiberglass, plaster, or precast) material by dipping in a bucket of cool water.
- ➤ Apply casting material to the posterior portion of the leg and ankle.
- ➤ Mold the casting material to the shape and angle of the limb ensuring a 90-degree flexion of the ankle.
- ➤ Wrap with elastic wrap proximally to distally. Sufficient elastic wrap should be used to hold the posterior splint snugly.
- ➤ Fold over the edge of stockinette and complete the elastic tape wrap. Secure end with tape.
- ➤ Allow casting material to dry.
- ➤ *Method 2*—Aircast technique
  - ➤ Position the ankle in neutral position ensuring adequate stretching of the Achilles tendon (90-degree angle).
  - ➤ Apply stockinette or cotton sock.
  - ➤ Apply Aircast splint and secure straps.
  - ➤ Inflate as directed.

KNEE IMMOBILIZATION

See Figure 36–2

- ➤ Position the client comfortably, and place a rolled towel underneath the knee sufficient to flex it 15 to 20 degrees.

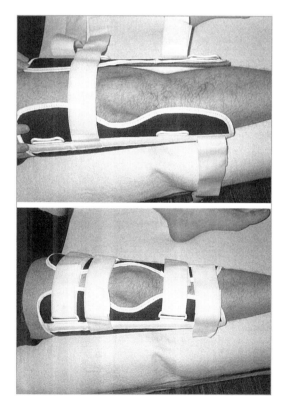

FIGURE 36 • 2 Knee immobilization.

➤ Optional—Apply stockinette extending to approximately 4 to 6 cm below the groin to midcalf (i.e., greater than the length of the immobilizer).
➤ Support pantyhose can be used in place of stockinette.
➤ Open the knee immobilizer and center the patellar notch of fabric.
➤ Close and secure the knee immobilizer with self-adhering straps.

WRIST SPLINTING

➤ *Method 1*—premade wrist splint (Fig. 36–3)
   ➤ Position the client comfortably with wrist in neutral position.
   ➤ Optional—Apply stockinette and cut a small hole to slide the thumb through in a glovelike fashion. It should extend to a length approximately equal to the splint itself.
   ➤ Position the splint to ensure adequate support of the joint structure.
   ➤ Secure with self-adhering straps.
➤ *Method 2*—volar splinting (Fig. 36–4)
   ➤ Position the wrist slightly hyperextended (5 to 10 degrees).
   ➤ Apply stockinette at least 6 to 8 cm longer than intended casting material, being sure to cut a hole to allow thumb through.
   ➤ Optional—Apply cotton web padding to a thickness of at least 2 inches.
   ➤ Select appropriate width of casting material (usually a 6-inch width).
   ➤ Cut the casting material to the length needed.
      • If not precast with preset thickness, fold in 10 to 12 overlapping layers equaling the length plus 4 cm of the projected splint.
   ➤ Moisten the plaster (fiberglass, plaster, or precast) material by dipping in a bucket of cool water.
   ➤ Apply the casting material to the forearm, wrist, and palm of hand.
   ➤ Apply casting material and mold it to the shape of the wrist.
   ➤ If necessary, trim the distal edge of the casting material to the middle interphalangeal joint.
   ➤ Fold excess stockinette over plaster.
   ➤ Using elastic wrap, wrap from distal to proximal. Ensure secure fit with the use of two or three layers of elastic wrap.
   ➤ Secure end with tape.
   ➤ Apply sling until dry.

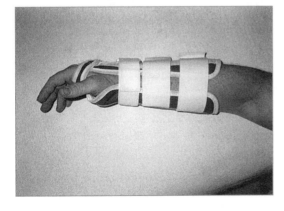

FIGURE 36 • 3 Premade wrist splint.

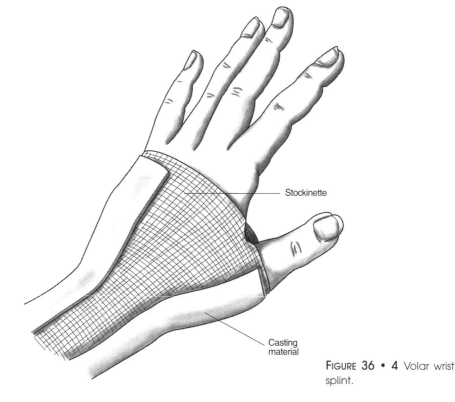

FIGURE 36 • 4 Volar wrist splint.

THUMB SPLINTING

- *Method 1*—premade wrist splint
  - See method 1, premade wrist splint application.
- *Method 2*—aluminum thumb splint (Fig. 36–5)
  - Position the wrist and hand comfortably, the thumb slightly flexed at the distal interphalangeal (DIP) joint. Have the client grasp an elastic wrap or 3-inch gauze roll in the web space of the hand.
    - Hyperflex the wrist approximately 5 to 10 degrees and in neutral radioulnar deviation position.
  - Measure the aluminum splint from the end of the thumb and 6 to 10 cm to the anatomic snuffbox of the forearm. Be sure to trim any sharp edges.
  - Optional—Apply stockinette to the thumb and forearm in the same length as the splint. Cut a hole in the stockinette to allow the thumb to slide through.
  - Optional—Apply cotton padding in 1- to 2-inch thickness.
  - Bend the aluminum splint to the position of the thumb and wrist.
  - Apply the splint to either the dorsal (most commonly performed) or the palmar side of the thumb.
  - Optional—Apply a single strip of tape to the aluminum splint at the DIP.

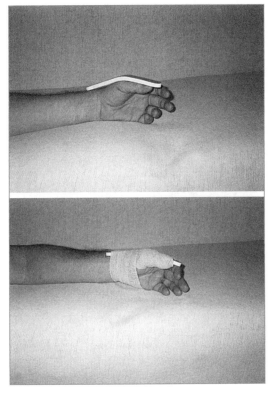

FIGURE 36 • 5 Aluminum thumb splint.

> Remove webbing used to maintain proper position.
> Wrap the aluminum splint distally to proximally with the elastic wrap including the thumb. A modified figure eight pattern of thumb, wrist, and metacarpals can be used.
> Secure with tape.
> *Method 3*—thumb spica (Fig. 36–6)
> Position the wrist and hand comfortably, the thumb slightly flexed at the DIP joint. Have the client grasp an elastic wrap or 3-inch gauze roll in the web space of the hand.
  • Hyperflex the wrist approximately 5 to 10 degrees and in neutral radioulnar deviation position.
> Measure the casting strips from just proximal to the distal palmar crease to mid forearm. Use narrower width of casting material for the thumb, with the length being measured from the tip of the thumb to mid forearm.
> Apply stockinette to the thumb and forearm.
> Optional—Apply cotton padding in 2-inch thickness, including the thumb.
> Moisten all casting material by dipping in a bucket of cool water.
> Apply wider casting material to the underside of the forearm.

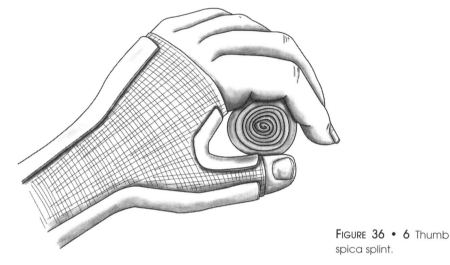

FIGURE 36 • 6 Thumb spica splint.

➤ Take narrower thumb strips and apply on lateral surface of thumb, molding them to the anatomic placement of the thumb.
➤ Apply elastic wrap distally to proximally, including the thumb. A modified figure eight pattern of thumb, wrist, and metacarpals can be used.
➤ Apply a sling until dry.

Taping

Equipment

➤ Soft padding material
➤ Elastic wrap tape (2-, 4-, or 6-inch widths)
➤ Tape adherent spray (e.g., tincture of benzoin)
➤ Zinc white (cotton) tape in various widths (1-, 2-, 3-, or 4-inch widths)
➤ Scissors—nonsterile
➤ Arm sling
➤ Foam-cushion foot insert

Procedure

ANKLE TAPING

➤ *Method 1*—Louisiana ankle wrap technique (Fig. 36–7)
  ➤ Position the ankle in a neutral position ensuring adequate stretching of the Achilles tendon (90-degree angle).
  ➤ Optional—Apply stockinette to the ankle with it extending approximately 2 to 3 inches above and below the projected wrap area.
  ➤ Spray tape adherent to the proposed taping site.
  ➤ Begin wrap by anchoring across the top of the foot.
  ➤ Continue wrap around instep, then proceed to around heel.
  ➤ Continue wrapping in a layer format until satisfactory reduction of movement has been achieved.
  ➤ Secure end of wrap with tape.

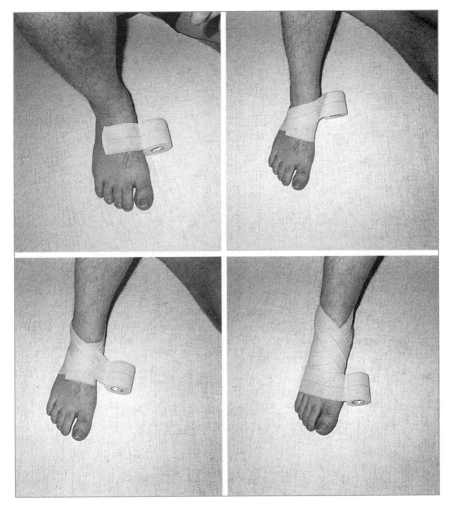

Figure 36 • 7 Louisiana ankle wrap technique.

➤ *Method 2*—open Gibney technique with heel lock (Fig. 36–8)
  ➤ Position the ankle in neutral position, ensuring adequate stretching of the Achilles tendon (90-degree angle).
  ➤ Optional—Apply stockinette to ankle, with it extending approximately 2 to 3 inches above and below the projected wrap area.
  ➤ Spray tape adherent to the proposed taping site.
  ➤ Using zinc (cotton) tape 1 or 2 inches wide (depending on ankle size), apply a tape anchor approximately 10 to 12 cm above the lateral and medial malleolus encircling the leg.
  ➤ Apply two to three overlapping stirrup strips in a continuous fashion medially and laterally. These stirrup strips should extend from the anchor tape on the lateral side of the ankle under the bottom of the foot and back up to the anchor tape on the medial side of the ankle.

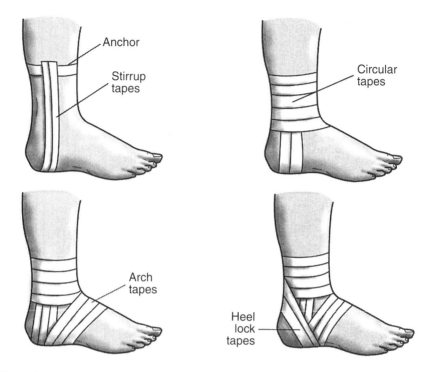

FIGURE 36 • 8 Open Gibney technique with heel lock.

> ➤ Apply five to six overlapping circular tape layers over the stirrup strips.
> ➤ Apply two to three diagonal overlapping circular tape layers to the arch region.
> ➤ Apply two to three overlapping diagonal tape layers to the heel.
> ➤ If using stockinette, fold the excess stockinette over the tape, anchor with tape, and trim.

➤ *Method 3*—open Gibney technique without heel lock (Fig. 36–9)
  > ➤ Position the ankle in neutral position, ensuring adequate stretching of the Achilles tendon (90-degree angle).
  > ➤ Optional—Apply stockinette to ankle with it extending approximately 2 to 3 inches above and below the projected wrap area.
  > ➤ Spray tape adherent to the proposed taping site.
  > ➤ Apply 6 to 10 overlapping semicircular tape strips to cover 50% of the posterior lower leg to approximately 1 to 2 cm above and 10 to 12 cm below the lateral and medial malleolus.
  > ➤ Apply four to six longer semicircular strips in an overlapping pattern to the long axis of the foot. Start at 2 cm proximal of the medial distal metatarsal head around the posterior heel extending to 2 cm proximal of the lateral distal metatarsal heads.
  > ➤ Apply four to six semicircular strips in an overlapping pattern in the arch region of the foot extending from the distal calcaneus to mid metatarsal region.

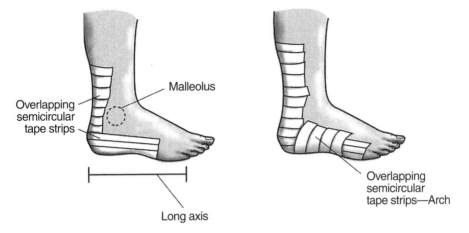

Malleolus

Overlapping
semicircular
tape strips

Long axis

Overlapping
semicircular
tape strips—Arch

FIGURE 36 • 9 Open Gibney technique without heel lock.

> If using stockinette, fold over the excess stockinette, anchor with tape, and trim.
> *Method 4*—basket-weave technique with heel lock (Fig. 36–10)
>> Position the ankle in neutral position ensuring adequate stretching of the Achilles tendon (90-degree angle).
>> Optional—Apply stockinette to ankle with it extending approximately 2 to 3 inches above and below the projected wrap area.
>> Spray tape adherent to the proposed taping site.
>> Apply two circular tape strips as follows
>>> • One strip at the top of the projected area of taping approximately 10 to 12 cm above the lateral and medial malleolus
>>> • One strip at the bottom of the projected area of taping approximately 2 cm above the distal metatarsal head
>> Apply longitudinal and vertical tape strips in an overlapping pattern.
>> Apply a layer of circular tape strips covering the vertical tape strips.
>> Apply five to six circular strips across the arch region to approximately mid metatarsal.
>> If using stockinette, fold over the excess stockinette, anchor with tape, and trim.

KNEE TAPING

See Figure 36–11.
> Position the client comfortably, and place a rolled towel underneath the knee sufficient to flex it 15 to 20 degrees.
> Optional—Apply foam pad over the popliteal space to reduce chafing.
> Optional—Apply stockinette extending to approximately 4 to 6 cm below the groin to midcalf.
> Spray tape adherent to the proposed taping site.

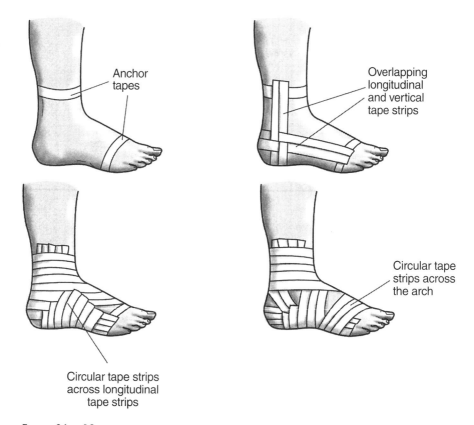

FIGURE 36 • 10 Basket-weave technique with heel lock.

➤ Apply overlapping circular strips of tape (2- or 3-inch tape suggested) beginning either proximally or distally depending on personal preference in a basket-weave pattern.
➤ Apply 3- to 4-inch elastic tape (4-inch tape recommended) in a larger figure eight pattern, crossing over the medial and lateral collateral ligaments. This may be repeated in a layered fashion for three to four layers.
➤ If using stockinette, fold over the excess stockinette, anchor with tape, and trim.

WRIST TAPING

See Figure 36–12.

➤ Position the client comfortably with the thumb slightly flexed. Position of the thumb can be maintained with a roll of elastic tape or gauze in the web space.
➤ Optional—Apply stockinette and cut a small hole to slide thumb through in a glovelike fashion. It should extend approximately 2 inches beyond the proposed taping area.

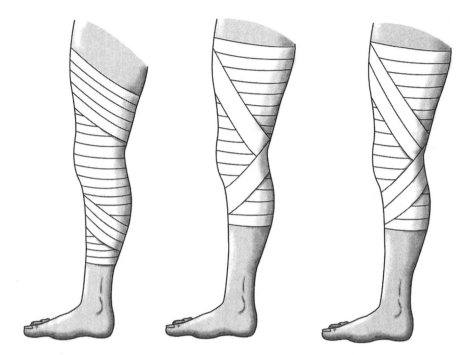

FIGURE 36 • 11 Knee taping.

➤ Spray tape adherent to the skin.
➤ Cut approximately four to six 2-inch tape strips, and apply along the medial portion of the forearm covering the location of the distal insertion of the adductor pollicis across the distal radial head and the extensor carpi radialis longus and extensor carpi ulnaris brevis.
➤ If using stockinette, fold over the excess stockinette, anchor with tape, and trim.

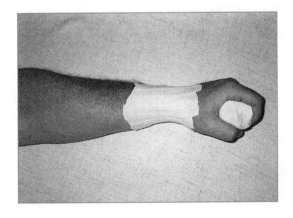

FIGURE 36 • 12 Wrist taping.

➤ Optional—Apply an elastic wrap in a figure eight pattern for further rigidity.

ELBOW TAPING—LATERAL EPICONDYLAR TAPING

See Figure 36–13.

➤ Position the client comfortably with the elbow flexed 90 degrees.
➤ Optional—Apply stockinette approximately 10 to 12 cm above and below the joint.
➤ Spray tape adherent to area to be taped.
➤ Apply 6-inch strips in an overlapping fashion over the lateral epicondylar process.
➤ If using stockinette, fold over the excess stockinette, anchor with tape, and trim.
➤ Apply an arm sling if only minimal relief was obtained from the taping.
  ➤ Use the sling no longer than 72 hours.

FOOT TAPING

➤ *Method 1*—figure eight technique (Fig. 36–14)
  ➤ Position the client comfortably with foot in neutral position (90-degree angle).
  ➤ Spray tape adherent to the area to be taped.
  ➤ Apply a circular figure eight pattern with inclusion of the heel from the base of the first metatarsal to the base of the fifth metatarsal.
  ➤ Continue in an overlapping pattern of at least three or four strips.
  ➤ Apply three to four transverse strips in an overlapping pattern across the plantar surface at the metatarsal heads. They should not extend into the arch unless relief is not obtained.
  ➤ Optional—Foam pad may be inserted in the shoe for added comfort.
➤ *Method 2*—full plantar taping technique (Fig. 36–15)
  ➤ Position the client comfortably with foot in neutral position (90-degree angle).

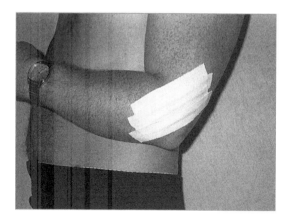

FIGURE 36 • 13 Lateral epicondylar elbow taping.

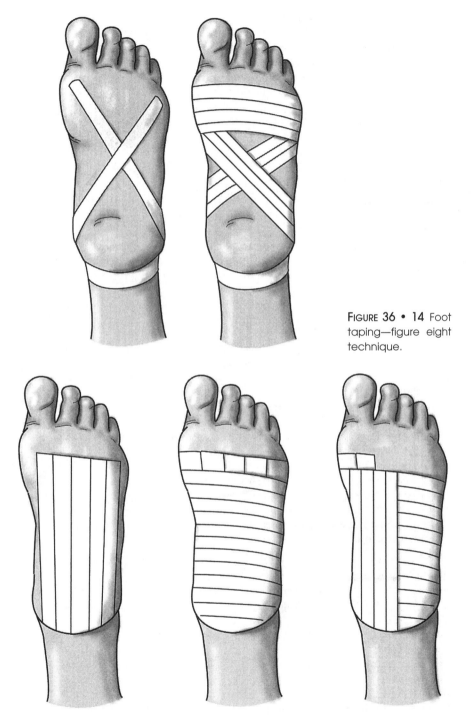

FIGURE 36 • 14 Foot taping—figure eight technique.

FIGURE 36 • 15 Foot taping—full plantar taping technique.

➤ Spray tape adherent to the area to be taped.
➤ Apply tape along the longitudinal axis of the plantar surface.
  • If necessary, reapply tape adherent spray if tape does not hold when using layering technique.
➤ Apply overlapping tape transversely.
➤ Apply overlapping tape longitudinally.
➤ If no improvement of the plantar fasciitis in 7 to 10 days, re-evaluation of the diagnosis should be considered.

Client Instructions

SPLINTING AND TAPING

➤ RICE—Rest, Ice, Compression (splinting or taping as indicated by injury), and Elevate the injured joint for at least 48 hours to minimize further trauma.
➤ Avoid weight bearing; use crutches for injuries of the knees or ankles.
➤ After 24 hours
  ➤ Remove splint at least four times a day and begin gentle range of motion.
  ➤ Remove taping once per day and begin gentle range of motion.
  ➤ If pain occurs when range of motion is attempted, delay for an additional 24 hours.
  ➤ If unable to resume gentle range of motion after 48 hours, return to the office for further evaluation of the injury.
➤ Observe for signs of neurovascular compromise including
  ➤ Pallor or decreased color of the fingers or toes
  ➤ Decreased sensation or numbness in the fingers or toes
  ➤ Increased pain
  ➤ If any signs of neurovascular compromise occur, remove the tape, and call health-care provider.
➤ To relieve pain and inflammation
  ➤ Use acetaminophen every 4 to 6 hours.
  ➤ Nonsteroidal anti-inflammatory drugs, such as ibuprofen, may be initiated 12 to 24 hours after injury.
  ➤ Elevate and rest the injured joint. This facilitates the effectiveness of medication.

BIBLIOGRAPHY

American Medical Association (1996). *Physicians' current procedural terminology.* Chicago: Author.

Birrer, R., and Poole, B. (1995). Athletic taping part 3: the knee. *J Musculoskeletal Med,* July, 43–45.

Cohen, M., and Lanigan, A. (1995) (2nd ed.). *Nurse practitioner protocols.* Tallahassee: Sunbelt Publishing, pp. 10-2–10-4.

Garrick, J., and Webb, D. (1990). *Sports injuries: diagnosis and management.* Philadelphia: Saunders.

Gould, J. (1988). *The foot book.* Baltimore: Williams & Wilkins.

Grana, W., and Kallenk, K. (eds.) (1991). *Sports medicine.* Philadelphia: Saunders.

Mercier, L. (1991) (3rd ed.). *Practical orthopedics.* St. Louis: Mosby.

Murtagh, J. (1995) (2nd ed.). *Practice tips.* New York: McGraw-Hill.

Netter, F. (1989). *Atlas of human anatomy.* Summit, NJ: Ciba-Geigy.

Pfenninger, J.L., and Fowler, G.C. (1994). *Procedures for primary care physicians.* St. Louis: Mosby.

Ramanmurti, C. (1979). *Orthopedics in primary care.* Baltimore: Williams & Wilkins.

Richard, J. (1995). Office orthopedics: thumb spica casting for scaphoid fractures. *Am Fam Physician,* 52(4), 1113–1119.

Ryan, J. (1995). Use of posterior night splints in the treatment of plantar fasciitis. *Am Fam Physician,* 52(3), 891–898.

37

TRIGGER POINT INJECTION

ANN GREEN

CPT Code

20550   Injection; tendon sheath, ligament, trigger points, or ganglion cyst

Trigger points are areas of localized pain in various muscle groups, often near bony attachments. Focal tender areas are located by palpating the various muscle groups to determine the trigger point and the corresponding area of pain. Common points of maximum tenderness often are located at moving parts and sliding surfaces.

OVERVIEW

➤ Incidence unknown
➤ More common with myofascial pain syndromes and fibromyalgia

HEALTH PROMOTION/PREVENTION

➤ Although exacerbations are not predictable, avoiding repetitive overuse of muscle groups might prevent occurrence.

RATIONALE

➤ To interrupt the pain cycle and provide immediate relief

INDICATIONS

➤ Areas of localized tenderness without other pathology

CONTRAINDICATIONS

➤ Irritation or infection at injection site
➤ Anticoagulant therapy or increased bleeding tendency
➤ **Septicemia**
➤ Emergency equipment not available

✓ *Informed consent required*

PROCEDURE

Trigger Point Injection

Equipment

➤ Alcohol wipes
➤ Gloves—sterile
➤ 4 × 4 gauze pads
➤ Skin-marking pencil
➤ Topical skin cleanser
➤ 0.25% to 1% lidocaine *without* epinephrine (single-dose vials, if possible)
➤ Choice of steroid (0.5 to 1 mL of selected steroid, such as methylprednisolone acetate if used with lidocaine)
➤ 25- to 27-gauge needle of length appropriate for site injected
➤ 3-, 5-, or 10-mL syringe

Procedure

➤ Position patient in comfortable, safe position in the event of a syncopal reaction.
➤ Mark the point of maximal tenderness with a marking pencil.
➤ Cleanse the skin with topical antiseptic.
➤ Identify the trigger point (maximal area of tenderness) with sterile gloved finger using sterile technique.
➤ Using the 25- or 27-gauge needle, draw 3 to 5 mL of lidocaine (if using only lidocaine, begin with 5 mL of 0.25% to 1% lidocaine).
➤ If using the additional steroid, draw 3 to 4 mL of the lidocaine first, then draw 1 mL of the steroid into the same syringe.
  ➤ *Note*—Change needles if drawing from both solutions because of dulling of the needle and contamination of multidose vials.
➤ Slowly advance the needle perpendicular to the skin until the point of tenderness is located.
➤ Aspirate for a blood return (relocate if identified).
➤ Inject 0.5 to 2 mL of the medication (the patient should have instant pain relief if properly located).
➤ Withdraw the needle slightly and inject the site two to four times at 30-degree angles from the first perpendicular injection (north, south, east, west).
➤ Remove the needle and wipe the skin with the disinfectant.
➤ Place an adhesive bandage over the injection site.

➤ Observe for immediate decrease in pain.
➤ Observe for light-headedness, tinnitus, peripheral numbness, slurring of speech, drowsiness, or seizures (may indicate reaction to the local anesthetic).

Client Instructions

➤ Observe for signs and symptoms of infection, such as
  ➤ Increase in pain after 24 hours
  ➤ Increase in temperature
  ➤ Redness or swelling
  ➤ Yellow or greenish drainage
  ➤ Foul odor
➤ If any signs or symptoms of infection are found, return to the office.
➤ Observe for the following problems
  ➤ Hematoma formation
  ➤ Reaction to local anesthetic
  ➤ Rebound pain
  ➤ Neuritis
➤ Trigger point injection may be repeated as needed if no steroids are used. If steroids are used, injections should be at least 6 weeks apart.

BIBLIOGRAPHY

Pando, J.A., and Klippel, J.H. (1996). Arthrocentesis and corticosteroid injections: an illustrated guide to technique. *Consultant*, 10, 2137–2148.

Ruoff, G.E. (1995). Technique of trigger point injection. In Pfenninger, J.L., and Fowler, G.C. (eds.). *Procedures for primary care physicians* (pp. 164–167). St. Louis: Mosby.

Genitourinary and Breast Procedures

38

BREAST BIOPSY
FINE NEEDLE ASPIRATION

MARGARET R. COLYAR

CPT Code

19000   Puncture aspiration of cyst of breast
19001   Puncture aspiration, each additional cyst
19100   Biopsy of breast, needle core
88170   Fine needle aspiration with or without preparation of smears; superficial tissue (e.g., thyroid, breast, prostate)

Fine needle aspiration is a method of obtaining samples of a solid or cystic mass for laboratory evaluation. Tissues commonly obtained by this method are
➤ Breast
➤ Thyroid
➤ Lymph node
Thyroid masses and lymph node biopsies are not currently within the scope of practice for nurse practitioners and should be referred to a physician for aspiration.

OVERVIEW
➤ Incidence is unknown.
➤ There are three common types of breast masses
  ➤ Fibroadenomas
  ➤ Cysts
  ➤ Breast carcinomas
Fibroadenomas are solid benign tumors usually found in younger women. Cysts are fluid-filled and usually are seen during midlife. Breast carcinomas are found as solid masses that increase in frequency with age and usually are not seen in women younger than 30 years old. To establish a definitive diag-

nosis, a mass must be drained or a sample of tissue obtained. Benign masses feel smooth, round, and freely movable. Carcinomas usually feel solid and unmovable with poorly defined or irregular edges. Some cancers can feel like benign masses, however. If there is a high suspicion of cancer, refer the patient to a surgeon to perform the **biopsy**. If the mass is thought to be benign, you may elect to perform the biopsy yourself.

RATIONALE

➤ To confirm etiology of a lesion for treatment
➤ To establish or confirm a diagnosis for treatment and/or intervention

INDICATIONS

➤ Palpable solitary breast mass
➤ Recurrent breast mass
➤ Anxiety concerning a mass

CONTRAINDICATIONS

➤ Coagulation disorder—REFER
➤ On anticoagulant therapy—REFER
➤ Bloody discharge from a nipple—REFER
➤ Definite cancerous breast—REFER

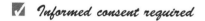 *Informed consent required*

PROCEDURE

Biopsy—Fine Needle Aspiration

Equipment

➤ Antiseptic skin cleanser
➤ 1% lidocaine
➤ 3-mL syringe
➤ 21-, 22-, or 23-gauge, $1^1/_2$-inch needle
➤ 12-mL syringe
➤ 4 × 4 gauze—sterile
➤ Gloves—sterile
➤ 27- to 30-gauge, $^1/_2$-inch needle
➤ Optional—EURO-Med FNA 21 for fine needle aspiration
   ➤ For solid core masses only
➤ Specimen jar with 10% **formalin**
   ➤ For fluid-filled cyst only
➤ Two sterile plain evacuated blood tubes
➤ Four microscope slides
➤ Fixative for slides
➤ Coverslips

Procedure

➤ Position the client with the mass easily accessible.
➤ Cleanse the mass and surrounding tissues with antiseptic skin cleanser.
➤ Inject 1% lidocaine around the mass, if desired (Fig. 38–1).
➤ If using a 12-mL syringe, aspirate one fifth of syringe full of air.
  ➤ Hold the mass immobile with nondominant hand.
  ➤ Using dominant hand with syringe held like a pen, insert the 12-mL syringe with 21- to 23-gauge needle into the mass and aspirate.
  ➤ Move needle around into all areas of the mass. Aspirate in each area.
  ➤ Before withdrawing the syringe, return the plunger to the position before aspiration to prevent withdrawal of sample while leaving the mass. This prevents seeding the needle tract with malignant cells.
➤ Eject cell material onto slides (if fluid) or into specimen jar containing 10% formalin (if solid core).
➤ To decrease the chance of hematoma formation, either apply pressure with 4 × 4 gauze for 5 to 15 minutes or apply an ice pack for 15 to 60 minutes.

Client Instructions

➤ To prevent hematoma formation
  ➤ Apply a pressure dressing and an ice pack for 24 hours.
➤ A moderate amount of pain, redness, and swelling are expected. Take acetaminophen (Tylenol) every 4 hours as needed.

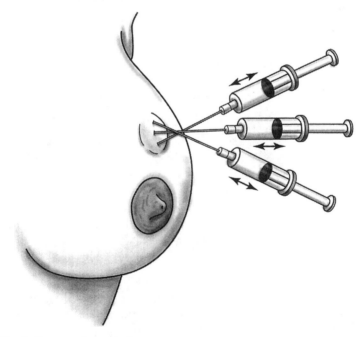

FIGURE 38 • 1 Fine needle aspiration.

➤ Observe for signs and symptoms of infection, such as
  ➤ Increase in pain after 24 hours
  ➤ Increase in temperature
  ➤ Redness or swelling
  ➤ Yellow or greenish drainage
  ➤ Foul odor
➤ If any signs or symptoms of infection are found, return to the office.

BIBLIOGRAPHY

Euro-Med, a division of Cooper Surgical. *FNA 21*. Belgium.
Kline, T.S. (1995). Fine-needle aspiration biopsy of the breast. *Am Fam Physician*, 52(7), 2021–2025.
Layfield, L.J., et al (1993). The palpable breast nodule. *Cancer*, 72(5), 1642–1651.
Pfenninger, J.L., and Fowler, G.C. (1994). *Procedures for primary care physicians*. St. Louis: Mosby.

39

COLPOSCOPY
ENDOCERVICAL CURETTAGE AND CERVICAL BIOPSY

MARGARET R. COLYAR

CPT Code

57452	Colposcopy
57454	Colposcopy with biopsy, single or multiple, of the cervix and/or endocervical curettage
57500	Biopsy, single or multiple, or local excision of lesion, with or without fulguration
57505	Endocervical curettage

A colposcopic examination is necessary after receiving an abnormal **Papanicolaou (Pap) smear**. Endocervical **curettage** and cervical biopsy are done when abnormalities are found on the colposcopic examination.

OVERVIEW

➤ The use of a colposcopic examination form is helpful in documenting findings (Fig. 39–1).

COLPOSCOPY

Date_____

Name_____ Age_____ DOB_____

Reason for colposcopy_____

LMP_____ Pap Smear date_____ Result_____

# of pregnancies___ # of children___ Type of contraception_____

History of STD's_____ Vaginal warts_____ Vaginal infections_____

Do you smoke?_____ How much?_____

Conclusions of the colposcopy

Vaginal vault_____ Urethra_____

Labia_____ Perineum_____ Rectum_____

Signs of vaginal infection_____

Complete transformation zone seen?_____

Biopsy site_____

Impressions_____

_____

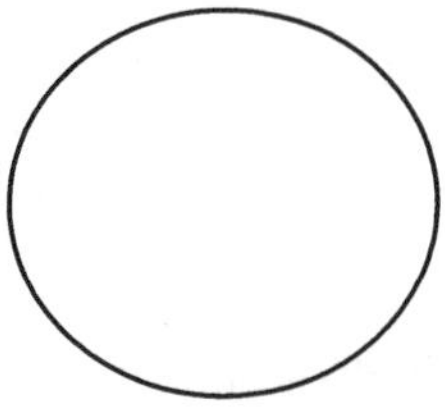

Recommendations: (Circle one)

Cryotherapy   Loop

Referral to_____

Signature_____

Key: WE - White epithelium

    L - Leukoplakia

    P - Punctation

    M - Mosaicism

    ATZ - Abnormal TZ

    AV - Abnormal vessels

    X - Biopsy sites

FIGURE 39 • 1 Sample colposcopic examination form.

- Questions to ask each client include
  - Menstrual history
  - Medications—especially hormones and anticoagulants
  - History of abnormal Pap smears
  - History of previous treatment for abnormal Pap smears
  - Signs of pelvic or vaginal infection
  - History of human papillomavirus (HPV) infection
  - History of diethylstilbestrol (DES) exposure
  - History of sexually transmitted diseases, sexual abuse, or partner with genital **condyloma acuminatum**
  - History of cervical, vaginal, or vulval cancer

RATIONALE

- To evaluate cervical abnormalities

INDICATIONS

- Abnormal Pap smear
- Observed cervical lesion
- HPV infection
- Unexplained vaginal bleeding
- History of DES exposure in utero

CONTRAINDICATIONS

- Pregnancy—REFER to gynecologist for testing
- Current heavy menses

☑ *Informed consent required*

Ask client to take 600 mg of ibuprofen 1 hour before the testing time to decrease uterine discomfort.

PROCEDURE

Colposcopy, Endocervical Curettage, Cervical Biopsy

Equipment

- Drape—sterile
- Gloves—nonsterile
- Syringe—3 mL
- Vaginal **speculum**—large
- Colposcope with
  - 3× to 20× power
  - Green light filter
- Ring **forceps**—sterile
- Cotton balls—sterile

➤ 0.9% sodium chloride—sterile
➤ Cotton-tipped applicators—small and large—sterile
➤ White vinegar—5% acetic acid solution
➤ Containers with 10% **formalin**
➤ Cervical biopsy punch forceps—sterile
➤ Cervical brush or broom
➤ Monsel's solution

Procedure

COLPOSCOPY

➤ Have the client void immediately before the procedure.
➤ Position the client in the lithotomy position.
➤ Drape the perineum.
➤ Put on gloves.
➤ Insert the warmed speculum into the vagina and bring the cervix into view.
➤ Inspect the cervix with the naked eye.
➤ Wash the cervix and vagina gently with large cotton-tipped swab or cotton balls soaked in sterile saline.
➤ Remove mucus with ring forceps and cotton balls.
➤ Position the colposcope. Visualize the cervix and vaginal walls using the 5× setting.
➤ Switch to green filter light (enhances visibility of blood vessels) and visualize.
➤ Using cotton balls soaked in vinegar for 3 to 5 minutes, wash the cervix with warm vinegar.
  ➤ *Note*—Vinegar dissolves mucus, constricts blood vessels, and allows better visualization of the cervix.
  ➤ Reapply vinegar every 5 minutes to maintain acetowhiteness during the procedure.
➤ Systematically examine the cervix for the squamocolumnar junction, **transformation zone,** and abnormalities using
  ➤ Low power and white light
  ➤ Higher power and white light
  ➤ Lower power and green filter light
  ➤ Higher power and green filter light
➤ Document findings.

CERVICAL BIOPSY

➤ Biopsy areas that show (Fig. 39–2)
  ➤ Acetowhite after application of vinegar
    • Shiny white indicates a low-grade lesion.
    • Dull grayish white indicates a high-grade lesion.
  ➤ **Mosaicism**—abnormal chicken wire, cobblestone, or tile-floor pattern
  ➤ **Punctation**—abnormal stippled appearance
➤ To biopsy

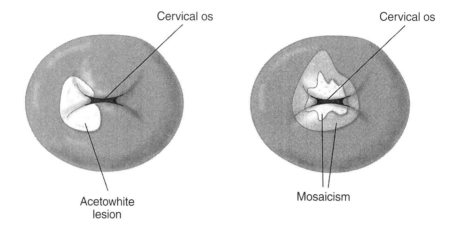

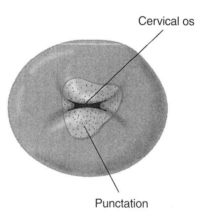

FIGURE 39 • 2 Abnormalities found on cervical biopsy that must be biopsied.

> Using the cervical biopsy punch forceps, start at the bottom of the cervix and work upward, taking 3-mm specimens (Fig. 39–3).
> Apply Monsel's solution to areas of bleeding.
> Put each specimen in a different specimen jar and label with location.

ENDOCERVICAL CURETTAGE

> After the cervical biopsies are completed, take a specimen from the endocervical canal.
> Insert the cervical brush or broom into the cervical os, and make a complete 360-degree turn.
> Remove and place scrapings into a container with 10% formalin and label.
> Remove the speculum.

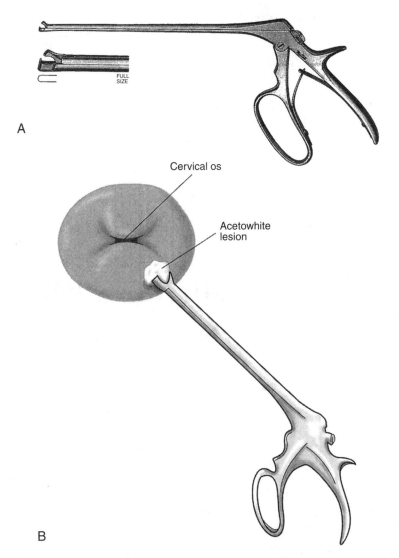

Cervical os

Acetowhite
lesion

A

B

FIGURE 39 • 3 *(A)* Cervical biopsy forceps. (Reproduced with permission from Miltex Instrument Company, Inc.) *(B)* The forceps are used to biopsy all abnormal cervical lesions.

➤ After examination of the cervix, apply vinegar to the vagina and external genitalia. Take biopsy specimens as necessary, when acetowhiteness appears.

Client Instructions

➤ You may have dark or black vaginal discharge for 2 days after the procedure.

➤ Observe for and report the following
  ➢ Heavy vaginal bleeding (greater than one sanitary pad change per hour)
  ➢ Low abdominal pain
  ➢ Fever, chills, or foul-smelling vaginal odor
➤ Do *not* use tampons for at least 1 week.
➤ Do *not* have sexual intercourse for 1 week.
➤ Do *not* douche for 3 weeks.

BIBLIOGRAPHY

Colodny, C.S. (1995). Procedures for your practice: colposcopy and cervical biopsy. *Patient Care,* June 15, 66–71.

Frisch, L.E., et al (1994). Naked-eye inspection of the cervix after acetic acid application may improve the predictive value of negative cytologic screening. *J Fam Pract,* 39(5), 457–460.

Johnson, B.A. (1996). The colposcopic examination. *Am Fam Physician,* 53(8), 2473–2482.

40 ENDOMETRIAL BIOPSY

MARGARET R. COLYAR

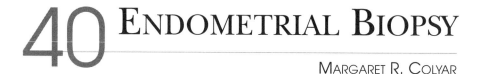

CPT Code
58100   Endometrial sampling

Endometrial **biopsy** is a procedure used to obtain cells directly from the lining of the uterus to evaluate dysfunctional uterine bleeding. If endometrial cancer is suspected, refer for diagnostic curettage.

OVERVIEW
➤ Incidence unknown

RATIONALE
➤ To diagnose
  ➢ Cancer
    • Take the specimen any time.
  ➢ Infertility (to determine corpus luteum function)
    • Take the specimen during the last half of the menstrual cycle (days 21 or 22).
  ➢ Menstrual disturbances (especially anovulatory bleeding)
    • Take the specimen immediately before menstruation. Get index of progesterone influence and ovulation.

INDICATIONS

➤ Suspicion of endometrial cancer
➤ Infertility
➤ Amenorrhea

CONTRAINDICATIONS

➤ Pregnancy

PROCEDURE

Endometrial Biopsy

Equipment

➤ Antiseptic skin cleanser
➤ Drape—sterile
➤ Light source
➤ Endometrial suction **curette** (Fig. 40–1)
➤ Vaginal **speculum**
➤ Water-soluble lubricant—K-Y jelly
➤ Gloves—sterile
➤ Ring **forceps** or **tenaculum**
➤ 4 × 4 gauze—sterile
➤ Container with 10% **formalin**

Procedure

➤ Have the client void immediately before the examination.
➤ In women of childbearing age, perform a urine pregnancy test.
➤ Place the client in the lithotomy position.
➤ Cleanse the perineum.
➤ Drape the perineum.
➤ Lubricate the vaginal speculum.

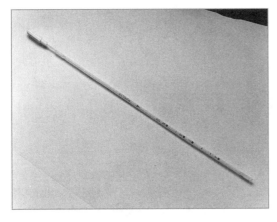

FIGURE 40 • 1 Pipelle endometrial suction curette. (Courtesy of Unimar Incorporated, Wilton, CT. Reproduced with permission.)

➤ Put on gloves.
➤ Insert the speculum into the vagina, and lock in place with the cervix and os in view.
➤ Using ring forceps or the tenaculum, cleanse the vagina and cervix with sterile gauze.
➤ Insert the endometrial suction curette into the cervical os 3 to 4 inches (7 to 10 cm) (Fig. 40–2).
➤ If entry is difficult, use the tenaculum to pull the bottom of the os gently down to increase the opening size (Fig. 40–3). The cervix has little nervous innervation up to the transformation zone. The client should feel no pain if you are careful not to grasp the os into the transformation zone.
➤ Pull back on the inner cannula of the suction curette to aspirate cells from the uterine lining.
➤ Withdraw the entire curette.
➤ Expel the specimen from the curette into the container with formalin.
➤ Label and send the specimen to the laboratory.

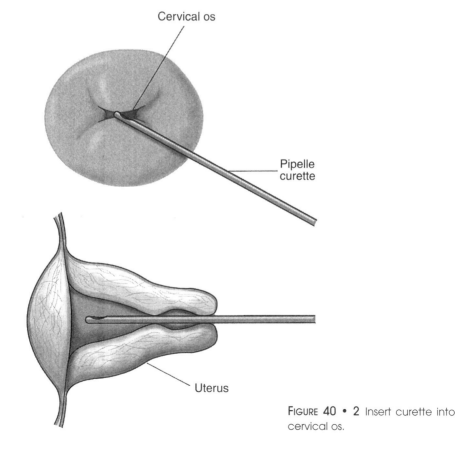

Cervical os

Pipelle curette

Uterus

FIGURE 40 • 2 Insert curette into cervical os.

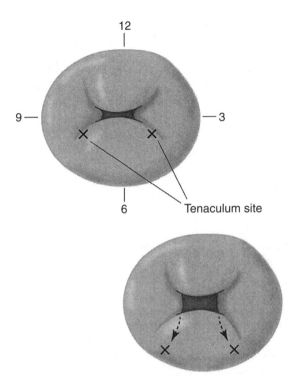

12

9

3

6   Tenaculum site

FIGURE 40 • 3 Pull the os down to increase the opening.

Client Instructions

➤ You may experience some cramping and bleeding after the procedure. If this occurs, take 400 to 600 mg of ibuprofen every 6 hours as needed.
➤ Observe for signs and symptoms of infection, such as
  ➤ Increase in pain after 24 hours
  ➤ Increase in temperature
  ➤ Foul odor
➤ If any signs or symptoms of infection are found, return to the office.

BIBLIOGRAPHY

Guido, R.S., et al (1995). Pipelle endometrial sampling: sensitivity in the detection of endometrial cancer. *J Reprod Med,* 40(8), 553–555.

Ignatavicius, D.D., et al (1995). *Medical-surgical nursing: a nursing process approach.* Philadelphia: Saunders.

Youssif, S.N., and McMellan, D.L. (1995). Outpatient endometrial biopsy: the pipelle. *Br J Hosp Med,* 54(23), 198–201.

SPECIMEN COLLECTION
GRAM'S STAIN, WET MOUNT (SALINE AND KOH)

41

MARGARET R. COLYAR

CPT Code	
87205	Gram's stain
87210	Wet smear
87220	KOH prep

Gram's stain technique is a procedure used to differentiate gram-positive and gram-negative organisms. The technique was named after Christian Gram, who developed it in 1884. Knowing if an organism is gram-positive or gram-negative helps the nurse practitioner determine the etiology of the infection.

The wet mount (wet prep, wet smear) is a tool used to evaluate the etiology of abnormal vaginal secretions. Saline and 10% potassium hydroxide (KOH) preparations are used. With the saline preparation, white blood cells, bacteria, trichomonads, and clue cells can be detected. With the 10% KOH preparation, hyphae and buds can be detected.

OVERVIEW

➤ Incidence is unknown.
➤ Potentially reportable vaginal infections include gonorrhea, syphilis, *Chlamydia trachomatis,* herpes genitalis, **condyloma acuminatum,** pelvic inflammatory disease, and nonspecific urethritis (male). Check the regulations for reporting sexually transmitted diseases in the state in which you practice.

HEALTH PROMOTION/PREVENTION

➤ To prevent vaginal, uterine, tubal, and ovarian infections, the use of condoms during intercourse is suggested.

RATIONALE

➤ To aid in assessment of all suspected vaginal infections.
➤ To assist in determination of disease etiology.

220

INDICATIONS

➤ Unusual foul-smelling vaginal discharge
➤ Lower abdominal pain
➤ Vaginal itching
➤ Dysuria

CONTRAINDICATIONS

➤ Recent douching
➤ Menses
➤ Intravaginal medications

PROCEDURE

Wet Smear (Saline and KOH)

Equipment

➤ Vaginal **speculum**—small, medium, or large
➤ Drape—nonsterile
➤ Two pairs of gloves—nonsterile
➤ Test tube with 1 mL 0.9% sodium chloride
➤ Cotton-tipped applicators—sterile
➤ 0.9% sodium chloride
➤ 10% KOH solution—two drops
➤ Two microscope slides
➤ Two coverslips
➤ Microscope

Procedure

➤ Place the client in the lithotomy position and drape.
➤ Insert the vaginal speculum and observe the vaginal wall and cervix for inflammation and/or infections, cysts, lesions, and bleeding.
➤ Using cotton-tipped applicators, collect specimen of vaginal secretions.
➤ Place one cotton-tipped applicator in the test tube with 1 mL 0.9% sodium chloride and mix well.
➤ Remove the speculum.
➤ With the cotton-tipped applicator, place a smear on each slide (Fig. 41–1).
  ➤ On one slide, add one or two drops of saline and cover with the coverslip.
  ➤ On the second slide, add one or two drops of 10% KOH and cover with the coverslip.
    • Gently heat the KOH slide for 2 to 3 seconds.
    • Allow the KOH slide to sit for 15 to 20 minutes at room temperature.
➤ Place the saline slide (Fig. 41–2) on the microscope at 10× (low power) and focus. Change to 40× (high power) and focus. Look for the following in five different fields

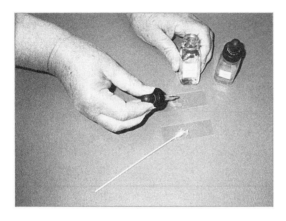

FIGURE 41 • 1 Slide preparation. Saline on one slide and KOH on the other.

➤ White blood cells
➤ Trichomonads
➤ Clue cells (large epithelial cells with indistinct borders with multiple cocci clinging to them)
  • Clue cells often are described as appearing like "pepper on a fried egg"; they indicate bacterial vaginosis.
➤ Place the KOH slide (Fig. 41–3) on the microscope at 10× and 40×. Look for the following in five different fields
  ➤ Hyphae
  ➤ Spores (buds, candidiasis)

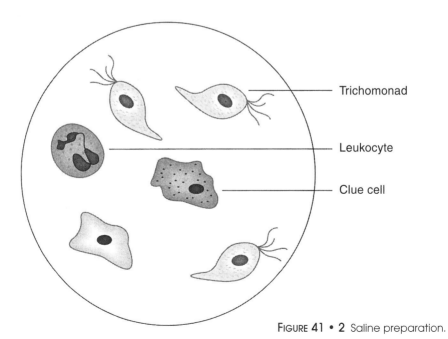

FIGURE 41 • 2 Saline preparation.

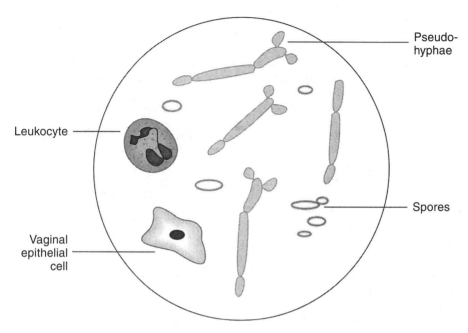

Pseudo-hyphae

Leukocyte

Spores

Vaginal epithelial cell

FIGURE 41 • 3 KOH preparation.

Client Instructions

➤ Based on the results of your vaginal smears, you have _____.
➤ You will need to take _____ for _____ days.
➤ Return to the office 1 week after you finish your medications for recheck or sooner if your symptoms worsen.

Gram's Stain

Equipment

➤ Vaginal speculum
➤ Drape—nonsterile
➤ Cotton-tipped applicators—sterile
➤ One microscope slide
➤ Gram's stain kit
➤ Microscope
➤ Gloves—nonsterile

Procedure

➤ Place client in lithotomy position and drape.
➤ Insert vaginal speculum, and observe vaginal wall and cervix (see Chapter 42).
➤ Using cotton-tipped applicators, collect specimen of vaginal secretions.
➤ Remove speculum.

➤ With cotton-tipped applicator, place drop of secretions on the slide, and follow the directions in the Gram's stain kit.
  ➤ Let specimen air dry.
  ➤ Apply solutions from the Gram's stain kit in the following manner
    • Stain with crystal violet and Gram's iodine solution.
      • All bacteria become blue-purple.
    • Rinse with a decolorizer (usually a 95% alcohol or alcohol-acetone mixture).
      • Gram-negative bacteria become transparent and lose their color.
      • Gram-positive bacteria retain the blue-purple color.
    • Apply safranin (a red dye) to the slide.
      • Gram-negative bacteria become red.
        • Gonorrhea bacteria are gram-negative.
      • Gram-positive bacteria remain blue-purple.

Client Instructions

➤ Based on the results of your vaginal smears, you have _____ .
➤ You will need to take _____ for _____ days.
➤ Return to the office 1 week after you finish your medications for recheck, or sooner if your symptoms worsen.

BIBLIOGRAPHY
Ferris, D.G., et al (1995). Office laboratory diagnosis of vaginitis. *J Fam Pract* 41(6), 575–581.

SPECIMEN COLLECTION
PAPANICOLAOU (PAP) SMEAR

42

MARGARET R. COLYAR

CPT Code

88150   Pap smear interpretation

Not used by the clinician; used by the pathologist who interprets the specimen

---

The **Pap smear** is a tool for screening of cervical cancer. Appropriate smear collection is paramount to detection of cancer cells. In addition, if a lesion is seen or palpated, other tests, such as ultrasound examination of the pelvis or **colposcopy,** should be performed in conjunction with the Pap smear.

OVERVIEW

➤ Incidence is unknown.
➤ Adequacy of the specimen is shown by the presence of
  ➢ Endocervical cells
  ➢ Squamous metaplasia (found in the **transformation zone**) (Fig. 42–1)
    • The transformation zone is found inside the cervical os; this is an area of replacement of endocervical columnar cells by squamous cells and varies with age. In perimenopausal women, the transformation zone is found high in the endocervical canal (Fig. 42–2).
➤ The nurse practitioner should be familiar with the classification of cervical smears
  ➢ Class I—Normal smear, no abnormal cells
  ➢ Class II—Atypical cells; no neoplasia
  ➢ Class III—Smear contains abnormal cells consistent with dysplasia
  ➢ Class IV—Smear contains abnormal cells consistent with carcinoma in situ
  ➢ Class V—Smear contains abnormal cells consistent with carcinoma of squamous origin

HEALTH PROMOTION/PREVENTION

➤ To detect cervical cancer, a yearly Pap smear is recommended.

RATIONALE

➤ To detect cervical carcinoma
➤ To detect early cervical dysplasia related to infection with HPV

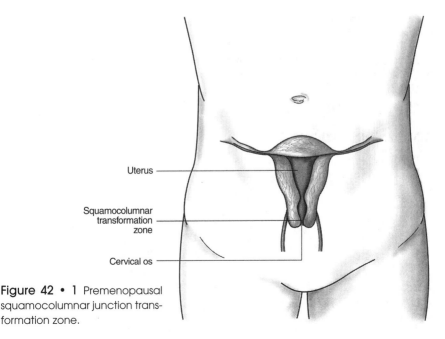

Uterus

Squamocolumnar transformation zone

Cervical os

Figure 42 • 1 Premenopausal squamocolumnar junction transformation zone.

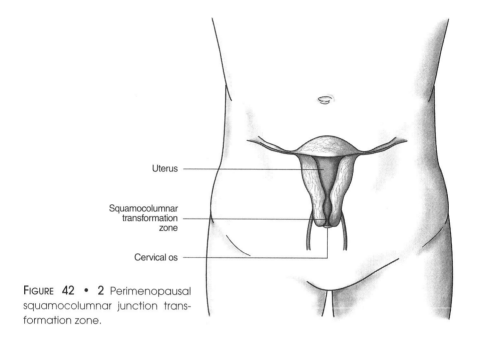

Uterus

Squamocolumnar
transformation
zone

Cervical os

FIGURE 42 • 2 Perimenopausal
squamocolumnar junction transformation zone.

INDICATIONS

➤ Abnormal vaginal bleeding or discharge
➤ Lower abdominal pain
➤ Yearly screening
➤ Visible or palpable cervical lesions
➤ Report of cervical dysplasia or malignancy on previous Pap smear
➤ DES-exposed female—REFER to gynecologist for treatment
➤ History of sexually transmitted disease
➤ History of multiple sexual partners

CONTRAINDICATIONS

➤ Pelvic inflammatory disease
➤ Active vaginitis
➤ Active cervicitis

PROCEDURE

Pap Smear

Equipment

➤ Vaginal speculum—small, medium, or large
➤ Drape—nonsterile
➤ Gloves—nonsterile

➤ Light source
➤ Pap smear kit with (usually provided by the reference laboratory)
  ➤ Wooden paddle and cotton-tipped applicator
  ➤ Optional—cytobrush (decreases the chance of a false-negative result)
  ➤ Cervical broom (Fig. 42–3)
  ➤ Microscope slides
  ➤ Fixative
➤ Water-soluble lubricant—K-Y jelly
➤ Large cotton-tipped swabs

Procedure

➤ Place the client in the lithotomy position and drape.
➤ Put on gloves.
➤ Examine the vulva and Bartholin's and Skene's glands.
➤ Warm the speculum with water or lubricate with water-soluble lubricant.
➤ Ask the client to relax and breath deeply (this may help the client to relax).
➤ Insert the speculum at a slight diagonal angle and rotate to a horizontal angle as inserting. Direct the speculum in a downward posterior direction, applying gentle pressure (Fig. 42–4).
➤ Open the speculum and adjust the position until the cervix is easily visible.
➤ Observe the cervix and vaginal wall for inflammation and/or infection, cysts, lesions, or bleeding.

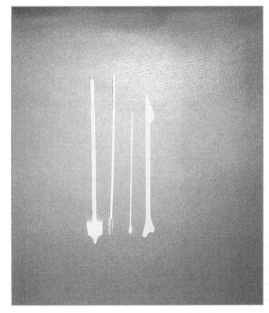

FIGURE 42 • 3 Four types of specimen collection tools. From *left to right:* cervical broom, cytobrush, cotton-tipped applicator, and wooden paddle.

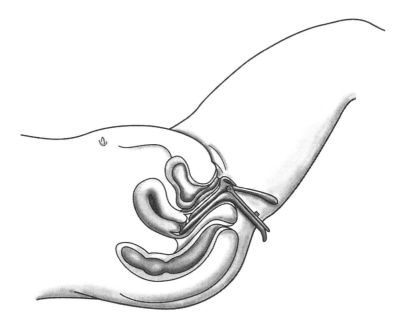

FIGURE 42 • 4 Direct the vaginal speculum in a downward posterior direction.

➤ If necessary, absorb discharge or blood with large cotton-tipped swab.
➤ Collect the specimen using the following procedure
  ➤ Insert the wooden paddle into the cervix and rotate 360 degrees.
  ➤ Place the smear on the slide indicated in the Pap smear kit (Fig. 42–5).

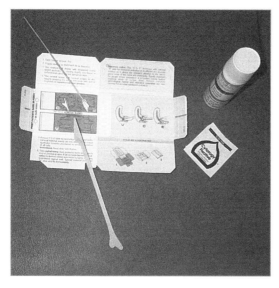

FIGURE 42 • 5 Pap smear kit.

> Insert other end of the wooden paddle and brush the ectocervix and vaginal wall.
> Apply this specimen to the slide indicated in the Pap smear kit.
> Next, insert the cytobrush, broom, or cotton-tipped applicator in the cervical os and rotate 360 degrees.
> Apply this specimen to the slide indicated in the Pap smear kit.
> Apply fixative provided to the slides.
> Label and send to reference laboratory.

> *Hint*—With postmenopausal and obese clients, the vaginal walls may prolapse into the open speculum, occluding your view of the cervix. To prevent this complication, a special splint (Fig. 42–6) using a glove and the speculum can be used. You can make this splint by
>> Inserting the speculum into the finger of a nonsterile glove
>> Removing the excess glove
>> Cutting off the fingertip
> The glove provides a splintlike effect when the speculum is opened in the vagina.

Client Instructions

> There may be minor bleeding after the examination. This is normal.
> If your Pap smear is class II through V, further testing is necessary.
> The nurse from the office will call you in 5 to 10 days with the results of your Pap smear.

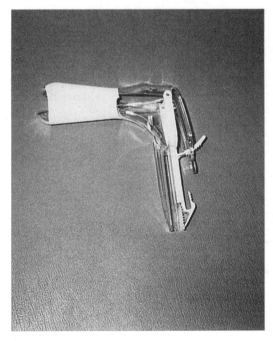

FIGURE 42 • 6 Speculum splint.

BIBLIOGRAPHY

Difco Laboratories (1994). *Gram stain sets and reagents.* Detroit: Author.

Helderman, G., et al (1990). Comparing two sampling techniques of endocervical cell recovery on Papanicolaou smears. *Nurse Practitioner,* 15(11), 30–32.

Lieu, D. (1996). The Papanicolaou smear: its value and limitations. *J Fam Pract,* 42(4), 391–399.

BARTHOLIN CYST ABSCESS

INCISION AND DRAINAGE

43

MARGARET R. COLYAR

CPT Code	
56420	Incision and drainage of Bartholin's gland abscess
56740	Excision of Bartholin's gland or cyst

Bartholinitis is inflammation of one or both of the Bartholin's glands at the opening of the vagina (Fig. 43–1). Obstruction of the main duct of these glands causes retention of secretions and dilation of the gland. Incision and drainage of abscessed Bartholin's glands is needed if the gland is swollen and painful. A culture of the abscess material should be taken to determine the etiology of the abscess and to provide treatment guidance.

OVERVIEW

➤ Approximately 2% of adult women develop an abscess of the Bartholin's glands.
➤ Recurrence rate is high.
➤ Most common causes are
  ➢ **Inspissated** mucus
  ➢ Congenital narrowing of the gland
  ➢ *Neisseria gonorrhoeae*
  ➢ *Staphylococcus*
  ➢ *Streptococcus*
  ➢ *Escherichia coli*
  ➢ *Trichomonas*
  ➢ *Bacteroides*

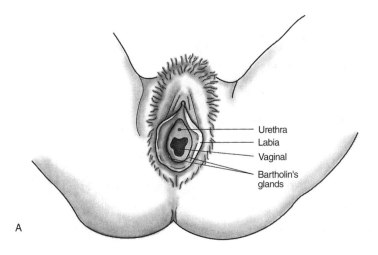

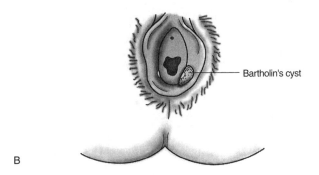

Figure 43 • 1 *(A)* Bartholin's glands are on either side of the vaginal orifice. *(B)* A Bartholin's cyst occurs when the gland becomes inflamed or infected.

➤ Symptoms of bartholinitis include
  ➤ Swelling of the labia
  ➤ Tenderness/pain in the labia when walking and/or sitting
  ➤ Enlarged inguinal nodes
  ➤ **Dyspareunia**
  ➤ Palpable mass
➤ Prevention includes
  ➤ Protected sexual intercourse
  ➤ Meticulous cleansing of the perineum

RATIONALE

➤ To relieve pain
➤ To determine the etiology and provide treatment guidance

INDICATIONS

➤ Infected Bartholin's glands

CONTRAINDICATIONS

➤ Pregnancy—REFER to a gynecologist

☑ *Informed consent required*

PROCEDURE

Bartholin's Cyst Abscess—Incision and Drainage

Equipment

➤ Antiseptic skin cleanser
➤ Drape—sterile
➤ Gloves—sterile
➤ 1% lidocaine—5 to 10 mL
➤ Two syringes—10 and 20 mL
➤ Two needles—18- and 25-gauge,$^1/_2$-inch needle
➤ 0.9% sodium chloride—250 mL
➤ No. 11 scalpel
➤ 4 × 4 gauze—sterile
➤ Iodoform gauze—$^1/_4$ or $^1/_2$ inch wide
➤ Scissors—sterile
➤ Curved **hemostats**—sterile
➤ Pickups—sterile
➤ Vaginal culture swab
➤ Peri pads—nonsterile

Procedure

➤ Instruct the client to empty her bladder.
➤ Position the client in the lithotomy position.
➤ Cleanse perineum with antiseptic skin cleanser.
➤ Open gauze, scalpel, needle, and syringes onto a sterile field.
➤ Put on gloves.
➤ Inject 5 to 10 mL of 1% lidocaine along the top of the abscessed Bartholin's gland using the 10-mL syringe with the 25-gauge needle.
➤ Incise the cyst along the top. Make the incision deep enough and long enough to allow drainage.
  ➤ A longer incision is considered better than a smaller incision.
➤ Culture the drainage.
➤ Insert a gloved finger into the vaginal orifice, and apply gentle pressure toward the abscess to express the exudate.
➤ After all exudate is expressed, inspect the wound with curved hemostats and break up any **loculations** (small cavities).
➤ Irrigate with 0.9% sodium chloride using the 20-mL syringe with the 18-gauge needle.

➤ Insert iodoform gauze into the wound, leaving approximately $^1/_2$ inch protruding from the wound.
➤ Cover with 4 × 4 gauze sponges and apply a peri pad.

Client Instructions

➤ To prevent further infection, the following antibiotic has been ordered: (doxycycline, erythromycin, or a cephalosporin)_____.
➤ Remove half of the gauze in 24 hours. Remove the remaining gauze in 48 hours.
➤ Change the 4 × 4 sponges and peri pad every 4 to 6 hours.
➤ Soak in a basin or tub of warm water four times per day for 1 week.
➤ Return to the office in 1 week for recheck, or sooner if your symptoms worsen.

BIBLIOGRAPHY

Apgar, B.S. (1994). Bartholin's cyst/abscess: word catheter insertion. In Pfenninger, J.L., and Fowler, G.C. (eds.). *Procedures for primary care physicians.* St. Louis: Mosby.

Rakel, R.E. (1997). *Conn's current therapy.* Philadelphia: Saunders.

Wolcott, M.W. (ed.) (1974). *Ferguson's surgery of the ambulatory patient.* Philadelphia: J.B. Lippincott.

Youngkin, E.Q., and Davis, M.S. (1994). *Women's health: a primary care clinical guide.* Norwalk, CT: Appleton & Lange.

CERVICAL CAP FITTING, INSERTION, AND REMOVAL

44

ANGELA DENERIS • JANE M. DYER

CPT Code
57170   Diaphragm/cervical cap fitting with instructions

A cervical cap is a helmet-shaped, rubber device that fits over the cervix. Some cervical caps have a removal strap. When used with spermicide, the cervical cap acts as a physical and chemical barrier to sperm. Cervical caps come in several sizes and must be fitted by a professional. It is a nonsystemic, nonhormonal, and reversible method of contraception.

OVERVIEW

➤ Incidence of use unknown
➤ Prevention of pregnancy—sources differ
  • Among nulliparous women, cervical caps are 80% to 91% effective; 9% to 20% become pregnant within the first year.
➤ Among parous women, cervical caps are 60% to 74% effective; 26% to 40% become pregnant within the first year.

Potential Complications

➤ Pregnancy
➤ Conversion from normal to abnormal cervical cytology
➤ Urinary tract infections
➤ Cervical or vaginal lesions with prolonged use
➤ Toxic shock syndrome
➤ Allergy to latex rubber or spermicide
➤ Sexually transmitted disease transmission

Assess

➤ Comfort with and ability (woman/partner) to insert, check placement, and remove cap
➤ Ability to understand instructions for proper use
➤ Length of cervix—a long or short cervix can compromise fit of cap
➤ Willingness to return after pregnancy or weight change of more than 10 lb

Types of Cervical Caps

➤ Latex helmet shaped with a groove inside of cap (Prentif)
➤ Latex helmet shaped with a wide rim and flatter dome (Vimule Lamberts)
➤ Latex dome without distinct rim (Dumas Lamberts)
➤ Silicone rubber, single use (Oves Veos)
➤ Silicone rubber with a brim, a dome, a groove between the dome and brim, and a removal strap (Femcap)

RATIONALE

➤ To provide a reliable, nonhormonal, nonsystemic, and reversible form of contraception

INDICATIONS

➤ Contraception
➤ Patient choice
➤ Contraindications to other methods of contraception

CONTRAINDICATIONS

➤ History of toxic shock syndrome
➤ Allergy to latex, rubber, or spermicide
➤ Suspected or known cervical or uterine malignancy
➤ Unusually long or short cervix
➤ Extensive cervical scarring or lacerations
➤ Unresolved abnormal Pap smear
➤ Inability to learn proper use

☑ *Informed consent required*

PROCEDURE
Cervical Cap Fitting, Insertion, and Removal

Equipment

➤ Cervical cap (Table 44–1)
  ➤ The clinician must order a set of cervical caps to use in the office for fitting the client. The caps are available in various internal rim diameter sizes. Sources include
    • Prentif Cap (latex)—Lamberts (Dalston) Ltd, Luton, England. The U.S. distributor is Cervical Cap Ltd, PO Box 38003-292, Los Gatos, CA 95031
    • Oves Veos (silicon rubber)—www.veos.france.com
    • Femcap (silicon rubber)—www.femcap.com
➤ Speculum
➤ Water-soluble lubricant—K-Y jelly
➤ Gloves—nonsterile

Procedure

CERVICAL CAP FITTING AND INSERTION

➤ Have client empty her bladder before fitting and insertion.
➤ Position the client in the lithotomy position.

TABLE 44•1 DIFFERENCES IN CERVICAL CAPS

TYPES	ADVANTAGES
Latex	
Prentif	Most often used
Vimule	Flatter and wider cap
Dumas	Specialized cap
Silicon Rubber	
Oves Veos	Light weight; single use only
Femcap	Reusable

➤ With a gloved hand, perform a bimanual examination to evaluate the size and position of the uterus and cervix.
➤ Apply K-Y jelly to a speculum.
➤ Insert the speculum to visualize the cervix to estimate the cap size, and note any scarring, lacerations, and length of the cervix. The cervix must be symmetrical, be long enough to apply the cap, and have a proper seal.
➤ Fold the rim of the cap and compress the cap dome to insert it into the vagina, and place it over the cervix. Unfolding the dome creates suction between the rim of the cap and the cervix.
➤ After applying the cap to the cervix, run a finger around the entire rim to check for gaps. Note the stability of the cap by determining how easily it is displaced with your finger. There should not be any gaps, and the cap must cover the cervix completely and fit snugly, but not tightly.
➤ After 1 to 2 minutes, check again for fit and suction. Try to rotate the cap, it should rotate with slight resistance and not come off the cervix.
➤ Try at least one other cap size, either smaller or larger, to determine which one fits best.
➤ Have the client feel the cap in place and give instructions for use.
➤ Provide a written prescription for the patient to fill at a pharmacy that carries cervical caps.

Cervical Cap Removal

➤ To remove the cap, insert one finger between the rim of the cap and the cervix to break the suction, then gently pull the cap down and out. If using a Femcap, remove with the removal strap.
➤ Have the client practice putting the cap on and off in the office.

Client Instructions

➤ Check cap for holes, tears, and cracks by holding the cervical cap up to a light.
➤ Apply a teaspoon of spermicidal cream to the dome of the cap before inserting.
➤ Empty bladder before insertion.
➤ Insert the cap in a squatting position.
➤ Do not remove the cap for at least 8 hours after last coitus.
➤ To reduce risk of toxic shock syndrome, the cap must be removed within 48 hours after use.
➤ To remove, push the rim away from the cervix to break the suction and pull the cap out.
➤ Use of additional spermicide with repeated intercourse is optional. Do not remove cap. Use a plastic introducer to insert fresh spermicide.
➤ Do not use during vaginal bleeding.
➤ After removal, clean the diaphragm with soapy water, rinse thoroughly in plain water, and air dry. Do not use powders, oils, or petroleum jelly (Vaseline) with the cap.
➤ Check fit yearly with annual examination and refit if client has had a pregnancy or gained or lost more than 10 lb.

B IBLIOGRAPHY
Hatcher, R., et al (1998) (17th ed.). *Contraceptive technology.* New York: Ardent Media.
(2002). http://www.cervcap.com/faqs.htm Cervical Cap LTD.
(2002). http://www.femcap.com/advantag.htm The Fem Cap.

45
CERVICAL LESIONS
CRYOTHERAPY

MARGARET R. COLYAR

CPT Code
57511   Cryocautery of cervix, initial or repeat

Cryotherapy is a technique in which the outermost layer of cervical cells is frozen. The **transformation zone** is destroyed. If the lesion is confined to the exocervix, cryotherapy is appropriate.

OVERVIEW

➤ Incidence is unknown.
➤ Depth of tissue destruction is 3 to 4 mm.
➤ Cryosurgery is not recommended if
  ➤ It is 5 to 7 days before menses.
    • Edema of cervical tissue may occur.
  ➤ The lesion cannot be entirely visualized.
    • You will be unable to cover with the cryoprobe.
  ➤ There is greater than grade II cervical dysplasia.
    • You will be unable to remove appropriate depth of tissue.
  ➤ The patient is immunocompromised or on high-dose steroids.
    • She may develop secondary infection.

OPTIONS

➤ Freeze options based on personal preference
  ➤ *Method 1*—freeze, thaw, freeze
  ➤ *Method 2*—freeze, thaw

RATIONALE

➤ To diminish pain
  ➤ To prevent further tissue destruction
  ➤ To prevent spread of the lesion

INDICATIONS

➤ Cervical dysplasia—grade I or II—if lesion can be covered by the cryoprobe
➤ Precancerous cervical lesions
➤ Carcinoma in situ

CONTRAINDICATIONS

➤ Pregnancy
➤ Cervical cancer
➤ Cervical dysplasia—greater than grade II
➤ Positive endocervical curettage
➤ Entire lesion cannot be seen
➤ Positive for sexually transmitted disease
➤ 5 to 7 days before menses
➤ Immunocompromised
➤ On high-dose steroids

☑ *Informed consent required*

PROCEDURE

Cervical Lesions—Cryotherapy

Equipment

➤ Methods 1 and 2
  ➤ Nitrous oxide cryoprobe unit
  ➤ Cryoprobes—flat or cone
  ➤ Water-soluble lubricant (K-Y jelly, Cryogel, lidocaine jelly)
  ➤ Drape—nonsterile
  ➤ Cotton-tipped applicators
  ➤ Vaginal **speculum** with retraction device (see Chapter 42)
  ➤ Light source
  ➤ Gloves—nonsterile
  ➤ Nonsteroidal anti-inflammatory drug

Procedure

METHOD 1—FREEZE, THAW, FREEZE

➤ Have the client take a dose of nonsteroidal anti-inflammatory drug 0.5 to 1 hour before the procedure.
➤ Position the client in the lithotomy position.
➤ Drape the client.
➤ Put on gloves.
➤ Select the appropriate cryoprobe (Fig. 45–1).
  ➤ Must cover the entire lesion
  ➤ Must be flat or slightly conical
➤ Apply a water-soluble lubricant to the cryoprobe tip.

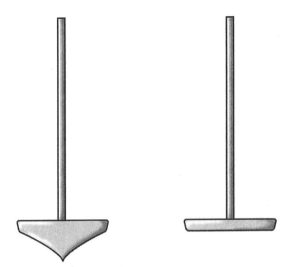

FIGURE 45 • 1 Cryoprobes.

➤ Activate the nitrous oxide unit according to the manufacturer's directions.
➤ Insert the vaginal speculum in the vaginal vault.
➤ Position the probe over the area to be treated and start the freeze (Fig. 45–2).
  ➤ Be sure the probe does not touch the vaginal wall (very sensitive).
  ➤ Freeze for 3 minutes or until 5-mm ice ball is beyond the lesion.

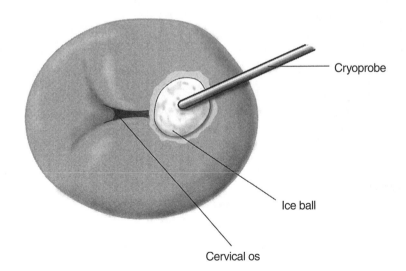

FIGURE 45 • 2 Cervical lesions. Freeze for 3 minutes or until a 5-mm ice ball surrounds the lesion. Thaw for 5 minutes, then refreeze.

➤ Thaw—wait 5 minutes.
➤ Refreeze for 3 minutes or until 5-mm ice ball is beyond the lesion.

METHOD 2—FREEZE, THAW

➤ Have the client take a dose of a nonsteroidal anti-inflammatory drug 0.5 to 1 hour before the procedure.
➤ Position the client in the lithotomy position.
➤ Drape the client.
➤ Put on gloves.
➤ Select the appropriate cryoprobe.
  ➤ Must cover the entire lesion
  ➤ Must be flat or slightly conical
➤ Apply a water-soluble lubricant to the cryoprobe tip.
➤ Activate the nitrous oxide unit according to the manufacturer's directions.
➤ Insert the vaginal speculum in the vaginal vault.
➤ Position the probe over the area to be treated and start the freeze.
  ➤ Be sure the probe does not touch the vaginal wall (very sensitive).
  ➤ Freeze for 5 minutes.
  ➤ Thaw.

Client Instructions

➤ You may expect some mild cramping and watery, foul-smelling discharge for 3 weeks.
➤ Take acetaminophen or ibuprofen as directed for abdominal cramping.
➤ Do not put anything inside the vagina for 3 weeks, such as
  ➤ Tampons
  ➤ Douching solutions
➤ Do not engage in vaginal intercourse for 3 weeks.
➤ You will need a follow-up Pap smear in 6 months. Your next appointment is _____.

BIBLIOGRAPHY
DeCherney, A.H., and Pernoll, M.L. (1994). Current obstetric and gynecologic diagnosis and treatment. Norwalk, Conn.: Appleton & Lange.
E.A. Conway Charity Hospital (1996). *Outpatient information—cryotherapy of the cervix.* Patient instruction sheet. Monroe, LA: Author.
Pfenninger, J.L., and Fowler, G.C. (1995). *Procedures for primary care physicians.* St. Louis: Mosby.
Youngkin, E.Q., and Davis, M.S. (1994). *Women's health: a primary care clinical guide.* Norwalk, CT: Appleton & Lange.

46

CIRCUMCISION AND DORSAL PENILE NERVE BLOCK

MARGARET R. COLYAR

CPT Code

54150   Circumcision (clamp); newborn
54152   Circumcision (clamp); child
54160   Circumcision, other (Plastibell); newborn
54161   Circumcision, other (Plastibell); child

Circumcision is a surgical procedure in which the prepuce of the penis is excised. It may be performed on newborns, boys, and men. Uncircumcised boys and men may require the procedure in treatment of phimosis and balanitis. For newborns, the American Academy of Pediatrics does not recommend circumcision as a routine procedure based on research published in the last 10 years concerning urinary tract infections, penile cancer, sexually transmitted diseases, analgesia, and complications of circumcision. They do note that parents should be allowed to make an informed choice taking into account cultural, religious, and ethnic traditions.

The three methods most often used to circumcise the penis of the newborn are Gomco clamp, Plastibell, and Mogen clamp techniques. There is no significant advantage of one device over the other. The Plastibell causes necrosis of the remaining foreskin by strangulation. The Gomco and Mogen clamps produce crushing of the nerve endings and blood vessels to promote hemostasis, while protecting the glans. The Gomco clamp and Plastibell techniques are outlined here. The Mogen clamp is not widely used, and it is not included in this chapter. The newborn to be circumcised should be at least 1 hour postprandial due to regurgitation and have had one documented void. Research has indicated that neonates who receive dorsal penile nerve block (DPNB) or local anesthesia cry less, have less tachycardia, are less irritable, and have fewer behavioral changes in the 24 hours after the circumcision procedure. Circumcision of the older child and man also is included.

INDICATIONS

➤ Cultural, religious, and ethnic traditions
➤ Phimosis

➤ Balanitis
➤ Condyloma
➤ Redundant foreskin

CONTRAINDICATIONS (CIRCUMCISION AND DPNB)

➤ Hypospadius
➤ Unusual-appearing genitalia (chordae, hypospadius, epispadius)
➤ Ambiguous genitalia, severe illness
➤ Less than 12 hours old
➤ Prematurity

☑ *Informed consent required*

PROCEDURE
Dorsal Penile Nerve Block

See Figure 46–1.

Equipment

➤ Restrainer board with padding
➤ 1% lidocaine without epinephrine
➤ 1-mL tuberculin syringe
➤ 27-gauge needle, 1 inch
➤ Gloves—nonsterile
➤ Alcohol

Procedure

➤ Restrain child.
➤ Inspect genitalia.
➤ Cleanse with antiseptic solution.
➤ Insert needle at 2:00 position 0.3 to 0.5 cm at base of penis beneath the skin surface.
➤ Aspirate. If no blood return, inject 0.2 to 0.4 mL of lidocaine without epinephrine.
➤ Repeat at 10:00 position.

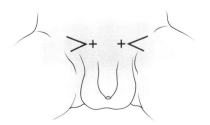

FIGURE 46 • 1 Dorsal penile nerve block injection sites. (From Colyar, M.R. (2003). *Well-child assessment for primary care providers.* Philadelphia: F.A. Davis.)

➤ Wait 4 minutes.
➤ Proceed with circumcision.

Circumcision—Three Methods

➤ Newborn—Gomco clamp
➤ Newborn—Plastibell
➤ Older boy and men
  ➤ Forceps-guided freehand method

Equipment

➤ Gomco clamp and Plastibell methods
  ➤ Restrainer board with padding
  ➤ Gloves—sterile
  ➤ Fenestrated drape
  ➤ Povidone-iodine (Betadine)
  ➤ Gauze pads
  ➤ Hemostats (2 curved/1 straight)
  ➤ Scissors
  ➤ Gomco clamp or Plastibell
  ➤ No. 11 scalpel
  ➤ Vaseline

Procedure

GOMCO CLAMP METHOD

See Figure 46–2.
➤ Restrain child.
➤ Inspect genitalia.
➤ Cleanse with antiseptic solution.
➤ Grasp foreskin with two hemostats at 10:00 and 2:00 position.
➤ Gently probe and lyse adhesions underneath the foreskin with a curved hemostat.
  ➤ Do not extend beyond the corona.
➤ Place the straight hemostat approximately two thirds of the distance from the foreskin to the opening of the corona.
  ➤ Keep in place for 1 minute.
  ➤ This crushes the skin and marks the area for placing the dorsal slit.
➤ Remove the hemostat.
➤ Cut through the middle of the crushed area.
➤ Peel the foreskin back with gauze, and remove any additional adhesions.
➤ Place the Gomco bell over the penis with the dorsal slit secured over the bell.
➤ Pull the foreskin over the bell.
➤ Bring the bell and foreskin through the Gomco clamp ring.
➤ Tighten the thumbscrew until snug.
➤ Remove visible foreskin with a No. 11 scalpel distal to the junction of the bell and clamp device.

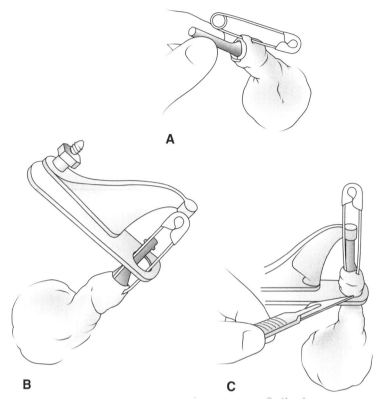

FIGURE 46 • 2 Steps of Gomco clamp method of circumcision. *(A)* After incising the dorsal slit, retract the foreskin, and place the Gomco bell. *(B)* Bring the bell, safety pin, and foreskin through the Gomco ring. Tighten the screw. *(C)* Trim the excess foreskin with a No. 11 scalpel. (From Colyar, M.R. (2003). *Well-child assessment for primary care providers.* Philadelphia: F.A. Davis.)

➤ Keep the Gomco clamp in place for 5 minutes to allow for hemostasis, which decreases the incidence of bleeding.
➤ Loosen the thumbscrew, and gently loosen the foreskin.
➤ Wrap the penis in Vaseline gauze.
➤ First void after the procedure should be documented.

PLASTIBELL METHOD

See Figure 46–3.
➤ Restrain child.
➤ Inspect genitalia.
➤ Cleanse with antiseptic solution.
➤ Grasp foreskin with two hemostats at 10:00 and 2:00 position.
➤ Gently probe and lyse adhesions underneath the foreskin with a curved hemostat.
    ➤ Do not extend beyond the corona.

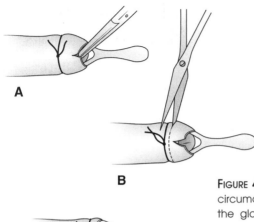

A

B

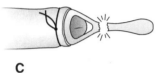

C

FIGURE 46 • 3 Steps of Plastibell method of circumcision. *(A)* Place the Plastibell over the glans, and place the string over the Plastibell indention. *(B)* Trim the foreskin. *(C)* Break off the Plastibell shaft, leaving the bell in place. (From Colyar, M.R. (2003). *Well-child assessment for primary care providers.* Philadelphia: F.A. Davis.)

➤ Place the straight hemostat approximately two thirds of the distance from the foreskin to the opening of the corona.
   ➤ Keep in place for 1 minute.
   ➤ This crushes the skin and marks the area for placing the dorsal slit.
➤ Remove the hemostat.
➤ Cut through the middle of the crushed area.
➤ Peel the foreskin back with gauze, and remove any additional adhesions.
➤ Place Plastibell over the glans.
➤ Pull foreskin over the Plastibell.
➤ Place Plastibell so that indentation is below the apex of the incision.
➤ Place 2-inch string over indention of the Plastibell and tighten until in place but not firm.
➤ Check placement of the string and bell.
   ➤ Make sure Plastibell moves freely over the glans.
➤ Tighten the string and hold tension for 30 seconds.
➤ Tie a square knot (right over left; left over right).
➤ Remove hemostats.
➤ Cut foreskin using scissors $^1/_8$ to $^3/_{16}$ inch distal to the string.
➤ Hold the Plastibell and gently snap the shaft off.
➤ Wrap the penis in Vaseline gauze.
➤ First void after the procedure should be documented.

Parent Instructions

➤ Yellow film will develop on the glans in the next few days. This is normal granulation tissue and disappears in the next few days.
➤ Keep penis clean and dry.

➤ Apply Vaseline on circumcised area after each diaper change until healed.
➤ Plastibell should fall off in 10 to 14 days. If it does not, call the health-care provider.

Circumcision—Older Boy and Man

Equipment

➤ 1% lidocaine without epinephrine
➤ 1-mL tuberculin syringe
➤ 27-gauge needle, 1 inch
➤ Locking forceps
➤ Scalpel
➤ Scissors
➤ Antiseptic skin cleanser
➤ Gloves—nonsterile
➤ Alcohol
➤ Silver nitrate sticks
➤ Vaseline gauze
➤ Kling

Procedure

➤ Consider giving preprocedure mediation to decrease anxiety.
➤ Inspect genitalia.
➤ Cleanse with antiseptic skin cleanser.
➤ Perform DPNB. Inject 0.5 to 1 mL of lidocaine without epinephrine.
➤ Grasp across foreskin with locking forceps parallel to corona of the glans. Pull out in front of the glans.
➤ Gently probe and lyse adhesions underneath the foreskin with a curved hemostat.
  ➤ Do not extend beyond the corona.
➤ Cut across the forceps furthest from the glans.
➤ Remove the excised foreskin.
➤ Snip frenulum.
➤ Unclamp foreskin.
➤ Cauterize with silver nitrate as necessary.
➤ Wrap with Vaseline gauze and Kling.

Client Instructions

➤ Monitor signs of infection, such as
  ➤ Red streaks
  ➤ Yellow-green drainage
  ➤ Foul odor from wound
  ➤ Elevated temperature
➤ If bleeding occurs, apply pressure dressing.
➤ If swelling occurs and unable to urinate within 8 hours, return to clinic or go to emergency department at local hospital for urinary catheterization.

➤ Give acetaminophen with codeine (Tylenol No. 3) every 6 hours as needed for severe pain; give ibuprofen 600 mg orally every 6 hours as needed for moderate-to-mild pain.
➤ Return to clinic in 1 week for recheck.

BIBLIOGRAPHY

American Academy of Pediatrics (2001). *Policy statement—circumcision.*
Fink, K.S., et al (2002). Adult circumcision outcomes study. *J Urol,* 167(5), 2113–2116.
Gilgal Society (2000). http://www.circinfo.com.
Hashmat, A.I., and Das, S. (1993). *The penis.* Philadelphia: Lea & Febiger.
Holman, J.R., et al (1995). Neonatal circumcision techniques. *Am Fam Physician,* 52, 511–517.
McMillian, J.A., et al (1999). *Oski's pediatrics: principles and practice.* Philadelphia: Lippincott Williams & Wilkins.
Pfenninger, J.L., and Fowler, G.C. (1994). *Procedures for primary care physicians.* St. Louis: Mosby.

47

CONDYLOMA ACUMINATUM REMOVAL

CYNTHIA EHRHARDT

CPT Code	
54050	Destruction of lesion(s), penis; simple, chemical
54054	Destruction of lesion(s), penis; simple, cryosurgery
54065	Destruction of lesion(s), penis; extensive, any method
56501	Destruction of lesion(s), vulva; simple, any method
56515	Destruction of lesion(s), vulva; extensive, any method

Condyloma acuminatum (or HPV genital infection) is a viral infection of the human host that is responsible for causing genital warts. These warts usually are located in the dermal layers of the body. Currently, 60 types of HPV have been identified. These viruses can be classified in three categories

➤ Viruses causing benign and low-risk lesions
➤ Viruses causing lesions with a moderate oncogenic risk
➤ Viruses causing lesions with a high oncogenic risk
  Genital warts typically have a hypertrophic or cauliflower-type appearance.
In the male, most of the lesions are located on the prepuce, glans, urethra,
penile shaft, and scrotum. In the female, most lesions are found on the vulva,
perianal area, vagina, and cervix.

OVERVIEW

➤ Incidence
  ➤ It is estimated that 1 million individuals are newly diagnosed with
    condyloma acuminatum in the United States each year.
  ➤ Incidence of success of treatment modalities is broken down into sever-
    al categories (Table 47–1).
➤ Complications of condyloma acuminatum include
  ➤ Increased risk for skin, cervical, and urethral cancers
  ➤ Bladder, testicular, and prostate cancers in men
➤ General principles
  ➤ Universal precautions should be followed.
  ➤ If uncertain about the malignancy of the lesion, perform a biopsy
    before attempting a treatment modality.

TABLE 47•1 INCIDENCE OF SUCCESS OF TREATMENT MODALITIES FOR CONDYLOMA ACUMINATUM

CATEGORY OF TREATMENT MODALITY	TREATMENT MODALITY	PERCENTAGE OF SUCCESS (WHERE KNOWN)
Destruction of lesion	Cryosurgical techniques	83
Surgical techniques	Electrocautery	93
	CO_2 laser ablation	89
	Excision	93
	Curettage by loop electrosurgical excisional procedure (LEEP)	90
Immunotherapy with local intralesional injection	Interferon	52
Antiviral agents*	Cimetidine (Tagamet)	
	Acyclovir (Zovirax)	
	Famciclovir(Famvir)	
	Zidovudine(Retrovir)	
Chemotherapy techniques	Acid treatment (trichloroacetic and dichloroacetic)	81
	Podophyllin	65
	Podofilox(Condylox)	61
	5-Fluorouracil	71
	Silver nitrate	60

*Effectiveness of oral agents is still under study.

HEALTH PROMOTION/PREVENTION

➤ Regular self-examination of the genital region
➤ Regular **Pap smear** examinations by all sexually active women and women
  with a history of HPV
➤ Prevention of the contraction of the infection by
  ➤ Avoidance of multiple sexual partners
  ➤ Use of condoms with new sexual partners to reduce the likelihood of
    disease transmission
➤ If infection has been acquired
  ➤ Prompt treatment of all visible lesions
  ➤ Regular screening examination by androscopy (male) and **colposcopy**
    (female) with cytologic testing
  ➤ Regular use of condoms during intercourse
  ➤ Regular self-examination of perianal area for new lesions and early
    treatment when the lesions are small

OPTIONS

➤ *Method 1*—intralesional injection (Table 47–2)
➤ *Method 2*—topical agent administration
➤ *Method 3*—cryosurgery

TABLE 47•2 TREATMENT OPTIONS

METHOD OF TREATMENT	ADVANTAGES	DISADVANTAGES
Intralesional injection	None	Painful, expensive, limited effectiveness
Topical agents Fluorouracil	Can be done at home	Not FDA approved
	Relatively inexpensive	High risk of skin irritation and ulceration
		Increased risk of dyspareunia
		Cannot use during pregnancy
Podophyllin and podofilox	Inexpensive	Prolonged treatment
	Low systemic absorption rate	Skin irritation
		Must abstain from sexual activity during treatment
		Cannot use during pregnancy
Trichloroacetic and dichloroacetic acid	Relatively inexpensive	Difficult to control skin penetration rate
	Shorter treatment period	Skin irritation
		Requires special kit for treatment[*]
		Requires special membership by the pharmacy to purchase[†]

[*]Professional Compounding Pharmacies of America, Houston; 800-331-2498.
[†]Glenwood, Inc, 83 N Summit St., Tenafly, NJ 07670; 800-542-0772.

RATIONALE

➤ To reduce the risk of the occurrence of oncogenic changes in tissue
➤ To promote cosmetic improvement

INDICATIONS

➤ All visible condyloma acuminatum
➤ Symptomatic condyloma acuminatum
➤ Documented abnormal Pap smear with or without suggestion of HPV infection

CONTRAINDICATIONS

➤ Lesions treated by ablation, which require biopsy to determine malignancy
➤ Prior history of adverse reaction to treatment regimen
➤ Pregnancy

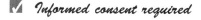 *Informed consent required*

PROCEDURE

Condyloma Acuminatum Removal

Equipment

➤ Methods 1 and 2
  ➤ Povidone antiseptic or antiseptic skin cleanser
  ➤ Gloves—sterile
  ➤ Cotton-tipped applicators—sterile
  ➤ 4 × 4 gauze—sterile
➤ Method 1 only
  ➤ Tuberculin syringes
  ➤ Interferon
➤ Method 2 only
  ➤ Silver nitrate sticks
➤ Method 3 only (see Chapter 14)

Procedure

METHOD 1—INTRALESIONAL INJECTION

➤ Position the client in a comfortable position with lesions easily accessible.
➤ Cleanse the lesions with povidone antiseptic or other antiseptic skin cleanser.
➤ Put on gloves.
➤ Draw up 0.05 mL of interferon in a tuberculin syringe for each lesion.
➤ Insert the needle into the wart, and inject the solution. A wheal should be noted in the lesion.
➤ Repeat the procedure for each lesion treated.
➤ Repeat intralesional injection twice a week for 8 weeks.

METHOD 2—TOPICAL AGENT ADMINISTRATION

➤ Position the client in a comfortable position with lesions easily accessible.
➤ Cleanse the lesions with povidone antiseptic or other antiseptic skin cleanser.
➤ Put on gloves.
➤ Apply the fenestrated drape.
➤ Using two digits, apply tension to the skin surrounding the lesion.
➤ Apply the chemically impregnated silver nitrate stick to the desired site for approximately 15 seconds.
➤ Remove the silver nitrate stick, and release the skin.
➤ Repeat this procedure to each wart.

METHOD 3—CRYSURGERY

See Chapter 14.

Client Instructions

➤ Use "safe sex" behaviors to reduce the risk of disease transmission.
➤ Observe for signs and symptoms of infection. If any of the following signs and symptoms of infection are found, return to the office
    ➤ Increase in pain after 24 hours
    ➤ Increase in temperature
    ➤ Redness or swelling
    ➤ Yellow or greenish drainage
    ➤ Foul odor
➤ Keep follow-up treatment appointments.
➤ Closely follow instructions on self-administered medication.
    ➤ Fluorouracil (topical 5-FU, Efudex, Fluoroplex)
        • Apply a thin coat of 5% cream to the lesion at bedtime once or twice a week for up to 10 weeks.
        • Leave on overnight.
        • For penile lesions, apply thin film over the lesion and wrap penis in gauze or condom three times a week for 3 to 4 weeks.
        • Rinse off in 3 hours.
    ➤ Podophyllum and podofilox agent
        • Apply Vaseline approximately 3 to 5 mm away from the lesion to reduce irritation of normal tissue and prevent running of the liquid.
            • Do not get any Vaseline on the lesion because it reduces the effectiveness of treatment.
        • Apply the liquid drop in sufficient quantity to cover the entire lesion.
        • Leave the chemical on for 4 to 6 hours.
        • Rinse off agent gently with soapy water.
        • Repeat the procedure twice a week until full resolution has occurred (usually 4 to 8 weeks).
        • Treat promptly if warts recur.
    ➤ Trichloroacetic acid (Tri-Chlor) and dichloroacetic acid (Bichloroacetic Acid) agents

- Apply petroleum jelly approximately 3 to 5 mm away from the lesion to reduce irritation of normal tissue and prevent running of the liquid.
- Apply to the affected lesion three times per week with maximum treatment of 4 weeks.
- Optional—Apply once or twice daily for 3 consecutive days per week for a maximum of 4 weeks.

BIBLIOGRAPHY

American Medical Association (1996). *Physicians' current procedural terminology.* Chicago: Author.

Carson, S. (1997). Human papillomatous virus infection update: impact on women's health. *Nurse Practitioner,* 22(4), 24–27.

Habif, T. (1996) (3rd ed.). *Clinical dermatology: a color guide to diagnosis and therapy.* St. Louis: Mosby.

Matzen, R., and Lang, R. (1993). *Clinical preventive medicine.* St. Louis: Mosby.

Mayeaux, E., et al (1995). Noncervical human papillomavirus genital infections. *Am Fam Physician,* 52(4), 1137–1150.

Miller, D., and Brodell, R. (1996). Human papillomavirus infection treatment options for warts. *Am Fam Physician,* 53(1), 68–74.

Pfenninger, J.L., and Fowler, G.C. (1994). *Procedures for primary care physicians.* St. Louis: Mosby.

48

DIAPHRAGM FITTING, INSERTION, AND REMOVAL

SANDRA KUHN

CPT Code	
57170	Diaphragm/cervical cap fitting with instructions

A **diaphragm** is a contraceptive barrier device that consists of a soft latex rubber dome supported by a round metal spring on the outside. Diaphragms come in various sizes and must be fitted to each individual. A diaphragm is a nonsystemic and reversible method of contraception. A diaphragm is not a 100% effective method of contraception, and it does not protect against sexually transmitted diseases.

OVERVIEW

➤ Incidence unknown
➤ Prevention of pregnancy
  ➤ Among first-year users: 2.2 pregnancies per 100 women
  ➤ Among established users: 1.9 to 2.4 pregnancies per 100 women per year
  ➤ Among women older than age 35: Fewer than 1.9 pregnancies per 100 women per year
➤ Potential complications include
  ➤ Pregnancy
  ➤ Increased risk of urinary tract infections
  ➤ Increased risk of cervicitis and vaginal infections
  ➤ Increased incidence of toxic shock syndrome
  ➤ Associated with a slightly increased risk of abnormal **Pap smears**
➤ Assess
  ➤ Comfortable (self or partner) in examination and insertion of fingers and diaphragm in vagina
  ➤ Has physical dexterity (self or partner) to use a diaphragm
  ➤ Able to inform the health-care provider and return for refitting should weight change of greater than 5 lb occur
  ➤ Muscle tone of the vaginal vault must be adequate to retain diaphragm
➤ Types of diaphragm kits
  ➤ Arching spring (most common)
  ➤ Coil spring
  ➤ Flat spring
  ➤ Wide spring

RATIONALE

➤ To provide a reversible form of contraception

INDICATIONS

➤ Contraception protection during sexual intercourse
➤ Other methods of contraception ruled out

CONTRAINDICATIONS

➤ Allergy to latex rubber products
➤ Allergy to spermicide gel
➤ Prior history of toxic shock syndrome
➤ **Cystocele**
➤ Rectocele
➤ Uterine retroversion
➤ Uterine prolapse
➤ History of frequent lower urinary tract infections

PROCEDURE

Diaphragm Fitting, Insertion, and Removal

Equipment

➤ Diaphragm kit with sizes ranging from 50 to 105 mm
➤ Lubricant (diaphragm gel or K-Y jelly)
➤ Gloves—nonsterile
➤ Light source
➤ Mirror for patient to watch—optional

Procedure

DIAPHRAGM FITTING

➤ Have the client empty her bladder before fitting.
➤ Place the client in the lithotomy position with feet in stirrups.
➤ Put on gloves and lubricate finger with gel.
➤ Insert a finger (usually middle) into the vaginal vault until it is deep in the posterior fornix.
➤ Using the thumb tip of the inserted hand, mark where the pubic bone touches the middle finger.
➤ Remove and match the width of the diaphragm to the distance measured on the middle finger.
   ➤ This is the approximate width of the diaphragm.

DIAPHRAGM INSERTION

➤ After lubricating the chosen diaphragm, hold it between the thumb and finger and gently squeeze the rim together.
➤ Separate the labia with the opposite hand, and use the free hand to insert a finger at the base of the vaginal os and apply pressure downward to open the os wider.
➤ Gently insert the diaphragm into the vagina with the diaphragm dome facing downward until it reaches the posterior fornix behind the cervix.
   ➤ A finger may need to be used to guide the diaphragm in place.
➤ As the diaphragm expands, feel that it fits snugly against the vaginal walls. The finger may be used as a guide.
➤ When fully in place, use the inserted finger to follow the edges of the diaphragm ring, feeling for gaps; if none are felt, remove finger.
➤ Several insertions and removals of different ring sizes may be required until the proper size is found.
➤ Have the client try the size larger and smaller before making a final selection.
➤ The diaphragm should be posterior to the symphysis pubis if inserted properly.
➤ Use the largest size that is comfortable for the client because the vaginal vault enlarges during sexual arousal.
   ➤ Too small a diaphragm may not cover the cervix properly and may increase the risk of trauma to the cervix and vaginal vault.

➤ Too large a diaphragm may cause vaginal pressure, abdominal pain and/or cramping, ulceration of the vaginal wall, and increased risk of urinary tract infections.
➤ With the diaphragm inserted, have the client squat and move around to ensure a proper fit.
➤ The client should not be able to feel the diaphragm.
  ➤ Sometimes during the fitting, the client may mistake the sensation of the fitting for the diaphragm.

DIAPHRAGM REMOVAL

➤ Place a finger behind the front rim of the diaphragm near the symphysis pubis, and pull it down and out.
  ➤ Have the client demonstrate the correct insertion, placement, and removal of the diaphragm at least three times in the office.

Client Instructions

➤ Preinsertion checklist includes
  ➤ Check diaphragm for holes, tears, and cracks by holding it up against a light.
  ➤ Apply a teaspoon of spermicidal gel or cream to the dome of the diaphragm.
  ➤ Apply additional spermicidal gel or cream to the ring of the diaphragm.
  ➤ If the diaphragm has been in place for 2 hours or more before intercourse, add spermicidal gel or cream into the vaginal vault.
  ➤ Check for proper placement before coitus.
➤ During coitus
  ➤ Use of condom increases contraceptive protection.
  ➤ Without removing the diaphragm, apply additional spermicidal gel or cream into the vaginal vault after each episode.
➤ Postcoitus care
  ➤ Do not remove for at least 6 hours after last coitus.
  ➤ Do not douche with diaphragm in place because it will wash away the spermicidal gel or cream barrier. Recheck for proper placement between acts of coitus.
  ➤ After removal, clean the diaphragm with soapy water, rinse thoroughly in plain water, and air dry. Avoid oil-based products because they can weaken the latex and accelerate deterioration.
  ➤ Avoid douching after removal of the diaphragm.
  ➤ Avoid wearing the diaphragm for 2 to 3 days before Pap smear testing.
  ➤ Refit
    • At annual visit
    • If increase or decrease in weight of 5 lb or more
    • After full-term pregnancy and delivery
    • After an abortion
    • If complaining of dyspareunia, cramping, bladder pain, or rectal pain or partner complains of penile pain
    • After pelvic surgery

BIBLIOGRAPHY

Hatcher, R., et al (1994) (16th ed.). *Contraceptive technology*. Philadelphia: Irvington.

Pernoll, M.L., et al (1999). *Current obstetrics and gynecologic diagnosis and treatment*. Los Altos, CA: Lange Medical Publications.

Pfenninger, J.L., and Fowler, G.C. (1994). *Procedures for primary care physicians*. St. Louis: Mosby.

49 INTRAUTERINE DEVICE (IUD) INSERTION

ANGELA DENERIS • JANE M. DYER

CPT Code	
58300	Insertion of intrauterine device (IUD)

An IUD is a small device that is inserted through the cervix and is retained in the uterus to prevent pregnancy. A string or strings hang from the IUD through the cervix and into the vagina to ensure the presence of the IUD and for removal. The exact mechanism of the IUD in preventing pregnancy is not known but may include prevention of fertilization and implantation. Some IUDs may contain copper or progestin. The IUD is a reversible form of contraception that does not offer protection against and may increase the risk of sexually transmitted infections. The Mirena IUD with levonorgestrel-releasing system thickens cervical mucus and alters the endometrial lining, which decreases the ability of sperm to enter the uterus and implant.

OVERVIEW

➤ Incidence of use unknown
➤ Prevention of pregnancy
➤ Treatment for menorrhagia

Potential Complications

➤ Increased risk of pelvic inflammatory disease
➤ Increased risk of infertility
➤ Increased risk of menorrhagia and dysmenorrhea with Copper-T-380 and ParaGard.

Assess

➤ Comfort with and ability of (woman/partner) to check IUD string(s) by inserting fingers in vagina.
➤ Ability to inform provider of absence of strings.

Types of IUDs

➤ IUDs consist of plastic devices
  ➤ Wrapped with copper wire (Copper T-380—ParaGard)
  ➤ With progesterone in the vertical stem (Progestasert)
  ➤ With a reservoir with a levonorgestrel-releasing system (LNS and Mirena)
➤ IUDs from other countries may be made of metal or plastic in a variety of shapes.

RATIONALE

➤ To provide a reliable and reversible form of contraception
➤ To treat menorrhagia (LNS and Mirena) due to progesterone effect

INDICATIONS

➤ Contraception
➤ Patient choice
➤ Menorrhagia (LNS)
➤ Contraindications to other forms of contraception
➤ Emergency contraception (Cu T insertion within 5 days of unprotected intercourse)

CONTRAINDICATIONS

➤ Pelvic inflammatory disease within the last 12 months or recurrent pelvic inflammatory disease (more than one episode in the past 2 years)
➤ Postabortal or postpartum endometritis or septic abortion in the past 3 months
➤ Known or suspected untreated endocervical gonorrhea, chlamydia, or mucopurulent cervicitis
➤ Undiagnosed abnormal vaginal bleeding
➤ Pregnancy or suspicion of established pregnancy
➤ Small uterine cavity with sounding less than 6.5 cm
  • A *sound* is a long narrow plastic disposable or metal calibrated rod that measures the internal length of the uterine cavity, including the length of the cervix.
➤ Suspected or known uterine perforation occurring with the placement of a uterine sound during the current insertion procedure
➤ History of ectopic pregnancy
➤ Human immunodeficiency virus/acquired immunodeficiency syndrome (HIV/AIDS)

➤ History of symptomatic pelvic actinomycosis confirmed by a culture (not asymptomatic colonization)
➤ Known or suspected allergy to copper or history of Wilson's disease (for copper IUD only)
➤ Acute liver disease or tumor—benign or malignant (levonorgestrel IUD only)
➤ Known or suspected breast cancer (levonorgestrel IUD only)
➤ Known or suspected cervical and uterine cancer

MEDICAL ELIGIBILITY CHECKLIST FOR IUDS/SYSTEMS

➤ Ask the client the following questions, before inserting an IUD or intrauterine system (IUS)
  ➤ Do you think you are pregnant, or have you had a recent pregnancy?
  ➤ When was your last menstrual period, and was it normal?
  ➤ Are your periods unusually heavy, or do you experience severe cramping?
  ➤ Do you have any abnormalities of the uterus?
  ➤ What contraception have you been using?
  ➤ Are you having any unusual bleeding between periods?
  ➤ Do you have multiple sexual partners, or does your partner have multiple partners?
  ➤ Have you ever had a sexually transmitted disease? If yes, which ones?
  ➤ Do you think you have HIV?
  ➤ Have you ever had pelvic inflammatory disease?
  ➤ Have you ever had cancer of the reproductive organs?
  ➤ Do you have any other medical conditions (i.e. bleeding disorders, anemia, steroid therapy, heart disease or murmur, hepatitis, leukemia)?
➤ Perform the following laboratory tests before insertion
  ➤ Urine pregnancy test
  ➤ Chlamydia and gonorrhea culture
  ➤ Offer HIV screening
  ➤ Pap smear

✔ *Informed consent required*

PROCEDURE
IUD Insertion
Equipment

➤ IUD
➤ Stabilizing rod (Mirena only)
➤ Insertion tube
➤ Gloves—nonsterile
➤ Gloves—sterile
➤ Speculum
➤ Uterine sound

➤ Light source
➤ K-Y jelly
➤ Povidone-iodine swabs
➤ Large cotton-tipped applicator
➤ Tenaculum
➤ 1% lidocaine—optional
➤ Silver nitrate—optional

Procedure

COPPER T-380 IUD (PARAGARD) OR PROGESTERONE IUD (PROGESTASERT SYSTEM)

See Figure 49–1.
➤ Screen client for copper sensitivity, if using the ParaGard IUD.
➤ Determine if the client is menstruating or in the follicular phase of the cycle.
➤ Advise client to take 400 to 800 mg of ibuprofen 1 to 2 hours before appointment.
➤ Have client read the medical checklist and sign consent form.
➤ Don nonsterile gloves.
➤ Apply K-Y jelly to second and third digits.
➤ Place client in the lithotomy position with feet in stirrups, and perform a bimanual examination to determine the size and position of the cervix and uterus.
➤ Change into sterile gloves.
➤ Using a sterile speculum, visualize the cervix.
➤ Wash the cervix three times with povidone-iodine swabs.
➤ Consider using a paracervical block with 1% lidocaine, if the patient has never had a full term pregnancy, has cervical stenosis, or has a history of vasovagal reactions.
  ➤ Place a tenaculum at the 2:00 and 10:00 position. Alert the patient that she will feel a sharp cramp with the placement of the tenaculum, if you have not used a paracervical block. The cramping subsides within 1 minute.
  ➤ With gentle traction on the tenaculum, sound the uterus. Alert the client she will feel another cramp when the sound reaches the uterine fundus.
    • Most uteri sound between 7 and 9 cm. Do not insert the IUD if the uterus sounds only to 6.5 cm or less, owing to increased expulsion rates.
➤ Using sterile technique, load the IUD into insertion tube, by bending the T arms of the device **downward**. The positioning rod is pushed back into the insertion tube when the IUD is loaded. The device has an approximate 5-minute memory to spring back into the T shape.
➤ Adjust the flange on the insertion tube to the depth measured by the sound. The flange is oval shaped, and the flattest part of the flange should be lined up with the T arms of the IUD to ensure proper positioning inside of the uterus.

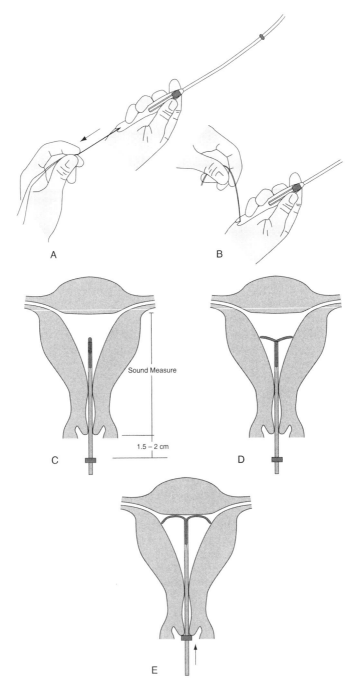

FIGURE 49 • 1 IUD insertion. *(A)* System being drawn in insertion tube. *(B)* Pull threads into the cleft tightly. *(C)* Insert into the cervix. *(D)* Release the arms of the IUD. *(E)* Release and withdraw the inserter.

➤ With gentle traction on the tenaculum, alert the client she will feel another uterine cramp as the IUD is being placed. Insert the IUD and insertion device into the cervix to the level of the flange, making sure the flange is in a horizontal orientation to the cervix.

➤ Holding the stabilizing rod in one hand and the insertion tube in the other, withdraw the insertion tube toward you.

  ➤ Never push the stabilizing rod deeper into the uterus; this would increase the possibility of uterine perforation.

➤ Withdraw the stabilizing rod with the insertion tube.

➤ Cut the string of the IUD to approximately 3 cm from the cervical os.

➤ Remove the tenaculum, and observe for bleeding at the tenaculum site on the cervix.

➤ Apply pressure to the site with a large cotton swab. If bleeding does not cease within 1 to 2 minutes, dab the site gently with silver nitrate or Monsel's solution.

➤ Give a piece of the IUD string to the client for her to feel and have her check her own cervix to feel the protruding IUD string.

Client Instructions

➤ Give client the card to have ParaGard Copper T removed after 10 years and the Progestasert after 1 year.

➤ Have the client take 400 to 800 mg of ibuprofen for several days if needed for cramping.

➤ Advise client that menstrual periods may be heavier, or she may experience severe cramping.

➤ Instruct client to return to the clinic in 6 weeks for a follow-up visit to check string length and side effects.

➤ Instruct client to check strings after each menstrual period and call immediately if unable to locate the strings.

➤ If client misses a menstrual period, have her perform a pregnancy test and come into the clinic immediately for removal of the IUD if she is pregnant.

Procedure

LEVONORGESTREL-RELEASING INTRAUTERINE SYSTEM (MIRENA)

➤ Determine if the client is menstruating or in the follicular phase of the cycle.

➤ Advise client to take 400 to 800 mg of oral ibuprofen 1 to 2 hours before appointment.

➤ Have client read the medical checklist and sign consent form.

➤ Don nonsterile gloves.

➤ Apply K-Y jelly to second and third digits.

➤ Place client in the lithotomy position with feet in stirrups, and perform a bimanual examination to determine the size and position of the cervix and uterus.

➤ Change into sterile gloves.

- Using a sterile speculum, visualize the cervix.
- Wash the cervix three times with povidone-iodine swabs.
- Consider using a paracervical block with 1% lidocaine, if the patient has never had a full-term pregnancy, has cervical stenosis, or has a history of vasovagal reactions.
  - Place a tenaculum at the 2:00 and 10:00 position. Alert the patient that she will feel a sharp cramp with the placement of the tenaculum, if you have not used a paracervical block. The cramping subsides within 1 minute.
  - With gentle traction on the tenaculum, sound the uterus. Alert the client she will feel another cramp when the sound reaches the uterine fundus.
    - Most uteri sound between 7 and 9 cm. Do not insert the IUD if the uterus sounds only to 6.5 cm or less, owing to increased expulsion rates.
- Carefully release the threads from behind the slider so that they hang freely.
- The slider should be in the furthest position away from you (positioned at the top of the handle nearest the IUS.
- The arms of the system must be horizontal, before loading the system.
- Without touching the IUS arms, load the IUS by pulling on both strings. This draws the IUS into the insertion tube, with the arms in an upward extended position.
- When the IUS is fully loaded, the end of the rounded knobs of the arms protrude from the end of the insertion tube.
- Fix the strings tightly in the cleft at the end of the handle.
- Set the flange to the depth measured by the sound.
- Advise the client she will feel a cramping sensation with the insertion of the IUS.
- Insert the IUS by using gentle traction on the tenaculum. **Stop advancing the IUS insertion tube when the flange is within 1.5 to 2 cm of the cervix.**
- While holding the inserter steady, release the arms of the IUS by pulling the slider back until it reaches the horizontal line on the handle. You will feel a popping sensation as the IUS is released.
- Push the inserter gently into the uterine cavity until the flange touches the cervix. The IUS now should be in the fundal position of the uterus.
- Holding the inserter firmly in position, release the IUS by pulling the slider down all the way. The strings release automatically.
- Remove the inserter from the uterus.
- Remove the tenaculum from the cervix.
  - Observe for bleeding, and apply pressure at the tenaculum site with a large cotton swab.
  - If the bleeding does not cease within 1 to 2 minutes, dab the site with silver nitrate.
- Cut the string to approximately 3 cm from the cervical os.
- Give a piece of the IUS string to the client for her to feel, and have her check her own cervix to feel the protruding IUS string.

Client Instructions

➤ Give client the card to have Mirena IUS removed after 5 years.
➤ Instruct her to return to the clinic in 6 weeks for a follow-up visit to check string length and side effects.
➤ Instruct client to check strings after each menstrual period and call immediately if she is unable to locate the strings.
➤ Advise the client that she may have some irregular menstrual bleeding for the first 3 to 6 months after insertion.
  ➤ These symptoms decrease over time; 90% of women have lighter periods in the future, and 20% will stop menstruating altogether.
➤ If the client does become pregnant on the IUS, she needs to have it removed as soon as possible.

Removal of an IUD/IUS

Equipment

➤ Gloves—nonsterile
➤ Speculum
➤ Light source
➤ K-Y jelly
➤ Pelvic ultrasound—optional

Procedure

➤ Put on gloves.
➤ With the patient in the lithotomy position, insert a speculum into the vagina.
➤ Grasp the IUD/IUS strings with a ring forcep, and with gentle traction withdraw the IUD/IUS from the uterus.
➤ If the strings are not present, obtain a pelvic ultrasound to determine the location of the IUD/IUS.

Client Instructions

➤ Client will feel slight cramping when the IUD/IUS is pulled. This should quickly abate.
  ➤ Only minimal bleeding should be experienced.
  ➤ If bleeding does not stop, contact health-care provider immediately.
➤ Fertility status returns immediately on removal of the IUD/IUS.

BIBLIOGRAPHY
Hatcher, R., et al (1998) (17th ed.). *Contraceptive technology.* New York: Ardent Media.
Hatcher, R.A., et al (1999). *Managing contraception.* Tiger, GA: Bridging the Gap Foundation.
Berlex Laboratories (2001). *The Contraception Report,* 12(2).

50 NORPLANT INSERTION

MARGARET R. COLYAR

CPT Code

11975   Insertion, implantable contraceptive
        capsules

Norplant is a mode of contraception that is reversible. Norplant is implanted under the skin of the upper arm, using daily release of progesterone to prevent pregnancy.

OVERVIEW

➤ Incidence is unknown.
➤ It is necessary to ensure that a woman who is to receive a Norplant implant is not pregnant at the time of implantation. The Norplant should be implanted 7 days after the menstrual cycle begins or right after an abortion.

RATIONALE

➤ To initiate the contraception process

INDICATIONS

➤ To prevent pregnancy

CONTRAINDICATIONS

➤ Active or history of thrombophlebitis
➤ Thromboembolic disorder
➤ Undiagnosed genital bleeding
➤ Known or suspected pregnancy
➤ Acute liver disease and/or benign or malignant liver tumors
➤ Known or suspected breast carcinoma
➤ Allergy to progesterone
➤ Nursing mother
➤ History of coronary artery disease
Client teaching includes advising of potential side effects such as
➤ Bleeding irregularities
➤ Ovarian cysts
➤ Ectopic pregnancy

- Foreign-body carcinogenesis
- Increase in thromboembolic disorder and other vascular problems if the client smokes
- Liver tumors
- Breast carcinoma
- Headache
- Nervousness and anxiety
- Nausea and vomiting
- Dizziness
- Rash
- Acne
- Pain in breasts
- Weight gain
- Hirsutism
- Scalp hair loss

Decreased efficacy of Norplant occurs with

- Phenobarbital
- Carbamazepine
- Rifampicin

✅ *Informed consent required*

PROCEDURE

Norplant Insertion

Equipment

The following equipment comes in package with Norplant.

- Trochar for Norplant system
- Scalpel
- **Forceps**
- Syringe
- Two syringe needles
- **Steri strips**
- Gauze sponges
- Stretch bandage
- One surgical drape (fenestrated)
- Two surgical drapes
- Antiseptic skin cleanser
- Gloves—sterile
- Drape—sterile
- 1% lidocaine

Procedure

- Position the client on her back with the left arm (if right-handed) or right arm (if left-handed) flexed at elbow and externally rotated.
- Draw a fan-shaped diagram of insertion (Fig. 50–1).

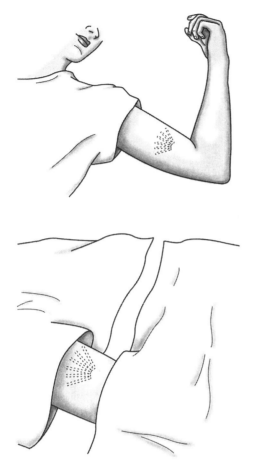

FIGURE 50 • 1 Draw a fan-shaped diagram on the inner aspect of the upper arm in which you plan to insert the Norplant.

➤ Prepare the upper arm with antiseptic skin cleanser. Norplant is inserted 8 to 10 cm above the elbow crease on the inside of the upper arm.
➤ Drape the arm above and below the insertion site.
➤ Open the sterile Norplant system onto a sterile drape and count the six capsules.
➤ Fill a 5-mL syringe with 1% lidocaine.
  ➣ Inject lidocaine into each of the six spokes of the fan about 4.5 cm in length.
➤ Using a No. 11 scalpel, make a small, shallow, 2-mm incision through the skin (Fig. 50–2).
➤ Insert the trochar, bevel up, under the skin to the first mark (about 4.5 cm) (Fig. 50–3).
➤ Remove the obturator (part of the trochar), and load the implant (Fig. 50–4).
➤ Replace the obturator, and advance the implant until resistance is felt.
➤ Hold the obturator steady, and back the trochar out (Fig. 50–5).

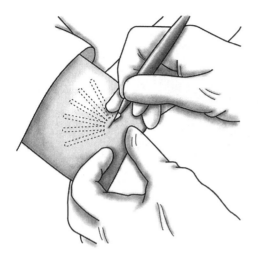

FIGURE 50 • 2 Make a shallow, 2-mm incision at the base of the insertion site.

➤ Repeat until all six implants are placed.
➤ Apply Steri strips across the wounds.
➤ Apply pressure with gauze.
➤ Secure with stretch bandage.
➤ Give postoperative instructions.

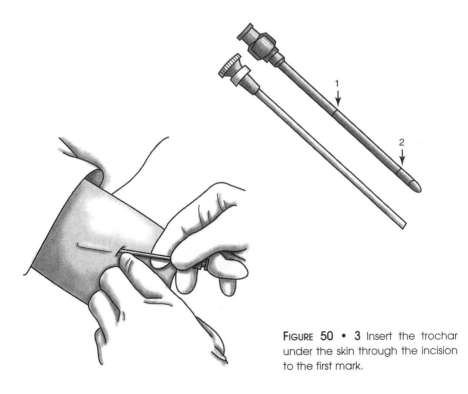

FIGURE 50 • 3 Insert the trochar under the skin through the incision to the first mark.

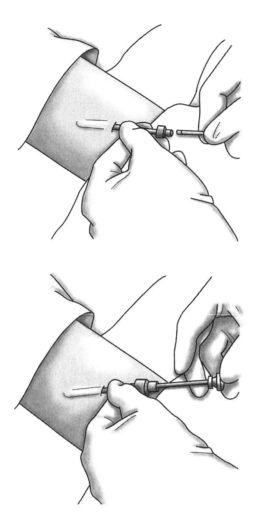

FIGURE 50 • 4 Remove the obturator, and load the implant. Insert the implant through the trochar.

Client Instructions

➤ Bruising may occur.
➤ Keep the incision clean and dry.
➤ You can expect some pain at the incision site.
   ➢ Take acetaminophen or ibuprofen every 4 to 6 hours as needed.
➤ To limit bruising
   ➢ Avoid heavy lifting for 2 to 3 days.
   ➢ Maintain the dressing in place for 24 hours.
➤ Observe for signs and symptoms of infection, such as
   ➢ Increase in pain after 24 hours
   ➢ Increase in temperature
   ➢ Redness or swelling

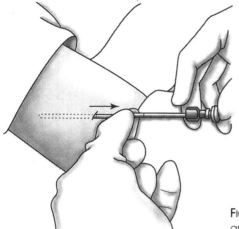

FIGURE 50 • 5 Hold the obturator steady and back the trochar out.

➤ Yellow or greenish drainage
➤ Foul odor
➤ If any of the signs and symptoms of infection are found, return to the office.

B I B L I O G R A P H Y
Medical Economics Data (1996). *Physician's desk reference* (pp. 2759–2764). Montvale, NJ: Author.
Wyeth-Ayerst Laboratories. *Norplant product information guide*. Philadelphia: Author.

51 NORPLANT REMOVAL

MARGARET R. COLYAR

CPT Code

11976 Removal, implantable contraceptive
        capsules
11977 Removal with reinsertion, implantable
        contraceptive capsules

Norplant removal consists of removing implanted contraceptive capsules that are used to prevent pregnancy. After removal of the implanted contraceptive capsules, fertility is returned immediately.

OVERVIEW
➤ Incidence unknown

RATIONALE
➤ To reverse the contraception process
➤ To diminish unwanted side effects

INDICATIONS
➤ Request of the client
➤ Five years elapsed since insertion
➤ Prolonged vaginal bleeding
➤ Pain at the implant site

CONTRAINDICATIONS
➤ None

 Informed consent required

PROCEDURE
Norplant Removal
Equipment

➤ Antiseptic skin cleanser
➤ Two drapes—sterile
➤ Gloves—sterile
➤ 1% lidocaine
➤ 10-mL syringe
➤ 25- to 27-gauge, $1^1/_2$-inch needle
➤ No. 11 scalpel
➤ **Hemostats**—sterile
➤ Topical antibiotic ointment (Bactroban, Neosporin, or Polysporin)
➤ **Steri strips**—$^1/_8$- to $^1/_4$-inch
➤ Tape adhesive (**benzoin**)
➤ Cotton-tipped applicators—nonsterile
➤ 4 × 4 gauze—sterile
➤ Kerlix or stretch bandage

Procedure

➤ Position the client's arm with the Norplant implant facing up.
➤ Locate the position of all six capsules by palpation.
➤ Cleanse the upper arm with antiseptic skin cleanser.
➤ Drape above and below the Norplant implant.
➤ Inject 1% lidocaine under the capsule ends.

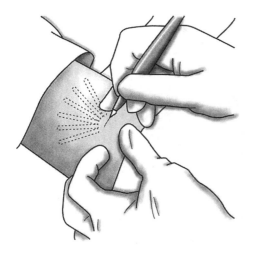

FIGURE 51 • 1 Make a small incision at the previous site. Do not incise the capsules.

➤ Make a small incision at the previous insertion site (Fig. 51–1).
  ➤ Do not incise the capsules.
➤ With hemostats, gently break away the tissue between the incision and the capsules (Fig. 51–2).
➤ Grasp one capsule with the hemostats and gently withdraw the capsule (Fig. 51–3).
➤ Repeat the procedure until all six capsules are removed.
➤ If you have difficulty withdrawing the capsule, gently break away the tissue around the capsule, then pull it out.
➤ Apply topical antibiotic.
➤ Apply Steri strips (see Chapter 20).
➤ Apply a pressure dressing and secure with Kerlix or stretch bandage.

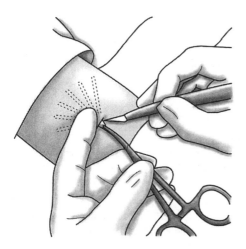

Figure 51 • 2 Gently break away the tissue between the incision and the capsules.

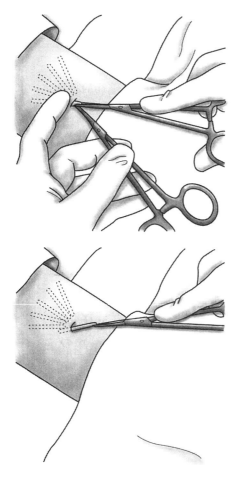

FIGURE 51 • 3 Grasp each capsule with the hemostats, and gently withdraw the capsule.

Client Instructions

➤ Bruising may occur.
  ➤ To avoid bruising, avoid heavy lifting for 2 to 3 days.
  ➤ Keep the dressing in place for 24 hours.
➤ Watch for signs and symptoms of infection.
  ➤ Keep incision clean and dry.
  ➤ Return to the clinic if any yellow or greenish drainage occurs.
➤ You can expect some pain at the incision site.
  ➤ Take acetaminophen every 4 hours or nonsteroidal anti-inflammatory drug as needed.

BIBLIOGRAPHY

Medical Economics Data (1996). *Physician's desk reference* (pp. 2759–2764). Montvale, NJ: Author.
Wyeth-Ayerst Laboratories. *Norplant product information guide*. Philadelphia: Author.

52

PARACERVICAL NERVE BLOCK

MARGARET R. COLYAR

CPT Code

64435 Injection, anesthetic agent; paracervical (uterine) nerve

The **paracervical** nerve block is a technique used to anesthetize the uterus, cervix, and upper vagina during cervical conization. The cervical block is of short duration (30 to 60 minutes). This procedure previously was used in the first stage of labor, but it no longer is considered safe during labor.

OVERVIEW

➤ Incidence unknown

RATIONALE

➤ To anesthetize the uterus, cervix, and upper vagina
➤ To diminish pain

INDICATIONS

➤ Cervical conization
➤ Cervical biopsy

CONTRAINDICATIONS

➤ Presence of infection or inflammation
➤ Pregnancy

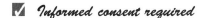 *Informed consent required*

PROCEDURE

Paracervical Block

Equipment

➤ Topical antiseptic cleanser
➤ Syringe with ring plunger—10 mL
➤ Iowa trumpet

- 22-gauge, $1^1/_2$-inch needle
- 1% lidocaine—10 mL
- Gloves—sterile
- 4 × 4 gauge—sterile
- K-Y jelly

Procedure

- Position the client in the lithotomy position.
- Cleanse the perineum with antiseptic skin cleanser.
- Put on gloves.
- Lubricate fingers and insert into the vagina.
- Locate the cervicovaginal junction.
- Insert the Iowa trumpet into the vagina at the cervicovaginal junction (Fig. 52–1).

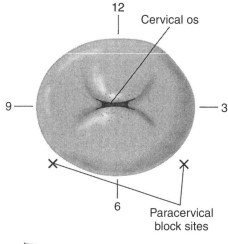

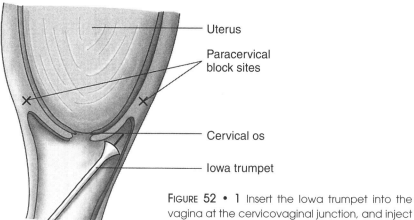

FIGURE 52 • 1 Insert the Iowa trumpet into the vagina at the cervicovaginal junction, and inject 1% lidocaine at the paracervical block sites.

➤ Insert the needle and syringe in the end of the trumpet outside the vagina.
➤ Insert the needle 0.5 cm into the tissue.
➤ Aspirate for the presence of blood.
➤ Inject 5 to 10 mL of 1% lidocaine.
➤ Repeat the procedure on the opposite side of the cervix.

BIBLIOGRAPHY
DeCherney, A.H., and Pernoll, M.L. (eds.). (1994). *Current obstetric and gynecologic diagnosis and treatment.* Norwalk, CT: Appleton & Lange.

53 PESSARY INSERTION

MARGARET R. COLYAR

CPT Code
57160   Pessary insertion

A pessary is a hard rubber or plastic prosthetic device that serves to elevate the uterus in the vaginal vault. Pessaries are indicated for women who have uterine **prolapse** or **cystocele**. Elderly women most commonly use pessary devices, especially if surgery is contraindicated or undesirable.

OVERVIEW

➤ Incidence unknown
➤ Used to maintain
  ➢ Uterine position
    • Prevention of uterine prolapse
    • Alleviation of **menorrhagia, dysmenorrhea,** or **dyspareunia**
  ➢ Bladder and rectum position
    • Prevention of incontinence
  ➢ Support of the pelvic floor in genital hernias because pessaries increase the tension of the pelvic floor
➤ Frequent complications
  ➢ Vaginal infection
    • Urinary tract infections
➤ Symptoms associated with pessary use
  ➢ Vaginal burning
  ➢ Vaginal itching

> Urinary retention
> Urinary frequency
> Urinary urgency
> Dysuria

OPTIONS

There are several types of pessaries to choose from (Fig. 53–1).
> For cystocele only
  > Gehrung
> For cystocele and/or rectocele
  > Ring
  > Doughnut
  > Ball

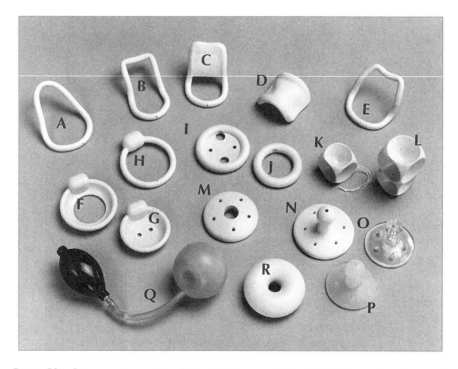

FIGURE 53 • 1 Types of pessaries. (A) Smith (silicone, folding). (B) Hodge without support (silicone, folding). (C) Hodge with support (silicone, folding). (D) Gehrung with support (silicone, folding). (E) Risser (silicone, folding). (F) Incontinence dish without support (silicone, folding). (G) Incontinence dish with support (silicone, folding). (H) Incontinence ring (silicone). (I) Ring with support (silicone, folding). (J) Ring without support (silicone, folding). (K) Cube (silicone, flexible). (L) Tandem cube (silicone, flexible). (M) Shaatz (silicone, folding). (N) Gellhorn (silicone, flexible, multidrain). (O) Gillhorn (acrylic, rigid, multidrain). (P) Gillhorn (95% rigid silicone, multidrain). (Q) Inflatoball (latex). (R) Donut (silicone). (Reprinted with permission from Milex Products, Inc, Chicago, IL.)

- Bee cell
- Inflatable
- For uterine prolapse
  - Gellhorn
  - Hodge
  - Napier

RATIONALE

- To elevate the uterus in the vaginal vault
- To provide relief with cystocele, rectocele, and uterine prolapse
- To assist in fertility

INDICATIONS

- For women who have one of the following problems but are unable or do not wish to have surgery
  - Uterine prolapse
  - Menorrhagia, dysmenorrhea, or dyspareunia caused by retroposition of the uterus or adnexa prolapse
  - Cystocele
  - Rectocele
  - Bladder or rectal incontinence
  - Hernia of the pelvic floor
  - Obstetric reasons
    - To tilt the cervix into the midline if indicated in infertility

CONTRAINDICATIONS

- Acute genital tract infection
- Adherent retroposition of the uterus

PROCEDURE

Pessary Insertion

Equipment

- Pessary—sterile
- Drape—nonsterile
- Gloves—nonsterile
- Povidone-iodine solution
- Basin—sterile
- Ring **forceps** or claw forceps—sterile
- Light source
- K-Y jelly

Procedure

- Position the client in the lithotomy position.
- Drape the lower half of the client's torso.

- ➤ Put on gloves.
- ➤ Measure the client for a pessary by
  - ➢ Length—measure from the introitus to the top of the posterior vaginal vault and subtract 1 cm.
  - ➢ Width—insert ring forceps into the vagina to the level of the cervix, and open until the blades touch the walls of the vagina.
    - Note the distance between the handles of the forceps.
    - Remove the forceps and open again the same distance.
    - Measure between the tips of the blades.
  - ➢ Average the two measurements. This is the diameter of the pessary.
- ➤ Soak the pessary in a sterile basin filled with povidone-iodine before insertion.
- ➤ Lubricate the pessary with K-Y jelly.
- ➤ Depress the perineum with the opposite hand to widen the introitus.
- ➤ Grasp the pessary with the forceps and squeeze together (Fig. 53–2).
- ➤ Insert the pessary toward the posterior of the vagina.
- ➤ When resistance is met, remove forceps.
- ➤ Using gloved finger, push the pessary into place behind the suprapubic bone.
- ➤ Have the client urinate to determine adequacy of placement.
- ➤ Have the client ambulate and squat to evaluate if the client has pain or discomfort or if the pessary gets displaced with position changes.

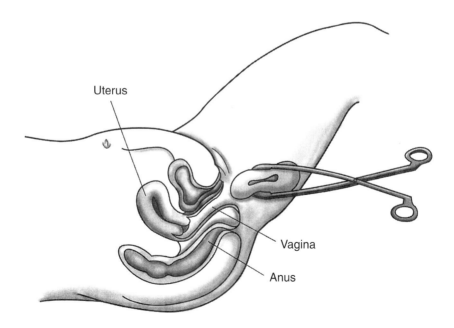

FIGURE 53 • 2 Squeeze the pessary with forceps, and insert toward the posterior vagina.

Client Instructions

➤ You have a _____ type of pessary inserted to maintain the position of the   uterus   bladder   rectum   pelvic floor.
➤ Your pessary should be removed   daily   weekly   monthly and cleaned with soap and water.
➤ Vaginal douching with half water and half vinegar is suggested to decrease the chance of infection and vaginal odor.
➤ Report the following symptoms as soon as possible
  ➤ Urinary retention
  ➤ Urinary frequency
  ➤ Urinary urgency
  ➤ Difficulty urinating
  ➤ Foul vaginal odor
  ➤ Vaginal discharge
➤ Your next appointment to check your pessary placement is _____ .

BIBLIOGRAPHY

Davila, G.W. (1996). Vaginal prolapse: management with nonsurgical techniques. *Postgrad Med*, 99(4), 171–176, 181, 184–185.

DeCherney, A.H., and Pernoll, M.L. (eds.). (1994) (8th ed.). *Current obstetrical and gynecologic diagnosis and treatment*. Norwalk, CT: Appleton & Lange.

Nygaard, I. (1995). Prevention of exercise incontinence with mechanical devices. *J Reprod Med*, 40(2), 89–94.

Youngkin, E.Q., & Davis, M.S. (1994). *Women's health: a primary care clinical guide*. Norwalk, CT: Appleton & Lange.

Zeitlin, M.P., and Lobherz, T.B. (1992). Pessaries in the geriatric patient. *J Am Geriatr Soc*, 40(6), 635–639.

54 VASECTOMY

MARGARET R. COLYAR

CPT Code
55250   Vasectomy

Vasectomy is a one-time sterilization technique. It is simple and safe. Vasectomy closes the tubes in the scrotum so that sperm cannot be transported to the penis. It does not interfere with sexual relations or impair sexual functioning. Vasectomy is considered a permanent procedure and is not easily reversible. Approximately a 50% rate of pregnancy occurs after reversal of a vasectomy.

OVERVIEW

➤ Incidence
  ➤ More than 500,000 men have a vasectomy performed in the United States each year.
➤ Cost-effective method of contraception
➤ Procedure takes approximately 20 to 30 minutes to perform

RATIONALE

➤ To prevent transportation of sperm from the testes through the penis.

INDICATIONS

➤ Desire to prevent pregnancy
➤ Have all children that are desired
➤ Cannot or does not want to use other methods of contraception

CONTRAINDICATIONS

➤ Infection in the genital area
➤ Coagulation disorder

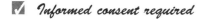 *Informed consent required*

PROCEDURE

Vasectomy

Equipment

➤ Towel—nonsterile
➤ Warm water—tap
➤ Antiseptic skin cleanser
➤ Fenestrated drape—sterile
➤ Nonfenestrated drape—sterile
➤ Gloves—sterile
➤ 10-mL syringe
➤ 27-gauge, $1^1/_2$-inch needle
➤ 1% lidocaine without epinephrine (10 mL)
➤ Battery-powered **cautery** pen
➤ Three **hemostats**—sterile
➤ **Forceps**—sterile
➤ Scissors—sterile
➤ Two vascular clamps or towel clamps—sterile
➤ No. 15 scalpel
➤ Needle holder—sterile
➤ 4-0 chromic suture
➤ **Steri strips**
➤ Container with 10% **formalin**

➤ Topical antibiotic ointment (Bactroban, Neosporin, or Polysporin)
➤ 4 × 4 gauze—sterile
➤ Tape

Procedure

➤ Position the client on his abdomen or on his side with knees drawn up to abdomen.
➤ Warm the scrotum with a warm, moist towel to promote relaxation of the scrotum.
➤ Clip scrotal hair.
➤ Cleanse the scrotum with antiseptic skin cleanser.
➤ Place the nonfenestrated drape underneath the scrotum.
➤ Place the fenestrated drape over the scrotum.
➤ Put on gloves.
➤ Locate and hold in place the vas deferens with three fingers and push it toward the top of the scrotum (Fig. 54–1).
➤ Anesthetize along both sides of the vas deferens using 3 to 5 mL of 1% lidocaine on each side.
➤ Incise the scrotum over the vas deferens—approximately 1 to 2 cm with the No. 15 scalpel (Fig. 54–2).
➤ Pull the vas deferens through the incision site with the vas clamp or towel clamp.
➤ Remove all the **fascia** from around the vas deferens using hemostats. You should have a loop of vas deferens held by the clamp (Fig. 54–3).
➤ Attach two curved hemostats to the vas deferens approximately 2 cm apart (Fig. 54–4).

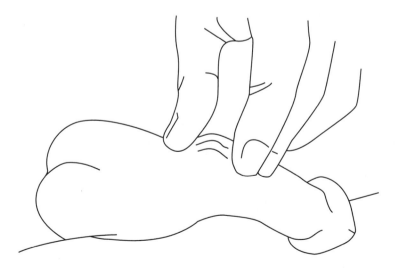

FIGURE 54 • 1 Locate and hold the vas deferens in place, and push it toward the scrotum.

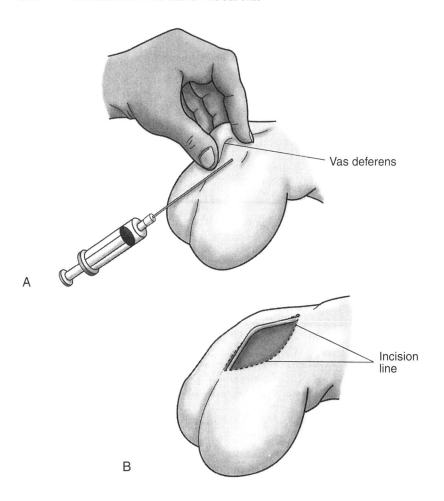

FIGURE 54 • 2 *(A)* Anesthetize along both sides of the vas deferens. *(B)* Incise the scrotum over the vas deferens.

➤ Clip the center of the vas deferens (Fig. 54–5).
➤ Cauterize each end of the partially clipped vas deferens.
➤ Apply Steri strips to the skin of the scrotum (see Chapter 20).

Client Instructions

➤ You may resume sexual intercourse as desired or wait 7 days.
➤ Another method of birth control must be used until the sperm are out of your system.
   ➤ You must flush the sperm out of the system. This takes approximately 20 ejaculations.
➤ Use condoms. A vasectomy does not protect against sexually transmitted diseases.

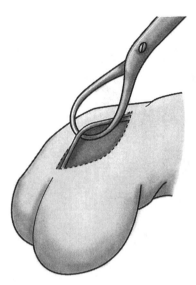

FIGURE 54 • 3 After removing all fascia from the vas deferens, pull it into view with a clamp.

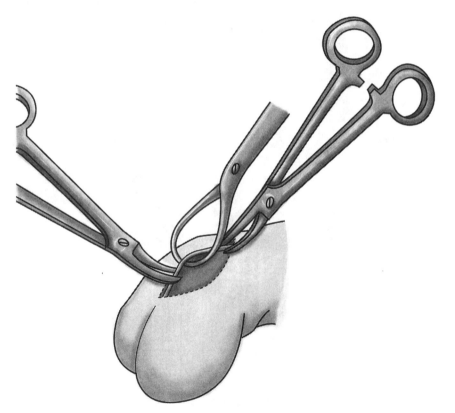

FIGURE 54 • 4 Attach two curved hemostats to the vas deferens approximately 2 cm apart.

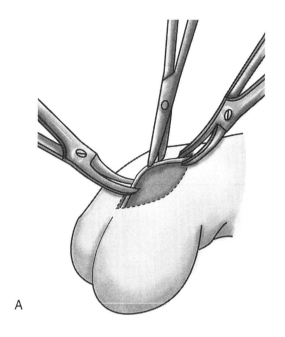

A

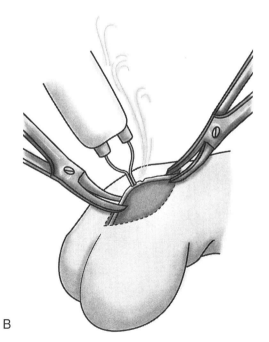

B

FIGURE 54 • 5 *(A)* Clip the center of the vas deferens halfway through in two areas 1 cm apart. *(B)* Cauterize the ends and complete the transection.

➤ Apply ice to the scrotum to prevent swelling.
➤ You may shower in 24 hours.
➤ Keep the area clean and dry.
➤ Return to the office in 6 weeks with a sample of semen taken within 12 hours of ejaculation.
  ➤ This sample is tested to ensure that there are no live sperm.
➤ Another sample of semen is required in 3 months to ensure the lack of sperm.

BIBLIOGRAPHY

Greenberg, M.J. (1989). Vasectomy technique. *Am Fam Physician,* 39(1), 131.

(1991). Vasectomy: Procedures for your practice. *Patient Care,* October, 116.

(2002). www.vasectomymedical.com.

Head: Eyes, Ears, Nose, and Mouth

55 AUDIOMETRY TESTING

CYNTHIA R. EHRHARDT

CPT Code
92551   Screening examination, pure-tone only

The **audiogram** is an objective assessment tool for the detection of hearing problems or loss in most age groups older than 6 months. The **audiogram** is not effective with children younger than 4 months of age. Hearing loss results in delayed speech and language development in infants and toddlers and poor academic progress in preschool-aged and school-aged children. Hearing loss in adults can be the cause of deterioration in interpersonal behaviors and social interactions.

OVERVIEW

➤ Incidence of hearing loss
  ➤ Approximately 1 in every 15 (16 million) Americans
  ➤ Infants—1 in 1000
➤ Average age of onset of hearing loss
  ➤ 55 to 75 years
➤ Suggested topics to discuss with the client
  ➤ Epidemiology of the cause of the dysfunction or hearing loss
➤ Environmental variables that contribute to the dysfunction (including allergies and smoking)
➤ Intervention variables that can improve the outcome of the problem

HEALTH PROMOTION/PREVENTION
Adults, Children, and Adolescents

➤ Avoid potential environmental circumstances that would produce severe loud sounds such as
  ➤ High-volume music with or without earphones
  ➤ Explosions
  ➤ Loud machinery
➤ Restrict agents that have ototoxic effects.
➤ Use decibel-reducing earplugs.

Infants and Toddlers

➤ Prevent factors such as
  ➤ Prenatal infections (cytomegalovirus, rubella, syphilis, human immun-odeficiency virus [HIV], herpes)
  ➤ Maternal drug and alcohol abuse
  ➤ Low birth weight
  ➤ Newborn jaundice
  ➤ Meningitis
  ➤ Head trauma
  ➤ Exposure to loud noises

RATIONALE

➤ To detect hearing problems or loss
➤ To prevent delayed speech and language development

INDICATIONS

➤ Evaluation of hearing loss
➤ Routine screening for infants and children
➤ Routine adult well-care screening
➤ Occupational screening for individuals in noisy work settings
➤ Speech and language development delays in infants and children
➤ Poor academic progress in school-age children
➤ High-risk infants for pre-existing hearing deficit
➤ Deterioration in interpersonal skills in home or work environment for the adult
➤ Unexplained behavior changes in the geriatric individual
➤ Complaints of tinnitus (ringing in the ears)

CONTRAINDICATIONS

➤ Cerumen obstruction
➤ Otitis externa
➤ Younger than 6 months (inaccurate readings)

PROCEDURE

Audiometry Testing

Equipment

➤ Audiometry tool with the recommended features (Fig. 55–1)
  ➤ Decibel frequencies 500 to 4000 Hz
  ➤ Correct size earpiece to ensure a good seal over the external canal opening
  ➤ Quiet room

Procedure

➤ Position the client in a comfortable sitting position.
➤ Ask the client to indicate hearing a tone by raising his or her hand.

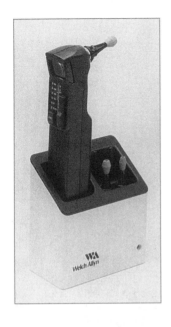

FIGURE 55 • 1 AudioScope 3. (Photo courtesy of Welch Allyn, Inc.)

➤ Inspect the ear canal for infection or cerumen obstruction.
➤ If using a hand-held model, select the proper ear probe for good seal of external canal (Fig. 55–2).
  ➤ Activate probe.
➤ If using a hand-held model, gently grasp the pinna and pull back (for children) or up and back (for adults) to obtain a good seal.
➤ If using an earphone or earplug model, position the equipment so that it covers the entire external os with a good seal.
➤ Begin testing as directed by the instrument manual.
➤ Record the results.
➤ Interpret the results (examples in Fig. 55–3 are from the AudioScope 3 by Welch Allyn).
  ➤ Note normal hearing screening range.
➤ If not within normal limits, suggest repeating at another time.
➤ If results are persistently not in normal range of screening (two or three testings), REFER to an audiologist for further testing.
➤ Review the results and implications of their interpretation in the management of the client's health problems with the client and/or parents. Suggested topics include
  ➤ Epidemiology of the cause of the dysfunction
  ➤ Environmental variables that contribute to the dysfunction (including allergies and smoking)
  ➤ Intervention variables that can improve outcome of the problem
  ➤ Referral to certified audiologist who can perform more detailed evaluation of hearing loss and recommend appropriate devices that can amplify sound and reduce hearing loss

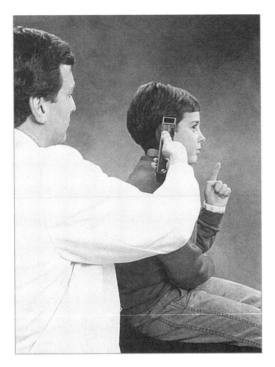

FIGURE 55 • 2 After obtaining a good seal, have the client indicate hearing a tone by raising a finger. (Photo courtesy of Welch Allyn, Inc.)

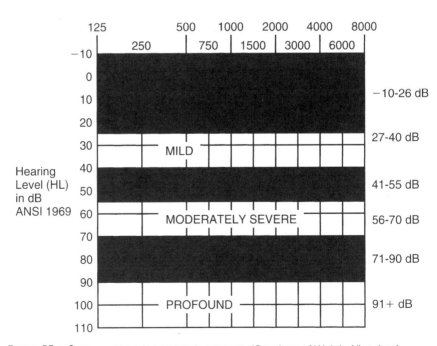

FIGURE 55 • 3 Normal hearing screening range. (Courtesy of Welch Allyn, Inc.)

Client Instructions

➤ Your hearing loss is caused by _____ .
➤ Some environmental variables that contribute to your hearing loss
  include
  ➤ Allergies
  ➤ Smoking
  ➤ Loud music
➤ To improve the outcome of your problem, do not allow smoking in the
  house.
➤ You should see a certified audiologist who can perform more detailed
  evaluation of hearing loss and recommend appropriate devices to amplify
  sound and reduce hearing loss.

MANUFACTURING COMPANIES

Micro Audiometrics
3749-B South Nova Road
Port Orange, FL 32019

Maico Hearing Instruments
7375 Bush Lane Road
Minneapolis, MN 55435

Aussco-Vasc
3421 North Lincoln Avenue
Chicago, IL 60657

Welch Allyn, Inc
4341 State Street Road
PO Box 220
Skaneateles Falls, NY 13153

BIBLIOGRAPHY
Baltross, S., et al (1995). Early identification and management of hearing impairment. *Am Fam Physician*, 51(6), 1437–1451.
Pfenninger, J.L., and Fowler, G.C. (1994). *Procedures for primary care physicians*. St. Louis: Mosby.
Roberts, R. (1995). Marriage of practice guidelines and outcomes research, screening for hearing impairments in newborns. *Am Fam Physician*, 51(6), 1452–1456.
United States Preventive Services Task Force. (1989). Screening for hearing impairment. In Guide to clinical preventative services: adult screening for hearing. *Nurse Practitioner,* 21(6), 106–116.
Welch Allyn. (1995). *AudioScope 3: instructions manual for portable audiometer instrument.* Skaneateles Falls, NY: Author.
Zozove, P., and Kileny, P. (1990). Devices for hearing impaired. *Am Fam Physician*, 46(3), 1876.

56

OCCIPITAL NERVE BLOCK

TRACY CALL-SCHMIDT

CPT Code

64405   Occipital nerve block, unilateral

64405–50   Occipital nerve block, bilateral

64640   Occipital nerve block, neurolytic

Occipital blocks are helpful in the treatment of occipital neuralgia and associated headaches. This type of nerve block is diagnostic and therapeutic. In general, injections can be provided with or without steroid. Without a steroid, a block may be performed when acute headaches occur, taking into account risk-to-benefit ratios. A general rule of thumb is that two injections using a steroid can be done over 2 weeks, then in 3 to 4 months, if necessary. The addition of steroid decreases inflammation at the nerve site. Magnetic resonance imaging and possibly radiographs of the cervical spine to rule out intracranial pathology or congenital abnormalities should be done unless a chronic intractable condition is present. Other treatment of this disorder includes massage, rest, and antidepressants.

OVERVIEW

➤ Incidence is unknown.
➤ It is crucial to be familiar with the anatomy at the injection site.
  ➤ Peripheral nerves can be located by anatomy related to structures they are next to or by nerve stimulators.
➤ Conditions that indicate injection include
  ➤ Occipital neuralgia of the lesser and/or greater occipital nerve. This can be caused by repetitive hyperextension or repeated muscle contraction of the neck or neck injury. These simple sensory nerves supply vascular sensation to the base of the neck resulting in headaches.
➤ Pain usually is described as a sudden-onset, sharp nervelike persistent pain at the skull base. Tension-type headaches can mimic occipital neuralgia pain and are more common in occurrence.

COMPLICATIONS

➤ Postblock ecchymosis
➤ Hematoma

- Pain increased
- Bleeding
- Immediate total spinal anesthetic (if needle enters the foramen magnum)—can lead to death
- Infection
- Nerve damage/paralysis

RATIONALE

- To decrease occipital neuralgia pain
- To restore function

INDICATIONS

- Occipital neuralgia

CONTRAINDICATIONS

- Infection at the site
- Hypersensitivity to the medications to be injected
  Use caution if on anticoagulation therapy (use a 27-gauge needle to avoid bleed).

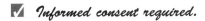 *Informed consent required.*

PROCEDURE

Occipital Nerve Block—Greater and Lesser Occipital Nerves

Equipment

- Alcohol prep pads
- Povidone-iodine prep pads
- Gloves—nonsterile
- Syringe—10- to 12-mL sterile syringes—one for unilateral/two for bilateral
- Needles—22-gauge $1^1/_2$- inch
- 10 to 20 mL of occipital block anesthetic of choice (amount used depends on unilateral or bilateral injection) (Table 56–1)
- Corticosteroid of choice—40 to 80 mg of methylprednisolone (80 mg if first block and 40 mg for subsequent blocks)—optional
- One 4 × 4 gauze—sterile
- Ice pack—optional

Procedure

- Draw 10 mL of anesthetic agent into the syringe (two 10-mL syringes if planning to do bilateral injections).
  - Add corticosteroid dose based on first block or subsequent blocks (see earlier).

TABLE 56•1 COMMON OCCIPITAL NERVE BLOCK AGENTS

TYPE/PACKAGING	DOSE
Anesthetics	
Bupivacaine (Marcaine) 0.25%	10 mL
6–8 hours of relief or headache resolution	
Lidocaine 1% or 2% (Xylocaine)	10 mL
$1^1/_2$ hours relief or headache resolution	
Corticosteroids	
Methylprednisolone	40 mg
Methylprednisolone 80 mg can be	
administered during the first block	
and 40 mg to blocks thereafter	
Triamcinolone acetonide (Kenalog) 10 mg/mL	5–10 mg
Triamcinolone diacetate (Aristocort) 25 mg/mL	12.5–25 mg

➤ If both agents are used, mix by rolling the syringe back and forth.
➤ Place the patient in a sitting position leaning forward over the examination table with chin to chest (can use a pillow for comfort).
➤ Identify anatomic landmarks by palpation. Identify the occipital artery, then palpate the superior nuchal ridge.
  ➤ Mark this area either unilateral or bilateral.
➤ Put on gloves.
➤ Cleanse the site with alcohol followed by povidone-iodine (allow to air dry).
➤ Insert needle medial to the occipital artery, advancing the needle in a perpendicular approach.
  ➤ **Do not inject facing toward the spinal cord.**
  ➤ Advance the needle to the periosteum of the occipital bone.
  ➤ **The patient should be warned that he/she might experience paresthesia at the needle insertion site.**
➤ Gently aspirate. If blood is obtained, remove the needle and apply pressure.
➤ Inject 4 to 5 mL of solution in a fanlike distribution (Fig. 56–1) being sure to avoid the foramen magnum.
  ➤ Next, turn the needle laterally.
  ➤ Aspirate and inject up to 4 mL to cover the lesser and superficial branches of the occipital nerve. You may be able to palpate a lump at the site of injection, which is normal.
➤ Remove needle, and apply pressure for at least 1 minute with sterile 4 × 4 gauze.
➤ Apply an ice pack to the area of injection, and monitor patient for swelling and immediate pain control at site.
➤ Monitor client for adverse reaction to medication procedure for approximately 20 minutes.

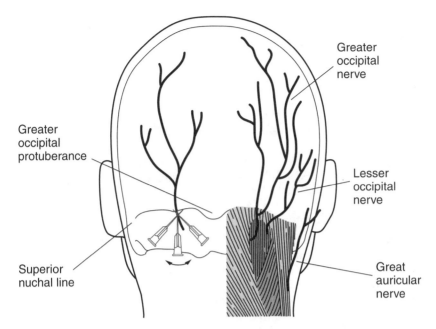

FIGURE 56 • 1 Anatomic landmarks for occipital nerve block insertion and fanlike distribution of medication.

Client Instructions

➤ Apply ice to area if pain persists after procedure.
➤ Report any signs or symptoms of infection such as
  ➤ Red streaks
  ➤ Yellow-green drainage
  ➤ Fever
➤ No bandage is necessary due to area being in the scalp/hair.
➤ Postprocedure pain may occur 36 hours after injection.
➤ Take ibuprofen 600 to 800 mg every 6 hours if needed.
➤ Call office if pain becomes severe or does not resolve in 36 hours.

BIBLIOGRAPHY

➤ Katz, J. (1985). *Atlas of regional anesthesia.* Norwalk, CT: Appleton-Century-Crofts.
➤ National Institute of Neurological Disorders and Stroke, National Institutes of Health. Bethesda, MD. Available at: http://accessible.ninds.nih.gov/health_medical/disorders/occipitalneuralgia.
➤ Waldman, S.D. (1996). *Interventional pain management.* Philadelphia: Saunders.
➤ Waldman, S.D. (2000). *Atlas of pain management injection techniques.* Philadelphia: Saunders.

57 TYMPANOMETRY

CYNTHIA R. EHRHARDT

CPT Code
92567 Tympanometry (impedance testing)
92568 Tympanometry with acoustic reflex

Tympanometry is an objective assessment tool for the mobility of the tympanic membrane, pressure within the middle ear, and volume of the external canal. This tool is used to measure resolution of otitis media and serous otitis media, determine the presence of eustachian tube dysfunction problems, and screen for causes of developmental delays.

OVERVIEW
- Incidence unknown

RATIONALE
- To assess mobility of the tympanic membrane, pressure in the middle ear, and eustachian tube dysfunction
- To determine causes of developmental delay

INDICATIONS
- Evaluation of hearing loss
- Evaluation of ear pain
- Establishing mobility of the tympanic membrane
- Detection of tympanic membrane perforation
- Assessment of middle ear function when audiometry is not possible
- Documentation of absence or presence of effusions of the middle ear
- Monitoring of effusions of the middle ear
- Evaluation of the effectiveness of pressure-equalization tubes
- Unexplained developmental delays in infants and children

CONTRAINDICATIONS
- Cerumen obstruction
- Otitis externa
- Younger than 4 months—leads to inaccurate readings

PROCEDURE

Tympanometry

Equipment

➤ Tympanometry tool with the recommended features (Fig. 57–1)
  ➤ 226-Hz probe tone
  ➤ Various-size ear tips that ensure a good seal over the external canal opening
  ➤ Air pressure range of (400 daPa (decaPascals) to +200 daPa (1.02 mm H$_2$O equals 1.0 daPa)
  ➤ Easy-to-use buttons to activate tool
  ➤ Readable numbers
  ➤ Printable results—optional

Procedure

➤ Inspect the ear canal for infection or cerumen obstruction.
➤ Adjust tympanometer device for altitude (usually not needed below 1280 feet) (Table 57–1).
➤ Position the client in a comfortable sitting position.
➤ Explain the procedure, including how the client will indicate hearing the tone.
➤ Select the proper ear tip for good seal of external canal.

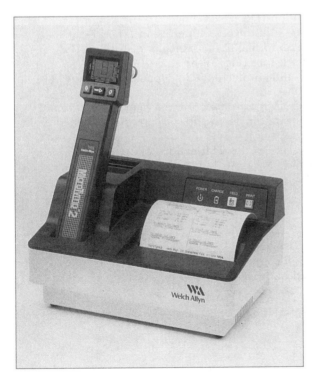

FIGURE 57 • 1 MicroTymp 2, portable tympanometric instrument. (Photo courtesy of Welch Allyn, Inc.)

TABLE 57•1 ALTITUDE ADJUSTMENTS

ALTITUDE, FT	ADJUSTMENT FOR 0.5 mL (mL)	ADJUSTMENT FOR 1.0 mL (mL)	ADJUSTMENT FOR 1.5 mL (mL)	ADJUSTMENT FOR 2.0 mL (mL)
1280	0.0	0.0	0.0	0.0
2530	0.0	0.1	0.1	0.2
3220	0.0	0.1	0.2	0.3
4757	0.1	0.2	0.3	0.4

➤ Activate.
➤ Gently grasp the pinna and pull back (for children) or up and back (for adults) to obtain a good seal.
➤ Apply the probe to the external canal with a good seal.
➤ When a good seal is achieved (machine indicates this), activate the test switch.
➤ Record the reading as directed by the instrument manual.
➤ Print out the results.
➤ Interpret the tympanogram results (examples are from the MicroTymp 2 by Welch Allyn).
  ➣ Normal tympanogram (Fig. 57–2)
  ➣ Too much artifact (Fig. 57–3)
  ➣ Ear canal occlusion (Fig. 57–4)
  ➣ Otitis media with effusion (Fig. 57–5)
  ➣ Oncoming or resolving otitis media with effusion (Fig. 57–6)
  ➣ Tympanic membrane abnormalities or ossicular disruption (Fig. 57–7)
  ➣ Negative middle ear pressure (Fig. 57–8)
  ➣ Patent **tympanostomy** tube or perforated tympanic membrane (Fig. 57–9)
➤ Review the results and their interpretation in the management of the client's health problems with the client and/or parents. Suggested topics include
  ➣ Epidemiology of the cause of the dysfunction
  ➣ Environmental variables that contribute to the dysfunction (including allergies, smoking, loud noises)
  ➣ Intervention variables that can improve outcome of the problem

Client Instructions

➤ You have the following problems: _____.
➤ Stay away from factors in the environment that cause your allergies to flare.
➤ No smoking is permitted in the house.

MANUFACTURING COMPANIES

Grason-Stadler, Inc
1 Westchester Drive
Milford, NH 03055–3056

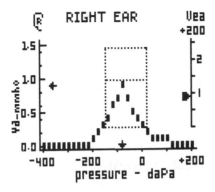

* Produces tympanogram within normal limits
A   relative to height and width

Tympanometric Measurement	Child's Ear (Under Age 10) 90% Range	Adult's Ear (Over Age 10) 90% range
Peak Ya	0.2 to 0.9 mmho	0.3 to 1.4 mmho
Gradient (GR) (Tympanometric Width)	60 to 150 daPa	50 to 110 daPa
Tympanometric Peak Pressure (TPP)	-139 to +11 daPa	-83 to 0 daPa
Equivalent Ear Canal Volume (Vea)	0.4 to 1.0 cc	0.6 to 1.5 cc

NOTE: For purposes of tympanometric norms, an adult is defined as a person 10 years of age or older, and a child as under age 10.
Normative data are taken from a study by Margolis and Heller (1987), and from the "Guidelines for Screening for Hearing Impairments and Middle
B   Ear Disorders" ASHA (1990).

FIGURE 57 • 2 The normal ear. (A) Tympanogram from a normal ear. (B) Normative tympanometric data. (Photo courtesy of Welch Allyn, Inc.)

Maico Hearing Instruments
7375 Bush Lane Road
Minneapolis, MN 55435

Micro Audiometrics
3749-B South Nova Road
Port Orange, FL 32019

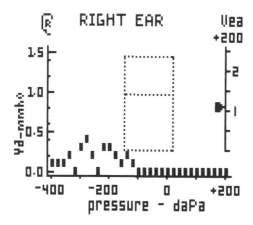

Tympanogram with Too Much Artifact
- Caused by patient or practitioner movement
- Requires repeating measurement

FIGURE 57 • 3 Conditions that cause too much artifact. (Photo courtesy of Welch Allyn, Inc.)

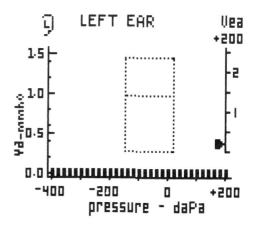

Ear Canal Occlusion
- Can produce flat tympanogram with ear canal volume lower than expected
- May also produce BLOCK message
- Requires repeating measurement

FIGURE 57 • 4 Conditions that artificially flatten the tympanogram. (Photo courtesy of Welch Allyn, Inc.)

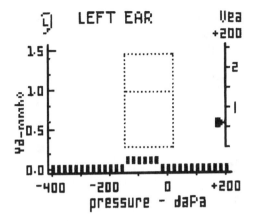

- Produces low static admittance
  (low peak height) tympanogram
- Tympanogram is also typical of tympanosclerosis, cholesteatoma, and middle ear tumor

FIGURE 57 • 5 Otitis media with effusion. (Photo courtesy of Welch Allyn, Inc.)

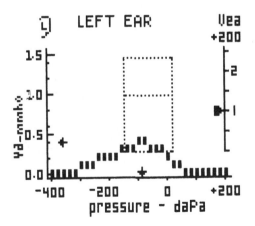

FIGURE 57 • 6 Oncoming or resolving otitis media with effusion. (Photo courtesy of Welch Allyn, Inc.)

- Produces normal peak height, but tympanogram
  which is too wide
- Tympanogram is also typical of tympanosclerosis

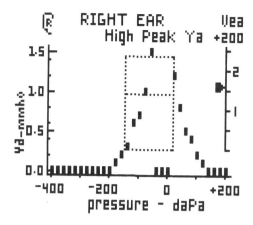

• Produces high static admittance
  (high peak height) tympanogram

FIGURE 57 • 7 Tympanic membrane
abnormalities or ossicular disruption.
(Photo courtesy of Welch Allyn, Inc.)

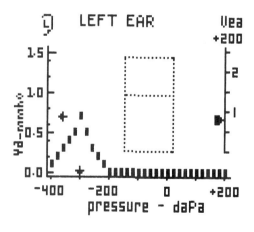

• Produces negative Tympanometric Peak
  Pressure (TPP) tympanogram
• Usually not associated with effusion when
  Peak Ya is normal
• Also associated with eustachian tube
  dysfunction, cold, or allergies

FIGURE 57 • 8 Negative middle ear
pressure. (Photo courtesy of Welch
Allyn, Inc.)

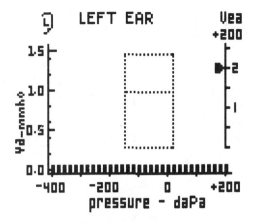

- Can produce flat tympanogram with ear canal volume higher than expected
- May also produce OPEN message

FIGURE 57 • 9 Patent tympanotomy tube or perforated tympanic membrane. (Photo courtesy of Welch Allyn, Inc.)

American Electromedics Corporation
13 Columbia Drive
Amherst, NH 03031

Welch Allyn, Inc
4341 State Street Road
PO Box 220
Skaneateles Falls, NY 13153

BIBLIOGRAPHY

American Medical Association (1996). *Physicians' current procedural terminology.* Chicago: Author.
Baltross, S., et al (1995). Early identification and management of hearing impairment. *Am Fam Physician,* 51(6), 1437–1451.
Bredfeldt, R. (1991). An introduction to tympanometry. *Am Fam Physician,* 44(6), 2113–2117.
Pfenninger, J.L., and Fowler, G.C. (1994). *Procedures for primary care physicians.* St. Louis: Mosby.
Welch Allyn (1995). *AudioScope 3: instructions manual for portable audiometer instrument.* Skaneateles Falls, NY: Author.

VISUAL FUNCTION—
EVALUATION

58
SNELLEN, ILLITERATE E

MARGARET R. COLYAR

CPT Code
Included in the office visit

Evaluation of visual function includes the testing of visual acuity, visual field defects, **strabismus,** and color vision. Visual acuity is tested using the Snellen eye chart. If the client is young or unable to read, the Illiterate E chart is more appropriate (Fig. 58–1). Visual field defects are tested by performing **confrontation**. Strabismus (squint, crossed eye) is tested in the ambulatory care setting using the cover/uncover test, corneal light reflex, and extraocular muscle movement tests. Color vision is tested using the Ishihara's or Hardy Rand Rittler's **polychromatic** cards.

OVERVIEW

➤ Incidence
  ➤ All yearly examinations and if an eye disorder is suspected
➤ The main causes of decreased visual acuity
  ➤ Diabetes mellitus
  ➤ Hypertension
  ➤ Cataracts
  ➤ Glaucoma
  ➤ Retinal detachment
➤ The main causes of visual field defects
  ➤ Glaucoma
  ➤ Retinitis
  ➤ Intracerebral tumors
  ➤ Detached retina
➤ The main causes of strabismus
  ➤ Hyperthyroidism
  ➤ Myasthenia gravis
  ➤ Cranial artery aneurysms
  ➤ Multiple sclerosis
  ➤ Neurologic disease
  ➤ Orbital disease
  ➤ **Amblyopia**

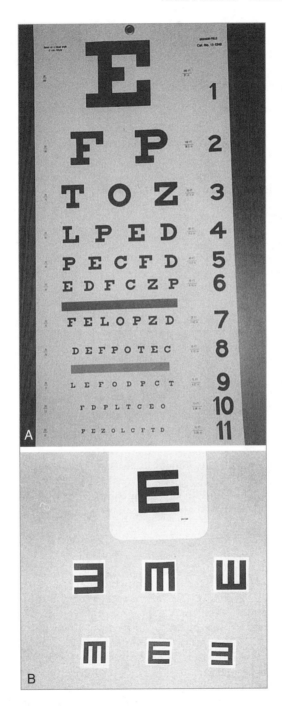

FIGURE 58 • 1 (A) Snellen and (B) Illiterate E eye charts.

Eight% of white males and 4% of black males inherit the recessive X-linked trait for color blindness. Although not disabling, a deficit in color vision may cause problems in learning and the ability to assess traffic lights.

HEALTH PROMOTION/PREVENTION

- Yearly eye examination
- Avoid stress and strain on the eyes

RATIONALE

- To evaluate visual function
- To determine the presence of visual defects

INDICATIONS

- Children
- Clients with visual complaints
- Ocular trauma
- Screening for school and employment
- Headache

CONTRAINDICATIONS

- None

PROCEDURE

Visual Examination

Equipment

- Penlight
- Snellen or Illiterate E eye chart
- 20-foot hall
- Color vision book—Ishihara or Hardy Rand Rittler set
- Near-vision chart or newspaper

Procedure

VISUAL ACUITY

- Have the client stand 20 feet from the chart.
  - Cover one eye and have the client read the smallest line. Do the same with the alternate eye. Then test with both eyes open.
  - If there is a difference of two or more levels between the eyes, suspect ambylopia. REFER to an ophthalmologist.
- If the client is age 40 or older, check near vision by having the client read at a distance of 14 inches.
- Record the results.
  - The first number indicates how far the client was standing from the eye chart. The second number indicates how far the person with normal sight could read the letters of a particular height.

- A measurement of 20/40 means the client can read at 20 feet what a normally sighted person can read at 40 feet.
- Always indicate if this measurement is with or without glasses.

VISUAL FIELDS—CONFRONTATION

➤ Stand 2 feet from the client.
➤ Have the client cover one eye with his or her hand and stare into your eye. The examiner also must cover the same eye.
➤ Hold an object (pencil, penlight) in each of the visual fields.
➤ Have the client indicate when he or she can see the object in each of the visual fields.
➤ The client's peripheral vision should match the vision of the examiner.
➤ Record the results.
   ➤ Document where a deficit occurs by using time on a clock or blackened circles (Fig. 58–2).

STRABISMUS

If discovered, REFER to an ophthalmologist.
➤ Observe both eyes to detect the deviation of one eye.
   ➤ Exotropia—lateral deviation
   ➤ Esotropia—nasal deviation

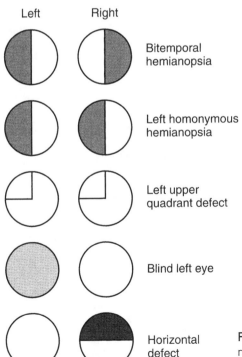

Left   Right

Bitemporal hemianopsia

Left homonymous hemianopsia

Left upper quadrant defect

Blind left eye

Horizontal defect

FIGURE 58 • 2 One method to document where a deficit occurs is to use blackened circles.

➤ To differentiate between paralytic and nonparalytic strabismus, check extraocular movement 2 to 3 feet away. Document deviation of the eyes.
➤ Perform corneal light reflex test.
  ➤ With strabismus, the light falls on different parts of the cornea.
➤ Perform cover/uncover test.
  ➤ With strabismus, the covered eye wanders and may or may not return to its position when uncovered.

COLOR VISION

➤ Using a color vision book, have the client read the numbers on each page of the book.
➤ Record on the chart the numbers that the client cannot read.
➤ Use the interpretive guidelines provided by the color vision book.

Client Instructions

➤ Based on the tests done in the office/clinic today, we observed the following problems:

_____

_____

_____

➤ An examination by an ophthalmologist is needed/not needed.
➤ Please make an appointment with your ophthalmologist within the next day/week/month for evaluation.

B IBLIOGRAPHY

Bates, B., et al (1995). *A guide to physical examination and history taking.* Philadelphia: Lippincott-Raven.

Jarvis, C. (1996). *Physical examination and health assessment.* Philadelphia: Saunders.

59

CORNEAL ABRASION AND FOREIGN BODY REMOVAL—EYE

CYNTHIA R. EHRHARDT

> ## CPT Code
> 65205   Removal of foreign body; external eye, conjunctival, superficial
>
> 65210   Removal of foreign body; external eye, conjunctival, embedded
>
> 65220   Removal of foreign body; external eye, corneal without slit lamp
>
> 99070   Eye tray: Supplies and material provided by physician over and above what usually is included in office visit

Corneal abrasions occur because of trauma to the anterior globe of the eye with or without penetration by a foreign object. Corneal foreign bodies result from superficial penetration by a foreign object to the anterior globe of the eye. The nurse practitioner should attempt to remove only foreign bodies that are superficial.

OVERVIEW

➤ Incidence
  ➤ 93% of injuries to the eye are nonperforating in nature.
  ➤ 72% involve the anterior chamber.
  ➤ 65% of injuries in children result from falls or sports.
  ➤ 5% of injuries to the eye are superficially perforating in nature.
➤ Complications
  ➤ Loss of vision
  ➤ Onset of corneal ulcer
  ➤ Loss of the eye organ
➤ Causes
  ➤ Adults
    • Foreign objects at work or home
  ➤ Children
    • BB-gun pellet fragments

311

- Projectile metallic objects
- Other foreign objects
- Falls
- Sports injuries
  - ➤ Any injuries involving children may require reporting to the responsible legal authorities. (Consult your local law enforcement officer.)
- ➤ General principles
  - ➤ Prolonged use of an eyepatch greater than 48 hours increases the risk of **amblyopia** for the client (especially children).
  - ➤ Tetanus booster: Needed if not received within 5 years.
- ➤ Perform an eye examination.
  - ➤ Document visual acuity with the use of the Snellen chart or eye card.
  - ➤ Visually inspect the eye and orbit region.
  - ➤ Inspect and palpate orbit rim for instability.
  - ➤ Verify equivocal sensation to orbit rim.
  - ➤ Verify presence or absence of corneal reflex (cotton wisp test).
  - ➤ Verify pupillary response.
  - ➤ Verify conjunctival status.
    - Absence or presence of subconjunctival hemorrhage
    - Injection
    - Chemosis
  - ➤ Note the location of any visible foreign body.
  - ➤ Note whether the foreign body is superficially embedded or not.
- ➤ Perform an ophthalmic examination.
  - ➤ Inspect anterior globe for
    - Clarity
    - Presence or absence of hyphema
    - Red reflex
    - Lens opacities
    - Vitreous appearance
    - Optic disc appearance
    - Retinal abnormalities (papilledema, vessel occlusion)

HEALTH PROMOTION/PREVENTION

- ➤ Protective eyewear is recommended for all ages while participating in sports.
- ➤ Protective eyewear is recommended when working around any machinery.
- ➤ Lessen the risk of BB-gun exposure through proper gun-handling education classes.
- ➤ Lessen the risk of falling accidents with the use of good safety habits.
- ➤ Wear correct protective eyewear against excessive and prolonged light exposure.

OPTIONS

- ➤ Corneal abrasion
- ➤ Removal of foreign body—eye

RATIONALE

➤ To diminish discomfort
➤ To promote healing
➤ To prevent loss of vision

INDICATIONS

➤ Onset of irritation and/or pain to the eye with a history of trauma
➤ Unilateral sensation of a foreign body present in the eye
➤ History of exposure to ultraviolet light, prolonged sunlight, or tanning beds
➤ History of wearing contact lens
➤ Mild chemical exposure
➤ Red eye
➤ In neonates and infants with unexplained crying, photosensitivity, unilateral tearing, and conjunctival inflammation

CONTRAINDICATIONS

➤ Emergent—REFER immediately to an ophthalmologist.
  ➤ Chemical acid or alkali exposure
    • *If not in the office*—Instruct the client to wash the eyes out immediately with water for a full 15 minutes, then go to the nearest emergency department for further treatment. Alkali chemicals have a more delayed presentation than acid chemicals.
    • *If in the office*—Apply ophthalmic anesthetic, and begin vigorous irrigation with the use of standard intravenous tubing and 0.9% sodium chloride solution or lactated Ringer's solution for 15 minutes or 2 L, whichever comes first.
  ➤ History of high-velocity injury
    • *If not in office*—Close the eyelid, and apply a nonpressure clean dressing to the eye and place sunglasses on.
    • *If in the office*—Apply a nonpressure eye patch and shield.
  ➤ Ruptured globe
  ➤ Corneal or sclera lacerations
  ➤ Lid lacerations
  ➤ Conjunctival lacerations
  ➤ Corneal ulceration
  ➤ Deeply embedded foreign object
  ➤ Unsuccessful removal of foreign body
  ➤ Uncooperative patient (adult, child, or infant) who requires sedation
➤ Urgent—REFER within 48 hours to an ophthalmologist.
  ➤ Onset of corneal opacities
  ➤ Presence of a "rust ring" at the former location of embedded foreign body
  ➤ Increasing pain
  ➤ Loss of vision
  ➤ Nonresolution of corneal abrasion

➤ Onset of preseptal cellulitis with periorbital cellulitis
➤ All children

☑ *Informed consent required*

PROCEDURE

Corneal Abrasion and Foreign Body Removal—Eye

Equipment

CORNEAL ABRASION AND FOREIGN BODY REMOVAL—EYE

➤ Penlight
➤ Direct ophthalmoscope
➤ Gloves—nonsterile
➤ Fluorescein strips
  ➤ Use individually packaged strips—multivial drops increase the risk of infection.
➤ Cobalt blue light **(Wood's light)**
➤ Eye patches
➤ Adhesive tape
➤ Intravenous tubing with sterile 0.9% sodium chloride or lactated Ringer's solution
➤ Tissue or 4 × 4 gauze—nonsterile
➤ Ophthalmic medication (Table 59–1)

FOREIGN BODY REMOVAL—EYE ONLY

➤ Cotton-tipped applicators—nonsterile
➤ 27- or 25-gauge, $^1/_2$- or 1-inch needle

Procedure

CORNEAL ABRASION

➤ Cover the lateral corner of the face with a drape or facial tissue to prevent drainage of dye onto another area of the face because dye can cause permanent stain to clothing.
➤ Provide tissue for client to wipe drips.
➤ Instill 1 to 2 drops of ophthalmic anesthetic or cycloplegic if no contraindications.
➤ Moisten strips with 2 to 3 drops of sterile 0.9% sodium chloride.
➤ Retract the lower lid and touch the moistened strip to the base of the globe until there is good fill.
➤ Allow the client to blink several times to disperse the dye.
➤ Turn off the overhead light and turn on cobalt blue light (Wood's light).
  ➤ Abrasions to the cornea are seen as bright yellow or yellow-green.
➤ Note the size, shape, and location of the abrasion.
➤ *If close to the central line of vision, consider REFERRING to an ophthalmologist because of a high incidence of permanent scarring in this area.*

TABLE 59•1 OPHTHALMIC DROPS THAT CAN BE USED TO TREAT CORNEAL ABRASION AND FOREIGN BODY REMOVAL

TYPE OF MEDICATION*	ONSET/DURATION
Anesthetic Ophthalmic Drops	
Tetracaine (Pontocaine) 0.5%	25 sec/15 min or longer
Proparacaine (Ophthaine) 0.5%	20 sec/10–15 min
Mydriatics†	
Phenylephrine (Neo-Synephrine)	
2.5% and 10% drops	5 min/2–3 hr
Cycloplegics/Mydriatics	
Cyclopentolate (Cyclogyl) 1%	5 min/24 hr
Tropicamide (Tropicacyl) 0.5% and 1%	5 min/6 hr
Homatropine (Homatrine) 2% and 5%	5 min/10–48 hr
Scopolamine (Isopto Hyoscine) 0.25%	5 min/3–5 days
Ophthalmic Antibiotics	
Erythromycin ophthalmic ointment	
Gentamicin (Garamycin) 3 mg/mL solution	
Tobramycin (Tobrex) 3 mg/mL solution or	
3 mg/g ointment	
Sulfacetamide (Sodium Sulamyd)	
10% and 30% solution or 10% ointment	

*To avoid allergic conjunctivitis, single-agent drops are suggested.
† Contraindications: narrow-angle glaucoma, hypertension, coronary artery disease.

➤ When completed, initiate a vigorous irrigation with 0.9% sodium chloride to remove all dye from the eye to lessen any further irritation. Always apply topical ophthalmic antibiotic of choice if an abrasion is found because of the avascular character of the cornea.
➤ Document—may be pictorial or description of location of abrasion.
➤ Apply a single or double eye patch (Fig. 59–1).
➤ Use of a patch should be considered in children older than age 5 years.
➤ The use of a single or double eye patch for all adults with corneal abrasion depends on the comfort of the client.
  ➤ Contraindicated in cases of conjunctivitis

REMOVAL OF FOREIGN BODY—EYE

➤ Have the client lie in a comfortable supine position.
➤ Put on gloves.
➤ Instill 1 to 2 drops of ophthalmic anesthetic.
➤ Spread the eyelids apart with the thumb and index finger.
➤ Have head positioned so that the foreign body is at the highest point on eye globe.
➤ Instruct the client to fix a gaze toward a certain point.
➤ *If not embedded,* use moistened sterile cotton-tipped applicator with gentle rolling motion to remove.

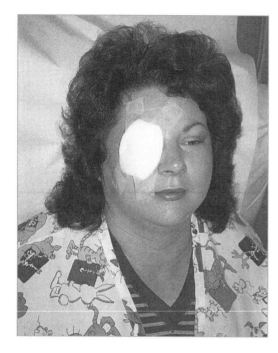

FIGURE 59 • 1 Apply an eye patch after the antibiotic is instilled in the eye.

➤ *If embedded*, use a 27- or 25-gauge needle bevel side up (Fig. 59–2) with pencil grip.
  ➤ Rest your lateral hand on side of the client's cheek for more stability in movement.
➤ Approach at a 90-degree angle to eye globe.
➤ Gently apply pressure across the surface to dislodge foreign body.
➤ After several unsuccessful attempts, apply antibiotic ointment, apply non-pressure patch, and REFER to an ophthalmologist.

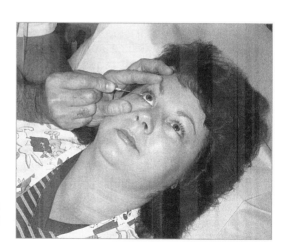

FIGURE 59 • 2 Remove the embedded foreign body using a 25- to 27-gauge needle.

➤ After removal of the foreign body, proceed to check for a corneal abrasion with fluorescein stain and patching.

Client Instructions

➤ *Do not drive yourself home.*
➤ To relieve pain—use acetaminophen with codeine (Tylenol No. 3) every 4 to 6 hours as needed for the first 24 hours. Then use plain or extra-strength acetaminophen (Tylenol) every 4 hours as needed.
  ➤ If the pain persists, call the office.
➤ *Avoid all topical ophthalmic anesthetics* because retardation in healing can occur.
➤ Avoid nonsteroidal therapy for 48 hours because retardation in healing can occur.
➤ Avoid removing the eye patch and rubbing the eye because this can slow the healing process.
➤ Return to the office in 24 and 48 hours to affirm that the healing process is occurring.
  ➤ The *absence* of pain does not guarantee complete resolution of the corneal injury.
➤ Return to the office sooner if
  ➤ Increasing pain without relief with medication
  ➤ Purulent (yellow or green) drainage from eye
  ➤ Loss of vision

BIBLIOGRAPHY

American Medical Association (1996). *Physicians' current procedural terminology.* Chicago: Author.
Berkow, R. (1994) (17th ed.). *The Merck manual.* Rahway, NJ: Merck.
Jones, N. (1989). Eye injury in sport. *Sports Med, 7,* 163–181.
Murtagh, J. (1995) (2nd ed.). *Practice tips.* New York: McGraw-Hill.
Pfenninger, J.L., and Fowler, G.C. (1994). *Procedures for primary care physicians.* St. Louis: Mosby.
Silverman, H., et al (1992). Treatment of common eye injuries. *Am Fam Physician, 45*(5), 449–456.

EYE IRRIGATION

CYNTHIA R. EHRHARDT

CPT Code

None—Billed as part of the office visit

Irrigation of the eye is a procedure done to rid the eye of irritants from chemical exposure. Strong precautions should be taken when working with acid and alkali chemicals because they are strong chemical irritants. Exposure to *alkali chemicals,* such as lye, lime, mortar, cement, plaster, and liquid ammonia, is highly damaging to the eye and *constitutes an ocular emergency.* Seek immediate emergency care.

OVERVIEW

➤ Incidence unknown
➤ Causes
   ➤ Accidental exposure by splashing of alkali or acid liquids into the eye
➤ Complicating factors
   ➤ Corneal injury
   ➤ Temporary or permanent loss of vision
   ➤ Delayed irrigation of alkali chemicals has a higher incidence of permanent vision loss.
   ➤ All alkali burns should be followed up by an ophthalmologist because of the high incidence of permanent injury to the cornea.
   ➤ A signed statement by the client indicating understanding of the importance of follow-up should be obtained because a high percentage of injuries caused by alkali burns have a delayed presentation.

HEALTH PROMOTION/PREVENTION

➤ Prevention is focused on eliminating situations that can result in the incidence of chemical splashing. This includes
   ➤ Use of safety glasses

RATIONALE

➤ To preserve vision

INDICATIONS

➤ Reported history of chemical splash injury to the eye

CONTRAINDICATIONS

➤ Suspected globe penetration or rupture injury

PROCEDURE

Eye Irrigation

Equipment

➤ Snellen chart
➤ Penlight
➤ Ophthalmoscope
➤ 9% sodium chloride, lactated Ringer's, or water—2 L
➤ Intravenous tubing
➤ Gloves—sterile

- 4 × 4 gauze—sterile
- Towels or absorbent pads
- Catch basin
- Eye irrigation kit—optional
  - Several companies offer apparatus to insert into eye for irrigation in place of intravenous tubing
  - Intravenous stand or hook to hang intravenous fluids
  - Ophthalmic anesthesia/antibiotics (Table 60–1)

Procedure

- Secure the client in a comfortable position.
- Perform an ophthalmic examination to ensure no globe perforation.
  - Although a thorough examination of the eye for defects should be undertaken, this should not unnecessarily delay the implementation of eye irrigation.
  - *Do not perform fluorescein examination until eye irrigation has been completed.*
- Administer ophthalmic anesthesia to the affected eye.
- Prepare the irrigation solution and hang the bag from the intravenous stand approximately 3 feet above the head of the client.
- Wrap protective garb (towels or absorbent pads) around the client.
- Position the catch basin to capture the used irrigation solution.
- Put on gloves.
- Gently retract the upper eyelid, and insert the tip of the irrigation tube into eye space (Fig. 60–1). Allow the eyelid to hold the intravenous tubing tip in place.
- Turn on the solution and administer at a rate of continuous flow for the irrigation to be completed in 15 to 20 minutes.
- Remove the irrigation tip on completion of irrigation.
- Perform a fluorescein stain examination (see Chapter 59).

TABLE 60•1 OPHTHALMIC ANESTHESIA AND ANTIBIOTICS

Ophthalmic Anesthesia*
- Tetracaine (Pontocaine) 0.5%
  - Onset of action within 25 sec
  - Duration 15 min or longer
- Proparacaine (Ophthaine) 0.5%
  - Onset of action within 20 sec
  - Duration of 10–15 min

Ophthalmic Antibiotics*
- Erythromycin ophthalmic ointment
- Gentamicin (Garamycin) 3-mg/mL solution
- Tobramycin (Tobrex) 3-mg/mL solution or 3-mg/g ointment
- Sulfacetamide (Sodium Sulamyd) 10% and 30% solution or 10% ointment

* To avoid allergic conjunctivitis, single-agent drops are suggested.

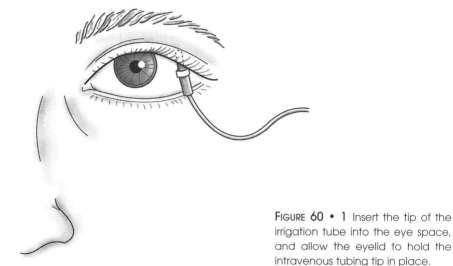

FIGURE 60 • 1 Insert the tip of the irrigation tube into the eye space, and allow the eyelid to hold the intravenous tubing tip in place.

Client Instructions

➤ *Do not drive yourself home.*
➤ Take acetaminophen or Tylenol No. 3 every 4 to 6 hours as needed for pain.
➤ Avoid topical ophthalmic anesthetics because they retard healing.
➤ Avoid nonsteroidal therapy for 48 hours because retardation in healing can occur.
➤ Antibiotics usually are not required. They may be used in presence of corneal abrasion.
➤ Follow-up care
  ➣ In alkali splashes, a follow-up appointment with ophthalmologist is scheduled for _____.
  ➣ If corneal abrasion present and eye patch applied, avoid removing the eye patch and rubbing eye because this can slow the healing process.
➤ Must keep follow-up appointments at 24 and 48 hours to affirm the healing process is occurring; if not, referred to ophthalmologist.
➤ Return to the office sooner if
  ➣ Eye pain increasing without medication relief
  ➣ Purulent drainage from eye
  ➣ Loss of vision

BIBLIOGRAPHY

American Medical Association (1996). *Physicians' current procedural terminology.* Chicago: Author.
Garcia, G. (1996). Management of ocular emergencies and urgent eye problems. *Am Fam Physician,* 53(2), 347–356.
Murtagh, J. (1995) (2nd ed.). *Practice tips.* New York: McGraw-Hill.
Silverman, H., et al (1992). Treatment of common eye injuries. *Am Fam Physician,* 45(5), 449–456.

61

EYE TRAUMA STABILIZATION

CYNTHIA R. EHRHARDT

> ## CPT Code
> None specific—part of the office visit

Eye trauma includes blunt or penetration injuries to the globe of the eye.

OVERVIEW

- ➤ Incidence unknown
  - ➤ Usually associated with blunt trauma, such as physical assault, or with situations that precipitate objects becoming projectiles, such as archery arrows and BB-gun pellets
- ➤ Complications
  - ➤ Fractures of the facial bones
  - ➤ Loss of sight in the affected eye
- ➤ Thoroughly examine the region for anatomic defects.
  - ➤ If possible, establish visual acuity.
  - ➤ *Avoid any pressure to the eyelid and the globe of the eye because it may precipitate a spontaneous and premature rupture and loss of the* **vitreous humor.** *Loss of vitreous humor results in permanent blindness.*
  - ➤ Inspect for disruption in the sclera.
    - Rotate the globe in an upward and downward motion.
    - This is important because when the eyelid closes, the globe automatically rotates upward.
  - ➤ Funduscopic examination
    - Note any iritis injection.
    - Note the absence of the anterior chamber.
    - Note wrinkling of anterior chamber (represents rupture of the chamber).
    - Note the presence or absence of macular edema.
    - Check the vitreous humor for clouding (represents hemorrhage).
    - Note the presence or absence of retinal detachment (i.e., changes in the color and shape of the retinal eye backgrounds compared with the uninjured eye).
  - ➤ Inspect the maxillary structures for loss of integrity.
  - ➤ Inspect the orbit structures for loss of integrity.
  - ➤ Perform a neurologic examination to exclude accompanying head injury.

HEALTH PROMOTION/PREVENTION

➤ Prevention is focused on eliminating situations that can result in the incidence of blunt trauma and penetration wounds. This includes
  ➤ The promotion of safety awareness habits
  ➤ Safety habits in gun and hunting situations
  ➤ Protection against projectile objects with the use of safety glasses
  ➤ Avoiding situations that produce projectile objects

RATIONALE

➤ To preserve eye function

INDICATIONS

➤ Visual inspection of the globe of the eye reveals laceration
➤ Projectile object embedded in the globe of the eye
➤ History of the injury suggests potential for eye globe injury

CONTRAINDICATIONS

➤ None

PROCEDURE

Eye Trauma Stabilization

Equipment

➤ Snellen visual acuity chart
➤ Ophthalmoscope
➤ Slit lamp—optional
➤ Plastic or Styrofoam cup or large eye shield
➤ Two rolls—4-inch gauze wrap
➤ Ophthalmic antibiotic ointment
➤ Eye patch
➤ Adhesive tape (1 or 2 inches)

Procedure

Do not perform the procedure for corneal abrasion (fluorescein stain) if a globe injury is suspected.

➤ Position the client in a comfortable position with the eye easily accessible.
➤ Make a donut ring using the 4-inch gauze wrap.
  ➤ Wrap loosely around the hand six to eight times in the approximate diameter to cover the eye (Fig. 61–1).
  ➤ Then, in a continuous motion, wrap the other 4-inch gauze wrap in a circular fashion around the loose gauze until a firm donut forms (Fig. 61–2).
  ➤ Cut and use tape to anchor edge of the gauze.
➤ Apply ophthalmic antibiotic ointment to the injured eye.

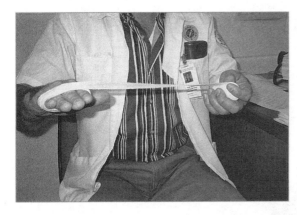

FIGURE 61 • 1 Wrap gauze loosely around the hand six to eight times.

➤ Apply the gauze donut over the orbit of the eye without coming in contact with the globe (Fig. 61–3).
➤ Place the plastic or Styrofoam cup or eye shield on the gauze donut (Fig. 61–4).
➤ Anchor the cup or shield with 4–in gauze around the head with several wraps (Fig. 61–5).
➤ Apply a double eye patch dressing to the unaffected eye, and continue wrapping the head to anchor both of the eye dressings (Fig. 61–6).
➤ Transport to the nearest emergency department in a slightly upright position for further evaluation by an ophthalmologist.

Client Instructions

➤ To prevent eye movement and further eye damage
  ➤ It is necessary for both eyes to be covered.
  ➤ Try not to cough, sneeze, or breathe deeply.

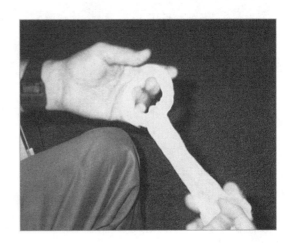

FIGURE 61 • 2 Wrap gauze in a circular fashion around the loose gauze until a firm donut forms.

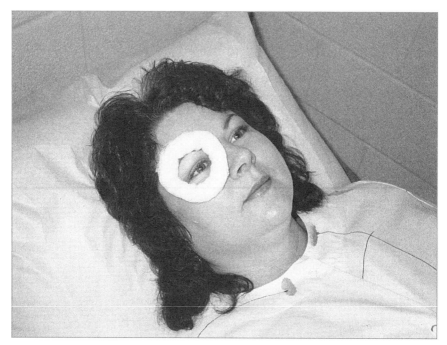

FIGURE 61 • 3 Apply the gauze donut over the orbit of the eye.

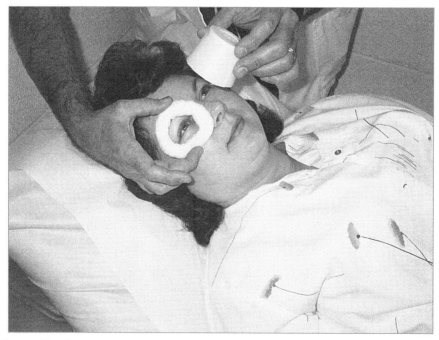

FIGURE 61 • 4 Place a plastic or Stryofoam cup or eye shield on the gauze donut.

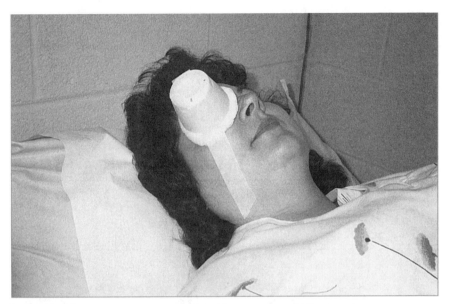

FIGURE 61 • 5 Anchor the cup or shield with gauze around the head.

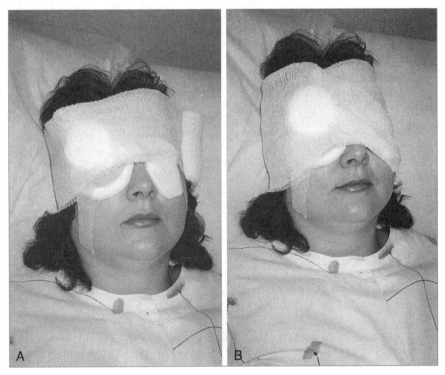

FIGURE 61 • 6 (A) Apply a double eye-patch dressing to the unaffected eye, and (B) continue wrapping the head with gauze.

BIBLIOGRAPHY
American Medical Association (1996). *Physicians' current procedural terminology.* Chicago: Author.
Garcia, G. (1996). Management of ocular emergencies and urgent eye problems. *Am Fam Physician,* 53(2), 347–356.
Murtagh, J. (1995) (2nd ed.). *Practice tips.* New York: McGraw-Hill.
Pfenninger, J.L., and Fowler, G.C. (1994). *Procedures for primary care physicians.* St. Louis: Mosby.

62

EYEBROW LACERATION REPAIR

CYNTHIA R. EHRHARDT

CPT Code	
12011	Simple repair of superficial wounds of face, ears, eyelids, nose, lips, or mucous membranes—2.5 cm or less
12013-18	Simple repair of superficial wounds of face, ears, eyelids, nose, lips, or mucous membranes—2.5 cm or greater

Eyebrow laceration repair may be required when there is trauma to the eyebrow. These lacerations most commonly are caused by blunt injury to the supraorbital area.

OVERVIEW

➤ Incidence unknown
  ➣ Usually associated with falls, contact sports, and other trauma
➤ Complications
  ➣ Fractures of the orbit and facial bones
  ➣ Globe injuries to the eye
➤ General principles
  ➣ Use contrasting suture material to allow easier removal of the sutures.
  ➣ Suturing beyond the ideal time of 6 hours postlaceration is considered because of cosmetic implications.
  ➣ Lacerations above and below the eyebrow may be closed with **Steri strips** if the wound is less than 0.25 cm in length and there is enough

room to anchor the tape. This is generally not recommended, however, because of poorer cosmetic healing.

➤ *Never shave the eyebrow.*

HEALTH PROMOTION/PREVENTION

➤ Eliminate situations that can result in laceration of the eyebrow.
➤ Promote safety habits when playing organized contact sports.
➤ Use safety devices such as protective headgear.
➤ Promote safety habits to prevent falls.

RATIONALE

➤ To promote healing of the laceration and prevent cosmetic complications

INDICATIONS

➤ Eyebrow laceration of greater than 0.25 cm
➤ Gaping eyebrow laceration

CONTRAINDICATIONS

➤ Multiple lacerations with involvement of the intramarginal lid of the eye
➤ Greater than 12 hours since the laceration occurred
➤ Suspected serious injuries, such as globe penetration and orbit fractures

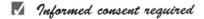 *Informed consent required*

PROCEDURE
Eyebrow Laceration Repair

Equipment

➤ Antiseptic skin cleanser
➤ Towels (fenestrated and nonfenestrated)—sterile
➤ Gloves—sterile
➤ 0.9% sodium chloride—sterile 3-mL syringe
➤ 25- to 27-gauge, $^1/_2$- to $1^1/_2$-inch needle for anesthesia administration
➤ Syringe—30- or 60-mL without needle for irrigation
➤ Lidocaine 1% or 2% with or without epinephrine
➤ 5-0 or 6-0 Ethicon suture material—contrasting color
➤ Topical antibiotic ointment (Bactroban, Neosporin, or Polysporin)
➤ Sterile suture kit (prepackaged or self-made) should include
  ➤ Curved and straight **hemostats**
  ➤ Needle holders ($4^1/_2$- and 6-inch)
  ➤ **Forceps** with teeth
  ➤ Iris scissors
  ➤ Cup to hold sterile 0.9% sodium chloride solution
  ➤ Cup to hold povidone-iodine (Betadine) solution
  ➤ 4 × 4 in sterile gauze

Procedure

➤ Thoroughly inspect the region.
  ➤ Anatomic defects to nasolacrimal duct and lacrimal canaliculus region
  ➤ Extraocular movements
  ➤ Orbit rim
  ➤ Eye for foreign bodies (see Chapter 59), hyphema, and globe injuries
➤ Drape the area to prevent any solution from draining into the eye.
➤ Infiltrate the borders of the laceration without accentuation of the margins (Fig. 62–1).
➤ Gently cleanse the skin around the wound with antiseptic skin cleanser, being careful to avoid getting the solution into the eye.
➤ Gently irrigate the wound with 30 to 60 mL of sterile 0.9% sodium chloride solution, being careful to avoid getting the solution into the eye.
➤ Carefully align the eyebrow margins (Fig. 62–2).
➤ If moderate maceration of the laceration, excise tissue in a parallel fashion to attain better margin alignment (Fig. 62–3).
➤ Use the suture technique of your choice (usually simple or running suture) (see Chapter 22).
➤ Apply topical antibiotic.
➤ Apply light pressure dressing for 1 to 2 hours.

Client Instructions

➤ Apply an ice pack to decrease pain and swelling to the area.
➤ Keep the area clean and dry for 24 hours.

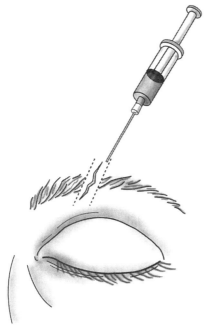

FIGURE 62 • 1 Infiltrate the borders of the laceration without accentuation of the margins.

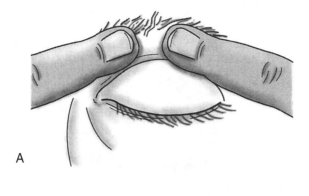

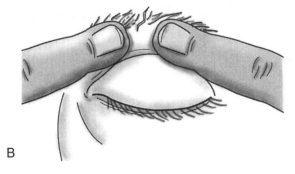

FIGURE 62 • 2 Align the eyebrow margins carefully. *(A)* Incorrect alignment; *(B)* correct alignment.

➤ Take the dressing off in 24 hours.
   ➤ Continuous covering of wound increases risk of infection.
➤ If a crust develops over the site, cleanse by gently rolling a cotton-tipped applicator saturated with hydrogen peroxide over the site. Gently rinse the area with warm water, and blot dry with clean towel or cotton gauze.
➤ Observe for signs and symptoms of infection, such as
   ➤ Increase in pain after 24 hours
   ➤ Increase in temperature
   ➤ Redness or swelling
   ➤ Yellow or greenish drainage
   ➤ Foul odor
➤ If any signs or symptoms of infection are found, return to the office.
➤ Bruising below the eye may occur in 24 to 48 hours.
➤ *Optional*—Return to the office in 48 hours for wound recheck.
➤ Return to the office in 3 to 5 days for removal of sutures (children and adults).
➤ Take acetaminophen every 4 to 6 hours as needed for pain.
   ➤ Tylenol No. 3 for pain is rarely needed.

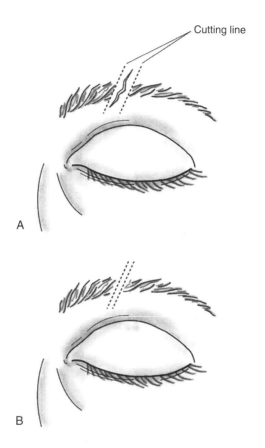

Cutting line

A

B

FIGURE 62 • 3 *(A)* Excise macerated tissue in a parallel fashion to *(B)* attain better margin alignment.

➤ Antibiotics generally are not recommended. Topical antibiotic ointment may be applied to the wound, however, to lessen scab formation.

BIBLIOGRAPHY

American Medical Association (1996). *Physicians' current procedural terminology*. Chicago: Author.
Murtagh, J. (1995) (2nd ed.). *Practice tips*. New York: McGraw-Hill.
Pfenninger, J.L., and Fowler, G.C. (1994). *Procedures for primary care physicians*. St. Louis: Mosby.
Trott, A. (1991). *Wounds and lacerations: emergency care and closure*. St. Louis: Mosby.

63

EYELID EVERSION

MARGARET R. COLYAR

CPT Code
None

Eversion of the eyelid is a technique used to inspect the conjunctiva of the upper eyelid.

OVERVIEW

➤ Incidence unknown
➤ Used to check for foreign bodies in the eye

RATIONALE

➤ To inspect the upper palpebral conjunctiva for
  ➢ Change in color
  ➢ Swelling
  ➢ Lesion
  ➢ Foreign body

INDICATIONS

➤ Eye trauma
➤ Complaints of eye irritation

CONTRAINDICATIONS

➤ Foreign body protruding through the eyelid
➤ Eyelid laceration
➤ Uncooperative client

PROCEDURE

Eyelid Eversion

Equipment

➤ Cotton-tipped applicator—nonsterile

Procedure

➤ Instruct the client to look downward.
➤ Get the client to relax the eye.

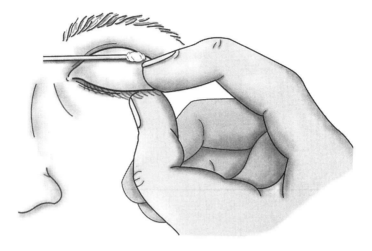

FIGURE 63 • 1 Place the tip of a cotton-tipped applicator on the upper eyelid. Grasp the upper eyelashes between the thumb and forefinger. Pull down and forward gently.

➤ Grasp the upper eyelashes between the thumb and forefinger and pull down and forward gently (Fig. 63–1).
➤ With the other hand, place the tip of the cotton-tipped applicator on the upper lid approximately 1 cm above the lid margin.
➤ Push down with the cotton-tipped applicator, and lift the lashes up gently. The lid turns inside out. Do not put pressure on the eyeball (Fig. 63–2).
➤ After inspection, gently pull the lashes outward as the client looks up. Eyelid returns to normal position.

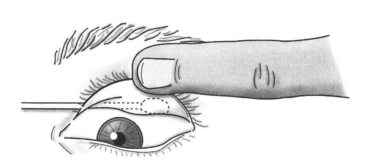

FIGURE 63 • 2 Push downward with the cotton-tipped applicator. Lift the lashes upward gently. The lid turns inside out.

BIBLIOGRAPHY
Bates, B., et al (1995). *A guide to physical examination and history taking.* Philadelphia: Lippincott-Raven.
Edmunds, M.W., and Mayhew, M.S. (1996). *Procedures for primary care practitioners.* St. Louis: Mosby.
Jarvis, C. (1996). *Physical examination and health assessment.* Philadelphia: Saunders.

AURICULAR HEMATOMA EVALUATION

64

MARGARET R. COLYAR

CPT Code
69000 Draining external ear; abscess or hematoma, simple
69005 Draining external ear; abscess or hematoma, complicated

An **auricular** hematoma is the accumulation of blood and serum between auricular cartilage and **perichondrium** (Fig. 64–1).

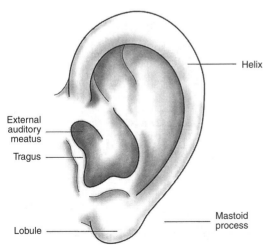

Helix

External auditory meatus

Tragus

Lobule

Mastoid process

FIGURE **64** • **1** Anatomy of the external ear.

OVERVIEW

➤ Incidence unknown
➤ Causes
  ➣ Direct blow to the external ear
  ➣ Indirect blow to the external ear

HEALTH PROMOTION/PREVENTION

➤ Apply ice to ear after trauma to decrease chance of hematoma formation intermittently for 24 hours.

RATIONALE

➤ To prevent
  ➣ Aseptic necrosis
  ➣ Loss of cartilage
  ➣ Secondary infection
  ➣ Perichondritis
  ➣ Cauliflower ear

INDICATIONS

➤ Local pressure
➤ Blood supply to ear decreased

CONTRAINDICATIONS

➤ Auricular laceration producing a hematoma

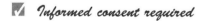 *Informed consent required*

PROCEDURE

Auricular Hematoma Evacuation

Equipment

➤ Antiseptic skin cleanser
➤ Drape—sterile
➤ Gloves—sterile
➤ Two syringes, 3 mL
➤ Two needles—27- to 30-gauge, $1^1/_2$-inch and 18- to 20-gauge, $1^1/_2$-inch
➤ 1% lidocaine
➤ No. 15 scalpel or scissors—sterile
➤ Curved **hemostat**—sterile
➤ **Forceps**—sterile
➤ Goggles
➤ 4 × 4 gauze—sterile
➤ Topical antibiotic ointment (Bactroban, Neosporin, or Polysporin)
➤ 2-inch gauze roll
➤ Suture—4-0 or 5-0 nylon

Procedure

➤ Position the client for comfort with the injured ear easily accessible.
➤ Cleanse the ear with topical skin cleanser.
➤ Drape the patient with the ear exposed.
➤ Put on gloves.
➤ Inject anterior and posterior to the hematoma using 1% lidocaine and a 27- to 30-gauge needle.
➤ Insert the syringe with an 18- to 20-gauge needle into the hematoma.
➤ Aspirate the hematoma.
➤ If the hematoma cannot be aspirated, incise the hematoma with the No. 15 scalpel.
➤ Using curved hemostats and digital pressure, explore the wound to remove remaining clots.
➤ Apply topical antibiotic.
➤ Roll 2-inch gauze into $1^1/_2$-inch-diameter pressure rolls.
➤ Apply a pressure roll over incision on each side of the ear and tape securely.
➤ If you cannot apply the pressure roll as described, using 4-0 or 5-0 nylon suture, insert the suture through one end of the roll, through the ear, into gauze roll on the posterior side of the ear, and back through the ear and anterior gauze (Fig. 64–2). Tie securely.

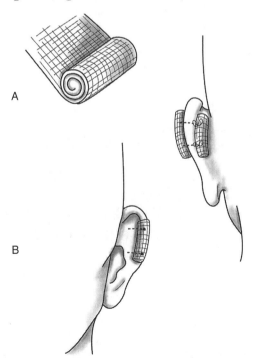

FIGURE 64 • 2 *(A)* Roll 2-inch gauze into $^1/_2$-inch-diameter pressure rolls; *(B)* apply the pressure rolls on both sides of the ear directly over the expressed hematoma, and suture in place.

Client Instructions

➤ Take cephalexin (Keflex) or cefadroxil (Duricef), 500 mg twice a day for 5 to 7 days.
➤ Observe for signs and symptoms of infection and perichondritis, such as
  ➤ Increase in pain after 24 hours
  ➤ Increase in temperature
  ➤ Redness or swelling
  ➤ Yellow or greenish drainage
  ➤ Foul odor
➤ If any signs or symptoms of infection are found, return to the office.
➤ To relieve pain
  ➤ Take Tylenol No. 3 every 4 to 6 hours for 24 hours.
  ➤ Take acetaminophen or ibuprofen every 4 to 6 hours for mild pain relief.
➤ Bleeding and oozing are normal for the first 24 hours. Apply an ice pack intermittently to the ear for 24 hours.
➤ Return to the office in 1 week for dressing removal.

BIBLIOGRAPHY

Forzley, G.J. (1994). Auricular hematoma evacuation. In Pfenninger, J.L., and Fowler, G.C. (eds.). *Procedures for primary care physicians* (pp. 184–187). St. Louis: Mosby.
Rakel, R.E. (ed.) (1997). *Conn's current therapy.* Philadelphia: Saunders.
Saunders, C.E., and Ho, M.T. (1992). *Current emergency diagnosis and treatment.* Norwalk, CT: Appleton & Lange.
Wolcott, M.W. (1988). *Ambulatory surgery and the basics of emergency surgical care.* Philadelphia: Lippincott.

CERUMEN IMPACTION REMOVAL
IRRIGATION OF THE EAR AND CURETTE TECHNIQUE

65

MARGARET R. COLYAR

CPT Code	
69210	Removal impacted cerumen, one or both ears

Cerumen impaction is the buildup of earwax in the auditory canal. Normal cerumen is sticky and honey-colored, hard and brown, or dry and scaly. Accumulation of cerumen can lead to pain and hearing difficulties. Irrigation of the ear is a technique used to cleanse the ear of large amounts of excess cerumen. To remove small amounts of cerumen, the curette technique can be used.

OVERVIEW

➤ Incidence unknown
➤ Need for removal of cerumen must be weighed against possible complications of
  ➤ Tympanic membrane perforation
  ➤ Vertigo
  ➤ Tinnitus
  ➤ Abrasions of the external canal
  ➤ Decreased or loss of hearing

HEALTH PROMOTION/PREVENTION

➤ Use earwax softeners periodically.

OPTIONS

➤ *Method 1*—curette technique
  ➤ Used for small amounts of cerumen that are easily visible
➤ *Method 2*—irrigation of the ear canal
  ➤ Used for cerumen impactions that occlude the tympanic membrane

RATIONALE

➤ To remove wax buildup
➤ To remove foreign bodies from the ear
➤ To reduce hearing impairment from occlusion of the ear canal
➤ To diminish pain

INDICATIONS

➤ Otalgia
➤ Hearing difficulty
➤ Unable to visualize the tympanic membrane

CONTRAINDICATIONS

➤ Drainage from the ear—yellow, green, or bloody exudate
➤ Tympanic membrane disrupted

PROCEDURE
Cerumen Impaction Removal

Equipment

➤ Methods 1 and 2
  ➤ Gloves—nonsterile
  ➤ Basin—nonsterile
  ➤ Absorbent drapes or towels
  ➤ Cotton-tipped applicators—nonsterile
  ➤ Alcohol
➤ Method 1 only
  ➤ Ear curette
➤ Method 2 only
  ➤ 60-mL syringe or Waterpik
  ➤ Hydrogen peroxide and water mixture 1:1

Procedure

METHOD 1—CURETTE TECHNIQUE

➤ Position the client sitting or lying with ear exposed.
➤ Drape client with absorbent pad or towels to protect clothing.
➤ Put on gloves.
➤ Grasp the pinna and straighten the ear canal.
  ➤ Down and back for children younger than 6 years old
  ➤ Up and back for individuals older than 6 years old
➤ Using an otoscope, visualize the position of the cerumen.
➤ Carefully insert the curette through the otoscope, and gently dislodge and remove the cerumen (Fig. 65–1).
➤ After the cerumen is dislodged, there may be slight bleeding in the ear canal. Cleanse the ear canal with alcohol applied to a cotton-tipped applicator.

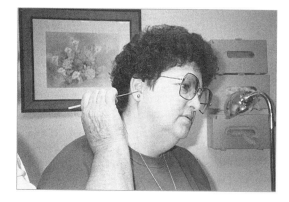

FIGURE 65 • 1 Curette technique.

METHOD 2—IRRIGATION OF THE EAR CANAL

➤ Position the client sitting up with ear to be irrigated tilted slightly downward.
➤ Mix hydrogen peroxide and water in basin or Waterpik basin at room temperature.
   ➤ Cold or excessively warm fluid may cause vertigo.
➤ Drape the client with absorbent pad or towels to protect clothing.
➤ Put on gloves.
➤ Hold basin snugly under the ear to be irrigated.
➤ Grasp the pinna and straighten the ear canal.
   ➤ Down and back for children younger than 6 years old
   ➤ Up and back for individuals older than 6 years old
➤ If using the 60-mL syringe to irrigate
   ➤ Aspirate the hydrogen peroxide and water mixture into the syringe, and inject the mixture into the ear. The stream should be directed toward the ear canal not the tympanic membrane.
   ➤ Gentle but vigorous irrigation may be necessary.
➤ Attaching a short section of intravenous tubing to the syringe allows you to reach further into the ear to irrigate (Fig. 65–2).
➤ If you are using the Waterpik for irrigation (Fig. 65–3)
   ➤ Insert the irrigation wand into the ear.
   ➤ Start the Waterpik using low pressure.
   ➤ Increase the water pressure as tolerated.
   ➤ Direct the water stream into the ear canal but not directly at the tympanic membrane.
➤ After the cerumen is dislodged, dry the ear canal with alcohol applied to a cotton-tipped applicator.

Client Instructions

➤ If cerumen was not dislodged, instill 2 drops of warmed glycerin, mineral oil, 0.5% acetic acid, or over-the-counter preparation four times per day for 4 days to soften the cerumen, then return to the office for a repeat irrigation.

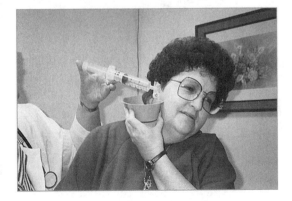

FIGURE 65 • 2 Irrigation with 60-mL syringe.

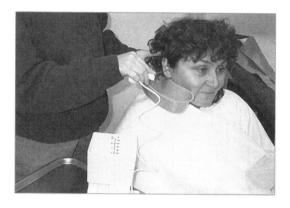

FIGURE 65 • 3 Irrigation with a Waterpik.

➤ If dizziness, pain in the ear, or drainage from the ear occurs, return to the office for evaluation.

BIBLIOGRAPHY

Ignatavicius, D.D., et al (1995). *Medical-surgical nursing: a nursing process approach.* Philadelphia: Saunders.

Smeltzer, S.C., and Bare, B.G. (1996). *Brunner and Suddarth's textbook of medical-surgical nursing.* Philadelphia: Lippincott-Raven.

EAR PIERCING

MARGARET R. COLYAR

CPT Code	
69090	Ear piercing

Ear piercing is a voluntary procedure that can be performed in the office on request.

OVERVIEW

➤ Incidence unknown

RATIONALE

➤ To promote esthetics as requested by the client

INDICATIONS

➤ Cosmetic desire of client

CONTRAINDICATIONS

➤ Diabetes mellitus
➤ Skin disorders
➤ Keloid prone
➤ Immunocompromised
➤ Coagulation problems

PROCEDURE

Ear Piercing

Equipment

➤ Antiseptic skin cleanser
➤ Surgical marking pencil
➤ Two 18-gauge, $1^1/_2$-inch needles
➤ Two 21-gauge, $1^1/_2$-inch needles
➤ Topical antiseptic skin cleanser
➤ 1% lidocaine or ice
➤ Gloves—nonsterile
➤ 14K gold or stainless-steel post earrings
➤ Basin—sterile
➤ Cotton-tipped applicator
➤ Alcohol

Procedure

➤ Position the client lying on his or her side.
➤ Cleanse the ear and surrounding tissue with topical antiseptic skin cleanser.
➤ Determine where the ears will be pierced, marking with the surgical pencil, and have the client approve of placement.
➤ Put on gloves.
➤ Anesthetize with 1% lidocaine *or* ice.
➤ Pierce the earlobe anterior to posterior with a 21-gauge needle (Fig. 66–1).
➤ Put an 18-gauge needle over the tip of the 21-gauge needle and pass back through the earlobe (Fig. 66–2).
➤ Remove the 21-gauge needle, and insert the post of the earring in the 18-gauge needle (Fig. 66–3).
➤ Pull back through the earlobe and remove the 18-gauge needle (Fig. 66–4).
➤ Apply the earring backing.
➤ Cleanse with alcohol.
➤ Repeat the procedure on the opposite ear.

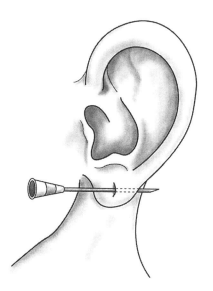

FIGURE 66 • 1 Pierce the earlobe with a 21-gauge needle.

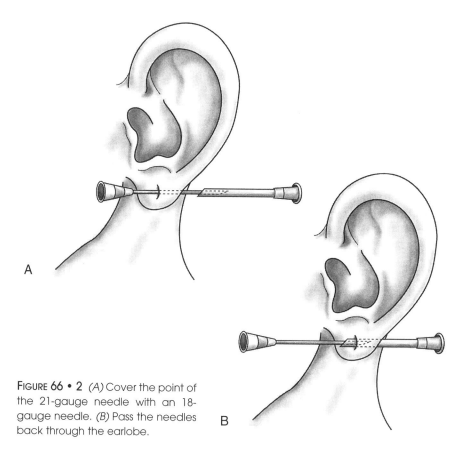

FIGURE 66 • 2 (A) Cover the point of the 21-gauge needle with an 18-gauge needle. (B) Pass the needles back through the earlobe.

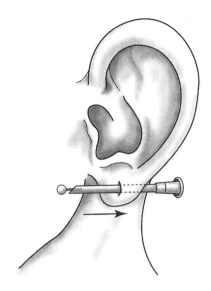

FIGURE 66 • 3 Remove the 21-gauge needle and insert the earring post into the 18-gauge needle.

Client Instructions

➤ Cleanse ears daily with soap and water or 70% isopropyl alcohol.
➤ Rotate the earrings three to four times daily.
➤ Apply mild antiseptic ointment around the earring posts daily.
➤ Leave the earring posts in place for 6 weeks or until healed.
➤ Avoid swimming.
➤ Complications are rare. Observe closely for the following
   ➤ Secondary infection—yellow or green drainage from the puncture site
    • Return to the office immediately.

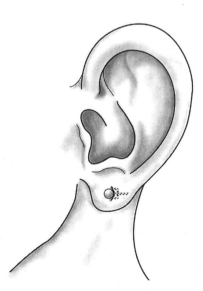

FIGURE 66 • 4 Pull the 18-gauge needle back through the earlobe. Remove the needle. Apply the earring backing.

- Premature closure
  - Return to the office if you desire to have the ear repierced.
- Keloid formation
  - Return to the office for evaluation.
- Hematoma (accumulation of blood at the site of the piercing)
  - Return to the office immediately.
- Cyst
  - Return to the office for evaluation.

BIBLIOGRAPHY

Edmunds, M.W., and Mayhew, M.S. (1996). *Procedure for primary care practitioners.* St. Louis, Mosby.

Forzley, G.J. (1994). Ear piercing. In Pfenniger, J.L., and Fowler, G.C. (eds.). *Procedures for primary care physicians* (pp. 202–205). St. Louis: Mosby.

67 EPISTAXIS CONTROL

CYNTHIA R. EHRHARDT

CPT Code	
30901	Control nasal hemorrhage, anterior, simple (limited cautery and/or packing); any method
30903	Control nasal hemorrhage, anterior, complex (extensive cautery and/or packing); any method. Control nasal hemorrhage, posterior, single; any method

Epistaxis is the onset of nasal hemorrhage with or without trauma. Because of potential complications, any client older than 40 years with a positive history of cardiovascular, pulmonary, hepatic, or renal disorder may receive anterior packing as a temporary stabilizing measure but should be referred to an emergency department as soon as possible.

OVERVIEW

- Incidence unknown
- Causes
  - Physical trauma to the nose

➤ Nasal mucosal irritation
  • Allergic rhinitis irritations
  • Bacterial infections
  • Chemical irritation
  • Climate (low humidity)
  • Drug induced (legal or illegal)
  • Foreign bodies (mostly with children)
  • Coagulopathies (aspirin, nonsteroidal drugs, warfarin)
  • Rhinoviruses
  • Tobacco smoking
➤ Disease pathology
  • Hypertension
  • Non–drug-induced coagulation disorders
  • Liver disorders (including alcohol abuse)
  • Cardiovascular disorders
  • Diabetes
➤ Location
  ➤ Anterior epistaxis
    • 90% frequency
    • Most common between 3 and 40 years of age
    • Low incidence of underlying abnormal pathology
    • Rarely require REFERRAL to ears, nose, and throat (ENT) specialist for consultation
    • Hospitalization rarely required
  ➤ Posterior epistaxis
    • 10% frequency
    • If in individuals older than age 40, must consider evaluation of local or systemic disease process
    • More difficult to control bleeding with packing
    • Usually requires ENT consultation
    • Higher incidence of hospitalization
➤ Complications include
  ➤ Rhinitis
  ➤ Sinusitis
  ➤ Otitis media
  ➤ Pressure necrosis of the nasal membranes from the packing
  ➤ Iatrogenic sleep apnea
  ➤ Hemotympanum
  ➤ Bacteremia with possible toxic shock presentation
  ➤ Respiratory distress
  ➤ Cardiac arrhythmia
  ➤ Rupture of the balloon with aspiration of saline if posterior packing is used

HEALTH PROMOTION/PREVENTION

➤ Prevention of epistaxis is focused on the causes.
  ➤ Minimize exposure to known allergens.
  ➤ Increase humidity through the use of humidifiers and normal saline nose drops applied to each nostril on a regular basis.

- Treat appropriately all nasal and sinus bacterial infections.
- Minimize the use of nasally administered chemicals.
- Avoid the use of medicines that produce coagulopathies, such as aspirin and nonsteroidal medications.
- Avoid tobacco and secondhand smoke.
- Prevent children from having unsupervised contact with small items such as beads, round seeds, and marbles.

OPTIONS

- *Method 1*—cotton applicator technique
  - Used for superficial anterior bleed
- *Method 2*—dental/tonsillar packing technique
  - Used for superficial anterior bleed
- *Method 3*—anterior nasal packing technique
  - Used for heavy anterior hemorrhaging
- *Method 4*—posterior nasal packing technique
  - Used for heavy posterior hemorrhaging

RATIONALE

- To control nasal hemorrhage
- To prevent hypovolemia

INDICATIONS

- Nontraumatic expistaxis not controlled by simple pressure to the nostril for 5 to 10 minutes

CONTRAINDICATIONS

- History of clotting disorder
- History of chronic obstructive pulmonary disease
- Suspected trauma
- Suspected foreign body
- Positive cardiovascular history

Informed consent required

PROCEDURE

Epistaxis Control

Equipment

- Methods 1, 2, 3, and 4
  - Good light source (head lamp with magnifying lens is ideal)
  - Gloves—nonsterile
  - Pharyngeal mirror
  - Nasal **speculums** (small, medium, large)—sterile

➤ Cotton applicators—sterile
➤ Suction machine with No. 5 Fraser tip
➤ Methods 2, 3, and 4 only
  ➤ Bayonet **forceps**—sterile
  ➤ Emesis basin—sterile
  ➤ Tongue blades
  ➤ Topical vasoconstrictor agent
➤ Methods 3 and 4 only
  ➤ Gloves—sterile
  ➤ Fenestrated sheets—sterile
➤ Method 2 only
  ➤ Dental/tonsil packing and expandable nasal packing—sterile
➤ Method 3 only
  ➤ Impregnated petrolatum and antibiotic (usually triple antibiotic oint-
    ment) gauze packings (prepackaged as $^1/_2$ inch × 72 inches)
➤ Method 4 only
  ➤ Iris scissors—sterile
  ➤ No. 14 Fr catheter (with 10- to 30-mL bulb)—sterile
  ➤ 30-mL syringe—sterile
  ➤ 0.9% sodium chloride—sterile
  ➤ Triple antibiotic ointment
  ➤ Portable pulse oximeter

Procedure

METHOD 1—COTTON APPLICATOR TECHNIQUE

➤ Secure the client in a comfortable position.
➤ Put on gloves.
➤ Locate the source of the bleed by using a nasal speculum to expand the
  nare.
➤ Gently suction the site clean.
➤ Dry the site with a cotton-tipped applicator.
➤ Select a vasoconstrictive agent.
➤ Saturate a cotton-tipped applicator with the vasoconstriction agent.
  ➤ In the case of silver nitrate, applicators are prepackaged.
➤ Place the applicator gently on the bleeding site for 5 minutes (Fig. 67–1).
  ➤ Caution should be taken not to damage any of the surrounding tissue;
    otherwise there is an increase in tissue necrosis. This is especially com-
    mon with the use of silver nitrate sticks.
➤ Keep the client upright for an additional 5 minutes.
➤ Inspect the site to ensure bleeding has halted.

METHOD 2—DENTAL/TONSILLAR PACKING TECHNIQUE

➤ Secure the client in a comfortable position.
➤ Put on gloves.
➤ Locate the source of the bleed by using a nasal speculum to expand the
  nare.
➤ Gently suction the site clean.

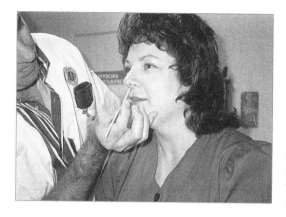

FIGURE 67 • 1 *Method 1.* Place the vasoconstriction agent gently on the bleeding site for 5 minutes.

➤ Dry the site with a cotton-tipped applicator.
➤ Select a vasoconstrictive agent (Table 67–1).
➤ Saturate the packing with the vasoconstriction agent of choice.
   ➤ *Silver nitrate cannot be used with this technique.*
➤ Insert the packing into nostril using the bayonet forceps through the nasal speculum.
➤ Have the client pinch his or her nose and hold for 5 to 10 minutes.
➤ Remove the packing, and inspect site to verify bleeding has halted.

METHOD 3—ANTERIOR NASAL PACKING TECHNIQUE

➤ Secure the client in a comfortable position.
➤ Put on nonsterile gloves.
➤ Locate the source of the bleed using a nasal speculum to expand the nare.
➤ Gently suction the site clean.
➤ Dry the site with cotton-tipped applicator.
➤ Select a vasoconstrictive agent.
➤ Apply the fenestrated drape.
➤ Put on sterile gloves.
➤ Prepare nasal packing by removing the $1/2$-inch impregnated petrolatum and antibiotic from packaging and folding it in half.
➤ Stabilize the nasal speculum with one hand resting on cheek, and expand the nare to visualize site (Fig. 67–2).

TABLE 67•1 TOPICAL VASOCONSTRICTOR AGENTS

➤ Topical 4% lidocaine mixed with 1:1000 epinephrine in a 1:1 ratio
➤ Topical tetracaine
➤ Topical phenylephrine hydrochloride (Neo-Synephrine) 0.05 to 1%
➤ Benzocaine spray
➤ Silver nitrate sticks
➤ Petrolatum jelly

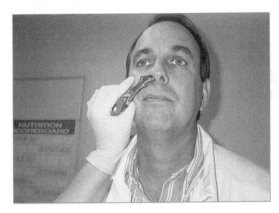

FIGUER 67 • 2 Expand the nares with the nasal speculum.

➤ Take the packing at the folded end and insert as far into the anterior chamber floor as possible using bayonet forceps (Fig. 67–3).
  ➤ Repeat the procedure in a layered fashion until no further packing can be inserted.
➤ Tie a large knot in the packing protruding from the nare to prevent a dislocation of the anterior packing (Fig. 67–4).
➤ Recheck vital signs after 5 to 10 minutes (especially pulse oximetry).
➤ Remove packing after 48 hours.

METHOD 4—POSTERIOR NASAL PACKING TECHNIQUE

➤ Secure the client in a comfortable position.
➤ Monitor with pulse oximetry if available.
➤ Put on nonsterile gloves.
➤ Locate the source of the bleed using a nasal speculum to expand the nare.
➤ Identify the presence of posterior hemorrhage using the pharyngeal mirror.

FIGURE 67 • 3 Insert the impregnated packing as far as possible into the anterior chamber.

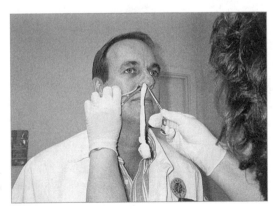

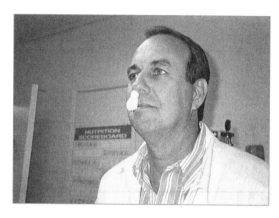

FIGURE 67 • 4 Tie a large knot in the packing to prevent dislocation.

➤ Gently suction the site clean.
➤ Spray the postpharyngeal wall with benzocaine.
  ➤ Advise the client about possible choking sensation and hoarseness from the medication.
➤ Apply the fenestrated drape.
➤ Put on sterile gloves.
➤ Verify an intact bulb of the No. 14 Fr catheter by expanding the balloon, then deflating it.
➤ Sever the tip distal of the No. 14 Fr catheter without losing balloon function (Fig. 67–5).
➤ Lubricate the catheter liberally with antibiotic ointment.

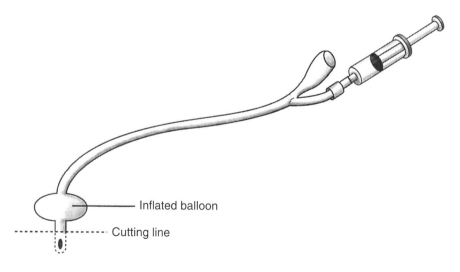

Inflated balloon

Cutting line

FIGURE 67 • 5 Verify an intact bulb of the No. 14 Fr catheter. Sever the distal tip without losing balloon function.

➤ Introduce the catheter until it contacts the choana (Fig. 67–6).
  ➣ Ask the client to open his or her mouth; visualize the catheter with a pharyngeal mirror.
➤ Inflate the balloon gently with 5 mL 0.9% sodium chloride.
➤ Inflate the balloon with a total of 10 to 15 mL 0.9% sodium chloride once proper position has been verified (Fig. 67–7).
➤ Stabilize the catheter with tape.
➤ Begin insertion of anterior packing to stabilize the catheter.
➤ Recheck in 5 to 10 minutes with the pharyngeal mirror to verify cessation of bleeding.
➤ Deflate the balloon, and reverify absence of bleeding.
➤ Leave catheter in place for 12 hours in case of recurrence of hemorrhage.
➤ Transport to ENT physician or emergency department for follow-up care and possible hospitalization.

Client Instructions

➤ Activities
  ➣ Avoid strenuous exercise and bending and lifting for 5 days.
➤ Hygiene
  ➣ Avoid sneezing, blowing nose, and rubbing nose.
  ➣ Do not insert anything into nose.
  ➣ Humidification may be used in low-humidity environments.

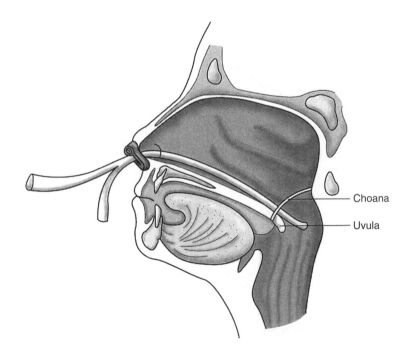

Choana

Uvula

FIGURE 67 • 6 Insert the catheter into the nares until the choana is reached.

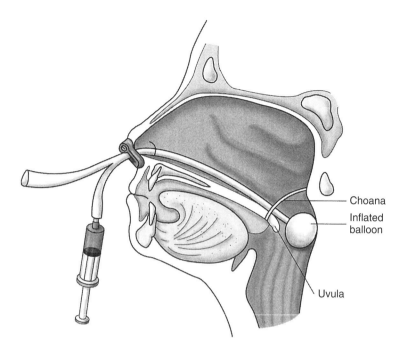

FIGURE 67 • 7 Inflate the balloon with 5 mL of 0.9% sodium chloride.

➤ Drugs to be avoided include aspirin, alcohol, and nonsteroidals for 5 days.
   ➤ Minimal amount of decongestant or antihistamines may be used to control severe nasal drainage.
➤ Avoid factors that led to the hemorrhage.
   ➤ Use either normal saline drops (3 drops each nostril three to four times a day) or petroleum jelly to nares (three to four times a day) to decrease friable nasal mucosa.
   ➤ If hemorrhage should recur, initiate pressure to the nares.
➤ If no relief has occurred, return for more aggressive treatment.
➤ *Anterior nasal packing*—as above except avoid sneezing or pulling packing out.
➤ Observe for signs and symptoms of infection and complications including
   ➤ Fever greater than 99.5°F
   ➤ Increased frequency of headaches
   ➤ Facial pain (especially below the eye)
   ➤ Malodorous breath or nasal discharge
   ➤ Change in level of consciousness (especially children)
   ➤ Increasing breathing difficulty
   ➤ Unexplained bleeding and/or bruising
   ➤ Recurrence of nasal bleeding
➤ Antibiotics
   ➤ Required with nasal packing to prevent stasis sinusitis.

- ➤ Drug of choice should be a broad-spectrum antibiotic that covers the flora normally found in the nasopharyngeal chamber.
- ➤ Frequently used are amoxicillin, amoxicillin with clavulanic acid (Augmentin), erythromycin, or second-generation cephalosporins.
- ➤ Give acetaminophen for appropriate age and/or weight for pain.
- ➤ Occasional use of Tylenol No. 3 can be considered in moderate and severe pain.
- ➤ Avoid nonsteroidal medication for 5 days.
- ➤ Children should not take ibuprofen.
- ➤ Decongestants and antihistamines may be used sparingly if excessive nasal drainage occurs.
- ➤ Return to the office before scheduled visit if bleeding recurs.
- ➤ Return to the office
  - ➤ *Anterior packing*—in 48 hours and recheck in 5 days
  - ➤ *Posterior packing*—requires immediate transport to hospital or ENT office for further evaluation and may be followed up if further diagnostic workup is required

BIBLIOGRAPHY

American Medical Association (1996). *Physicians' current procedural terminology*. Chicago: Author.

Murtagh, J. (1995) (2nd ed.). *Practice tips*. New York: McGraw-Hill.

Pfenninger, J.L., and Fowler, G.C. (1994). *Procedures for primary care physicians*. St. Louis: Mosby.

Randall, D., and Freeman, S. (1991). Management of anterior and posterior epistaxis. *Am Fam Physician*, 43(6), 214–221.

REMOVAL OF FOREIGN BODY
EAR AND NOSE

68

MARGARET R. COLYAR

CPT Code

69200 Removal of foreign body from external auditory canal without general anesthesia

30300 Removal of foreign body, intranasal; office-type procedure

Foreign bodies, such as vegetation, small solid objects, and insects, are found commonly in the external auditory canal and nose in young children.

OVERVIEW

➤ Incidence unknown
➤ Objects commonly found in ears and nose include
  ➣ Vegetation—beans, nuts, seeds, popcorn, paper balls, fabric, modeling clay
  ➣ Solid objects—beads, small toys, money, watch batteries, rocks
  ➣ Insects—roaches, flies, ticks, spiders

OPTIONS

➤ *Method 1*—irrigation technique
  ➣ Used for small solid objects, vegetation, and dead insects
➤ *Method 2*—light technique
  ➣ Used for live insects

RATIONALE

➤ To relieve pain
➤ To remove foreign bodies from the ears and nose
➤ To prevent infection

INDICATIONS

➤ Foreign body seen in ear or nose

CONTRAINDICATIONS

➤ Hard vegetation that has become swollen
➤ Foreign body in inner third of auditory canal in which easy access is occluded—REFER to a pediatrician or ENT specialist
➤ Child uncooperative—REFER to a pediatrician

PROCEDURE

Removal of Foreign Body—Ear and Nose

Equipment

➤ Methods 1 and 2
  ➣ Ear and nasal **speculum**
  ➣ Topical ear anesthetic (Auralgan or Otocain)
  ➣ 0.9% sodium chloride for irrigation
  ➣ Gloves—nonsterile
  ➣ Drape or towel—nonsterile
  ➣ Cotton-tipped applicator—nonsterile
  ➣ Alcohol
➤ Method 1 only

➤ Foreign body extraction tools (Fig. 68–1)
  • Nasal **forceps**
  • Alligator forceps
  • Ear **curettes** with hook
➤ Method 2 only
  • Flashlight or penlight

Procedure

METHOD 1—IRRIGATION TECHNIQUE

➤ Position the client for comfort.
➤ Apply a drape or towel to protect clothing.
➤ Put on gloves.
➤ Instill topical anesthesia into the ear canal or nose.
➤ Insert the speculum.
➤ Insert the appropriate tool through the speculum, grasp the object, and gently remove.
  ➤ If the auditory canal or nasal passage is only partially occluded, try the hooked curette.
  ➤ If the object is hard, try alligator forceps or nasal forceps.
➤ Irrigate the orifice with 0.9% sodium chloride to remove remaining debris.
➤ If there is bleeding present, cleanse the orifice with a cotton-tipped applicator saturated with alcohol.

METHOD 2—LIGHT TECHNIQUE

➤ Position the client for comfort.
➤ Apply a drape or towel to protect clothing.
➤ Put on gloves.
➤ Instill topical anesthesia into the ear canal or nose.
➤ Insert the speculum.

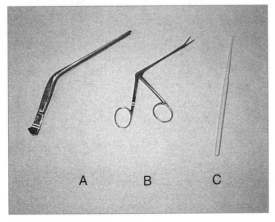

A   B   C

FIGURE **68** • **1** Foreign body extraction tools include *(A)* nasal forceps, *(B)* alligator forceps, and *(C)* ear curettes.

➤ Turn on flashlight or penlight, and shine the light into the ear canal or nasal passage.
  ➤ Many times the insect follows the light source and walks out of the orifice.
➤ Irrigate the orifice with 0.9% sodium chloride to remove remaining debris.
➤ If there is bleeding present, cleanse the orifice with a cotton-tipped applicator saturated with alcohol.

Client Instructions

➤ Take acetaminophen or ibuprofen every 4 to 6 hours for pain.
  ➤ If pain continues after 24 hours, notify the practitioner.
  ➤ Although slight, there is a chance of infection. Observe for signs and symptoms of infection, such as
  ➤ Increase in pain after 24 hours
  ➤ Increase in temperature
  ➤ Yellow or greenish drainage
  ➤ Foul odor
➤ If any of the signs and symptoms of infection are found, return to the office.

B I B L I O G R A P H Y
Ignatavicius, D.D., et al (1995). *Medical-surgical nursing: a nursing process approach.* Philadelphia: Saunders.
Smeltzer, S.C., and Bare, B.G. (1996). *Brunner and Suddarth's textbook of medical-surgical nursing.* Philadelphia: Lippincott-Raven.

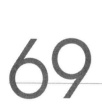

FRENOTOMY FOR ANKYLOGLOSSIA

CYNTHIA EHRHARDT

CPT Code
41010   Incision of a lingual frenulum

Frenotomy is a procedure used to release an abnormal attachment of **frenulum** to the tongue. This abnormal attachment is known as **ankyloglossia**. It can lead to poor feeding in infants and speech impairment in older children.

OVERVIEW

➤ Incidence unknown
➤ Causes unknown
  ➤ Hereditary predisposition suggested

RATIONALE

➤ To release the tongue and provide full range of motion for essential growth and development

INDICATIONS

➤ Difficulty sucking
➤ Difficulty breast-feeding
➤ Difficulty chewing
➤ Inhibits tongue protrusion
➤ Abnormal dentofacial growth and development
➤ Speech impairment

CONTRAINDICATIONS

➤ Severe ankyloglossia that interferes with lingual function should be REFERRED to a surgeon, dentist, or otolaryngologist.

PROCEDURE

Frenotomy

Equipment

➤ 3-mL syringe
➤ 25- to 27-gauge, $^1/_2$-inch needle
➤ 1% lidocaine with epinephrine
➤ Topical 20% benzocaine
➤ Tongue retractor
➤ Hemostat—sterile
➤ Gloves—sterile
➤ Iris scissors—sterile
➤ 4 × 4 gauze—nonsterile
➤ Cotton-tipped applicators—nonsterile
➤ Adequate light source

Procedure

➤ Position the client in a comfortable position with easy access to the mouth.
➤ Locate the frenulum.
➤ Apply a cotton-tipped applicator saturated with benzocaine to the lingual frenulum (Fig. 69–1).
➤ Retract and stabilize the tongue (Fig. 69–2).

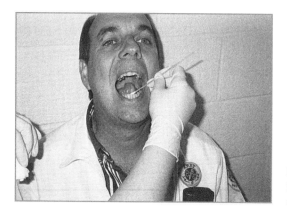

FIGURE 69 • 1 Anesthetize the lingual frenulum with benzocaine.

➤ Using the tip of the **hemostat,** grasp the area of the frenulum that is to be ligated, then clamp and crush to the depth required (Fig. 69–3).
  ➤ After a few seconds, release and remove the hemostat.
➤ Using the iris scissors, snip the tissue crushed by the hemostat.
➤ Apply pressure with a clean cotton-tipped applicator.
  ➤ If bleeding continues, apply a cotton-tipped applicator saturated with 1% lidocaine with epinephrine until bleeding is halted.

Client Instructions

➤ Infant may begin feeding immediately.
➤ Observe for signs and symptoms of infection, such as
  ➤ Increase in pain after 24 hours
  ➤ Increase in temperature
  ➤ Redness or swelling
  ➤ Yellow or greenish drainage
  ➤ Foul odor
  ➤ Decreased feeding
➤ If any signs or symptoms of infection are found, return to the office.

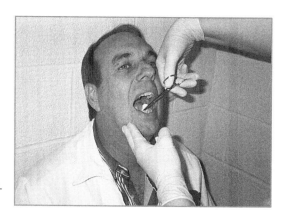

FIGURE 69 • 2 Retract and stabilize the tongue.

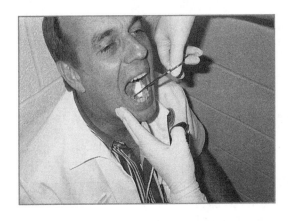

FIGURE 69 • 3 Clamp and crush the frenulum to the depth planned for ligation.

➤ Antibiotics generally are not required unless secondary infection occurs.
➤ To relieve pain
  ➢ Take acetaminophen every 4 to 6 hours as needed.
  ➢ No children's ibuprofen should be used.
➤ Return to the office in 2 weeks for recheck.

BIBLIOGRAPHY

American Medical Association (1996). *Physicians' current procedural terminology*. Chicago: Author.
Murtagh, J. (1995) (2nd ed.). *Practice tips*. New York: McGraw-Hill.
Paradise, J. (1990). Evaluation and treatment of ankyloglossia. *JAMA, 263,* 2371–2374.
Pfenninger, J.L., and Fowler, G.C. (1994). *Procedures for primary care physicians*. St. Louis: Mosby.

70

LIP LACERATION REPAIR

CYNTHIA R. EHRHARDT

CPT Code	
40650	Repair lip, full thickness; vermilion only
40652	Repair lip, full thickness; vermilion only—up to half vertical height
40654	Repair lip, full thickness; vermilion only—over one half vertical height, or complex

Lip lacerations usually are caused by trauma to the perioral area of the face resulting from blunt injury or falls. Suturing beyond the ideal time of 6 hours after laceration is considered because of the cosmetic implications.

OVERVIEW

➤ Incidence unknown; usually associated with falls and contact sports
➤ Complications
  ➤ Fractures of the facial bones

HEALTH PROMOTION/PREVENTION

➤ Eliminate situations that can result in laceration of the lip.
➤ Promote safety habits when playing organized contact sports.
➤ Use safety devices such as protective mouth gear.

RATIONALE

➤ To promote healing
➤ To promote esthetics

INDICATIONS

➤ Lip laceration of greater than 0.25 cm
➤ Gaping lacerations

CONTRAINDICATIONS

➤ Suspected injury of the orbicularis oris muscle
➤ Suspected facial bone fracture
➤ Need for extensive revision and/or debridement to the lip
➤ Laceration through the margin of the lip
➤ Vertical through-and-through laceration
➤ If more than 12 hours since the laceration occurred, the patient should be referred to a plastic surgeon for evaluation.

PROCEDURE

Lip Laceration Repair

Equipment

➤ Gloves—sterile
➤ Towels (fenestrated and nonfenestrated)—sterile
➤ 3-mL syringe
➤ 25- to 27-gauge, $1/2$-inch needle for anesthesia administration
➤ Syringes—30 or 60 mL without needle for irrigation
➤ 1% or 2% lidocaine without epinephrine
➤ No. 6-0 Ethicon suture material
➤ 0.9% sodium chloride—sterile

➤ Topical antibiotic ointment (Bactroban, Neosporin, or Polysporin)
➤ Cotton-tipped applicators—nonsterile
➤ Sterile suture kit (prepackaged or self-made) should include
  ➤ Curved and straight **hemostats**
  ➤ Needle holders ($4^1/_2$-inch and 6-inch)
  ➤ **Forceps** with teeth
  ➤ Iris scissors
  ➤ Cup to hold sterile normal saline solution
  ➤ 4 × 4 sterile gauze

Procedure

➤ Thorough inspection for anatomic defects to the following areas
  ➤ Lip region to determine whether the laceration is through the margin
  ➤ Structural defect in the musculature, including injury to the orbicularis oris muscle, by examination of the symmetry of the smile
  ➤ Maxillary structures for loss of integrity
  ➤ Mandible structure for loss of integrity and range of motion of the temporomandibular joint
  ➤ Teeth for stability
➤ Drape the area to prevent any solution from draining into mouth.
➤ Infiltrate the borders of the laceration, but avoid as much as possible distortion of the lip margins.
➤ Do not clean the wound with povidone-iodine.
➤ Gently irrigate the wound with 30 to 60 mL of sterile normal saline solution, being careful to avoid getting the solution into the mouth.
➤ Carefully align the lip margins (Fig. 70–1).
➤ Suture the wound.
➤ Apply topical antibiotic.

Client Instructions

➤ Apply an ice pack to decrease pain and swelling to the area.
➤ Keep the area as clean as possible.
➤ If a crust develops over the site, cleanse by gently rolling a cotton-tipped applicator saturated with hydrogen peroxide over the site. Then gently rinse the area with warm water and blot dry with clean towel or cotton gauze.
➤ Eat a clear liquid diet for the first 24 hours, then soft diet for 3 to 4 days.
➤ No sucking or straw usage until sutures are removed.
➤ To lessen the discomfort, avoid citrus or acid foods.
➤ Observe for signs and symptoms of infection, such as
  ➤ Increase in pain after 24 hours
  ➤ Increase in temperature
  ➤ Redness or swelling
  ➤ Yellow or greenish drainage
  ➤ Foul odor
➤ If any signs or symptoms of infection are found, return to the office.
➤ Return to the office in 3 to 5 days (children and adults) for suture removal.

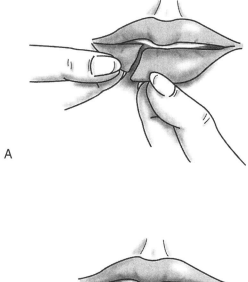

FIGURE 70 • 1 Align lip margins. (A) Incorrect alignment; (B) correct alignment.

➤ To relieve pain, take acetaminophen every 4 to 6 hours as needed.
  ➤ Tylenol No. 3 is rarely needed.
➤ Antibiotics generally are not recommended.

BIBLIOGRAPHY

American Medical Association (1996). *Physicians' current procedural terminology.* Chicago: Author.
Murtagh, J. (1995) (2nd ed.). *Practice tips.* New York: McGraw-Hill.
Pfenninger, J.L., and Fowler, G.C. (1994). *Procedures for primary care physicians.* St. Louis: Mosby.
Trott, A. (1991). *Wounds and lacerations: emergency care and closure.* St. Louis: Mosby.

71

TONGUE LACERATION REPAIR

CYNTHIA EHRHARDT

CPT Code

41250   Repair of laceration 2.5 cm or less; floor of mouth and/or anterior two thirds of tongue

41251   Repair of laceration 2.5 cm or less; posterior one third of tongue

Tongue laceration most commonly is caused by biting. Trauma to the face rarely involves fractured teeth except in instances of blunt trauma to the face.

OVERVIEW

➤ Incidence unknown
   ➤ Usually associated with falls and contact sports

HEALTH PROMOTION/PREVENTION

➤ Eliminate situations that can result in laceration of the tongue.
➤ Promote safety habits when playing organized contact sports, such as
   ➤ Use of tooth guards
   ➤ Prevention of falls

RATIONALE

➤ To promote healing

INDICATIONS

➤ Tongue laceration of greater than 1 cm
➤ Gaping tongue lacerations

CONTRAINDICATIONS

➤ If laceration is less than 1 cm and/or not gaping, suturing is not recommended.
➤ Through-and-through laceration should be sutured only on dorsal surface.

PROCEDURE

Tongue Laceration Repair

Equipment

➤ Gloves—sterile
➤ Towels (fenestrated and nonfenestrated)—sterile
➤ 3-mL syringe
➤ 25-gauge, $1^1/_2$-inch needle
➤ 30- or 60-mL syringe without needle for irrigation
➤ 1% or 2% lidocaine
➤ No. 5-0 chromic (Vicryl) suture
➤ No. 2-0 Ethicon suture—optional
➤ 0.9% sodium chloride—sterile
➤ Two bite blocks
➤ Sterile suture kit (prepackaged or self-made) should include
  ➤ Curved and straight **hemostats**
  ➤ Needle holders ($4^1/_2$- and 6-inch)
  ➤ **Forceps** with teeth
  ➤ Iris scissors
  ➤ Cup to hold sterile 0.9% sodium chloride solution
  ➤ 4 × 4 sterile gauze

Procedure

➤ Insert bite blocks on each side of mouth to prevent accidental biting by the client during the procedure.
➤ Stabilization of the tongue by either of the following methods is necessary for proper suturing of the tongue
  ➤ Have the assistant grasp the distal one third of the tongue with 4 × 4 gauze and extend until the laceration can be easily accessed
  ➤ Locally anesthetize with lidocaine the area of the tongue where two No. 2-0 Ethicon sutures can be placed temporarily to facilitate extension of the tongue by the assistant to expose the laceration (Fig. 71–1).
➤ Anesthetize the area by local infiltration of the laceration borders.
➤ Avoid vigorous irrigation of the laceration. Use gentle irrigation with 30 to 60 mL of 0.9% sodium chloride.
➤ Insert chromic (Vicryl) sutures for good approximation of the lacerated edges using a simple suture (see Chapter 22).
➤ Avoid long suture tails because they create increased irritation.

Client Instructions

➤ Do not eat or drink until the anesthetic has worn off (usually about 1 hour).
➤ Apply cool compresses (e.g., ice or Popsicle) to the tongue to decrease pain and swelling.
➤ Eat a clear liquid diet for the first meal after the suturing, then soft diet for 3 to 4 days.

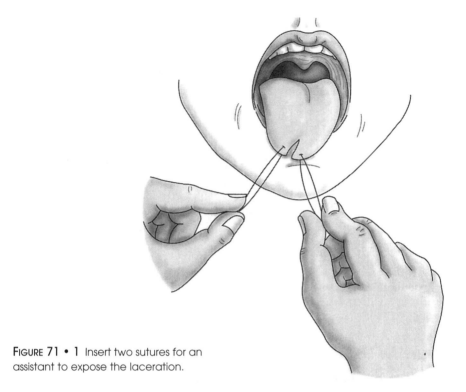

FIGURE 71 • 1 Insert two sutures for an
assistant to expose the laceration.

➤ Use a mixture of one half hydrogen peroxide and one half water as a
  mouth rinse as needed for 3 to 4 days (swish and spit).
➤ To relieve pain, take acetaminophen or Tylenol No. 3 every 4 to 6 hours
  as needed for pain.
➤ Antibiotics generally are not recommended.
➤ Observe for signs and symptoms of infection, such as
  ➤ Increase in pain after 24 hours
  ➤ Increase in temperature
  ➤ Redness or swelling
  ➤ Yellow or greenish drainage
  ➤ Foul odor
➤ If any signs or symptoms of infection are found, return to the office.
➤ Suture removal is not required because the sutures are absorbable.

BIBLIOGRAPHY

American Medical Association (1996). *Physicians' current procedural terminology*. Chicago: Author.
Murtagh, J. (1995) (2nd ed.). Practice tips. New York: McGraw-Hill.
Pfenninger, J.L., and Fowler, G.C. (1994). Procedures for primary care physicians. St. Louis:
Mosby.
Trott, A. (1991). Wounds and lacerations: emergency care and closure. St. Louis: Mosby.

72

TOOTH AVULSION AND FRACTURE

CYNTHIA R. EHRHARDT

CPT Code
873.63 Tooth injury
873.73 Complicated tooth injury

Tooth fracture is caused by trauma to the tooth with or without **avulsion** or **exarticulation** from the socket. Tooth avulsion is caused by trauma to a tooth resulting in complete displacement (avulsion or exarticulation) from the socket.

OVERVIEW

➤ Incidence unknown
➤ Causes
  ➢ Contact sports
  ➢ Blows to the face
  ➢ Poor dental hygiene
  ➢ Chewing hard objects (e.g., ice, hard candy, hard-shelled food, inanimate objects)
➤ Complications
  ➢ Laceration of the gum
  ➢ Partial or complete avulsion of the tooth
  ➢ Trauma and/or fracture of the facial bones
➤ General principles
  ➢ Key to successful preservation and restoration of the tooth is REFERRAL to the dentist for evaluation of the extent of the injury.
  ➢ If the fractured or avulsed tooth is found, preservation in transport medium should be undertaken.
  ➢ Time is the major factor in tooth preservation.

HEALTH PROMOTION/PREVENTION

➤ Eliminate situations that can result in tooth injury.
➤ Promote safety habits when playing organized contact sports, such as
  ➢ Use of tooth guards
  ➢ Teaching and promotion of safety habits

366

- ➤ Good dental hygiene
- ➤ Use of fluoridation
- ➤ Have tooth-saving equipment (Hank's solution kit) in first-aid kit.

RATIONALE

- ➤ To preserve the tooth and its function

INDICATIONS

- ➤ Presence of abnormal-appearing tooth after an incident, with or without pain
- ➤ Visualization of the fracture with or without partial displacement of tooth (permanent or immature) from the socket
- ➤ Total displacement of an intact tooth (permanent or immature) from the socket

CONTRAINDICATIONS

- ➤ Suspected facial fractures
- ➤ Laceration to the socket

PROCEDURE

Tooth Avulsion and Fracture

Equipment

- ➤ Transfer medium if unable to reinsert tooth (order of preference)
  - ➤ Hank's balanced salt solution (from local pharmacy)
  - ➤ Milk
  - ➤ 0.9% sodium chloride—sterile
  - ➤ Saliva
  - ➤ Water
- ➤ *Do not transport in tissue or towel because it will dry out the tooth cells.*

Procedure

- ➤ For fractured tooth with avulsion and less than 1 hour after injury
  - ➤ Locate the tooth and its fragments.
  - ➤ Inspect the tooth.
  - ➤ If tooth pulpal (root) appears totally intact and is not contaminated
    - • Irrigate the tooth socket with 0.9% sodium chloride or water to ensure that any clot has been removed.
    - • Grasp tooth at distal tip.
    - • Gently rinse with 10 to 30 mL of 0.9% sodium chloride.
    - • Gently set the tooth back into socket.
  - ➤ If tooth pulpal (root) has been contaminated
    - • Irrigate the tooth socket with 0.9% sodium chloride or water to ensure that any clot has been removed.
    - • Grasp tooth at distal tip.

- Gently rinse with 10 to 30 mL of 0.9% sodium chloride or water.
- Gently set tooth back into socket.
- Consult with a dentist.

➤ For fractured tooth with avulsion and more than 1 hour after injury
  ➤ Locate tooth and its fragments.
  ➤ Inspect tooth.
  ➤ Follow reimplantation instructions as given for injuries less than 1 hour old.
  ➤ If not possible to reimplant, place the fractured tooth in the transport medium.
  ➤ Contact dentist or endodontist as soon as possible for treatment.

Client Instructions

➤ If reimplantation is successful, do not dislodge the tooth from the socket.
➤ Gently clench the teeth. This may allow support of the tooth.
➤ Minimize activities such as talking, drinking, or chewing to prevent further trauma to the injured tooth and decrease the risk of dislodging from the socket.
➤ Seek dental attention (dentist or endodontist) as soon as possible. Delay in restoration can result in complete loss of the tooth.

BIBLIOGRAPHY

American Association of Endodontics (1995). Treating the avulsed permanent tooth: treatment guidelines. *Endodontics,* 1(1), 2–4.

American Medical Association (1996). *Physicians' current procedural terminology.* Chicago: Author.

Murtagh, J. (1995) (2nd ed.). *Practice tips.* New York: McGraw-Hill.

Pfenninger, J.L., and Fowler, G.C. (1994). *Procedures for primary care physicians.* St. Louis: Mosby.

Spatafore, C., and Jackson, R. (1989). Trauma: a simplified approach to treatment. Unpublished paper presentation at the American Association of Endodontics Meeting, April 1989.

Cardiovascular Procedures

73 DOPPLER TECHNIQUE

MARGARET R. COLYAR

CPT Code

93922   Noninvasive physiologic studies of upper or lower extremity arteries, single-level, bilateral (e.g., ankle/brachial indices, Doppler waveform analysis, volume plethysmography, transcutaneous oxygen tension measurement)

Doppler technique is the examination of artery function with an instrument that ultrasonically detects arterial blood flow. A good understanding of the anatomy of the arterial system is necessary (Fig. 73–1).

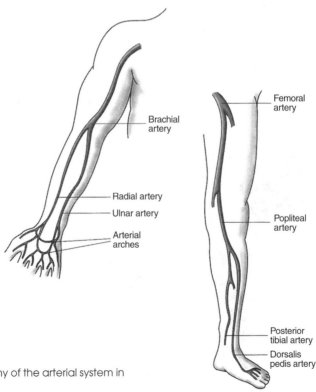

FIGURE 73 • 1 Anatomy of the arterial system in the extremities.

OVERVIEW

➤ Incidence unknown

RATIONALE

➤ To examine arterial function

INDICATIONS

➤ Extremity cool, edematous, pale, or cyanotic
➤ Arterial pulsation cannot be palpated in the extremity
➤ Determine placement for an arterial stick
➤ Assist in Allen's test

CONTRAINDICATIONS

➤ None

PROCEDURE

Doppler Technique

Equipment

➤ Ultrasound lubricant
➤ Doppler (Fig. 73–2)
➤ Marking pen

Procedure

➤ Position the client with the area to be assessed easily accessible.
➤ Apply ultrasound lubricant.

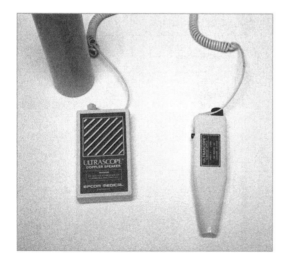

FIGURE 73 • 2 Doppler.

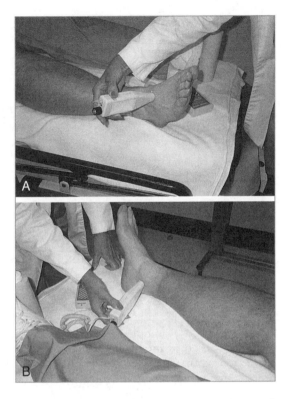

FIGURE 73 • 3 *(A)* Apply the Doppler probe to the lubricated area of expected arterial pulse. *(B)* Move the probe until the pulse is detected.

➤ Turn Doppler on.
➤ Apply Doppler probe to the area of expected arterial pulse (Fig. 73–3).
➤ Gently move the Doppler probe until the pulse is detected.
➤ Mark the area of pulse with a marking pen.

BIBLIOGRAPHY

Pfenninger, J.L., and Fowler, G.C. (1994). *Procedures for primary care physicians.* St. Louis: Mosby.
Potter, P.A., and Perry, A.G. (1994). *Clinical nursing skills and techniques.* St. Louis: Mosby.

ELECTROCARDIOGRAM (ECG) INTERPRETATION

74

MARGARET R. COLYAR

CPT Code

93000   Electrocardiogram (ECG) complete

93005   ECG technical component

The **ECG** is a unique tool used to assist the clinician in diagnosing or ruling out myocardial **infarction** (MI); potential life-threatening arrhythmias; and many cardiac problems caused by medications, electrolyte imbalance, or disease processes. Interpreting an ECG is not difficult. After learning the basic rules, you can understand and apply them easily.

OVERVIEW

➤ Incidence unknown
➤ Performed on almost every client presenting to the emergency department or ambulatory health-care facility with chest pain

RATIONALE

➤ To diagnose and rule out cardiac problems

INDICATIONS

➤ Chest pain
➤ Recent or remote MI follow-up
➤ Differential diagnosis of cardiac problems
➤ Baseline data if client is at risk for cardiac problems
➤ Preoperative workup
➤ Client starting an exercise program

CONTRAINDICATIONS

➤ None

PROCEDURE

ECG Interpretation

Basic Cardiac Information Needed

➤ **Depolarization**—electrical stimulation of the heart muscle causing the heart cells to contract
➤ **Repolarization**—resting or relaxation phase of the heart muscle
➤ ECG components
  ➤ **P wave**—depicts atrial stimulation or depolarization
  ➤ **P-R interval**—depicts the time it takes atrial stimulation to reach the atrioventricular (AV) node
    • During this time, blood flows from the atria through the AV valves into the ventricles. Normal time for this to occur is less than 0.2 second (Fig. 74–1).
  ➤ **QRS complex**—depicts the beginning of ventricular contraction or depolarization; normal time for this to occur is less than 0.12 second
    • **Q wave**—the first downward deflection of the QRS complex.
      • You may notice that sometimes the Q wave is absent from the QRS complex. *Don't be alarmed*. This is a physiologic variation and may happen occasionally.
    • **R wave**—the first upward deflection of the QRS complex
    • **S wave**—any downward deflection that first is preceded by an upward deflection of the QRS complex
    • **ST segment**—the pause after the QRS complex.
      • The line should be flat. If it is elevated or depressed, there is a major problem.
    • **T wave**—depicts ventricular repolarization or relaxation
➤ ECG paper
  ➤ 1 small square is 1 mm long and wide (0.04 second)
  ➤ 1 large square (from one heavy line to the next heavy line) is 5 mm long and wide (0.2 second)

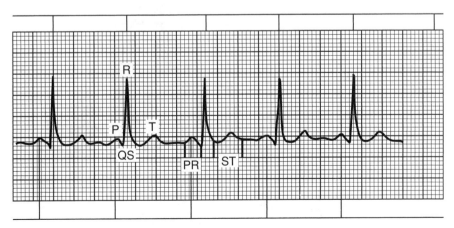

FIGURE 74 • 1 ECG components.

➤ Baseline ECG tracing—first tracing done on which further ECG changes are based

➤ Limb leads are measured in the frontal plane (Table 74–1). A pair of **electrodes** (one is + and one is −) forms a **limb lead**.

TABLE **74 • 1** 12 LEAD ECG TRACING: LIMB LEAD TITLES, LOCATION, AND NORMAL

LIMB HEADS	HEADS–FRONTAL PLANE	NORMAL CONFIGURATION
I	Left arm + → right arm −	Lead I
II	Left leg + → left arm −	Lead II
III	Left arm + → right arm −	Lead III
aVR	Right arm +; left arm and left leg −	AVR
aVL	Left arm +; right arm and left leg −	AVL
AvF	Left foot +; right and left arms −	AVF

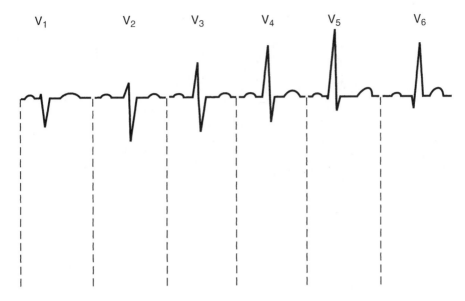

FIGURE 74•2 Normal chest leads.

➤ Chest leads are measured in the horizontal plane (Fig. 74–2). The chest leads normally produce a positive deflection in a progressive manner. The placement of the chest leads correlates with what area of the heart is measured (Table 74–2).

METHODOLOGIC INTERPRETATION

There are five general areas—rate, rhythm, axis, **hypertrophy,** and infarction.

➤ Rate—The following is the best method for measuring rate or beats per minute (beats/min) on the 12-lead ECG because it is based on 3 seconds of tracing (Fig. 74–3). Other methods are easier for measuring rate on a rhythm strip.

TABLE 74 • 2 ECG CHEST LEADS AND WHAT THEY MEASURE

LEAD	PLACEMENT	WHAT IS MEASURED
V_1	4th intercostal space (ICS) right sternal border (RSB)	Right side of the heart
V_2	4th ICS left sternal border (LSB)	Right side of the heart
V_3	Halfway between V_2 and V_4	Intraventricular septum
V_4	5th ICS midclavicular line	Intraventricular septum
V_5	Anterior axillary line lateral to V_4	Left side of the heart
V_6	Midaxillary line lateral to V_5	Left side of the heart

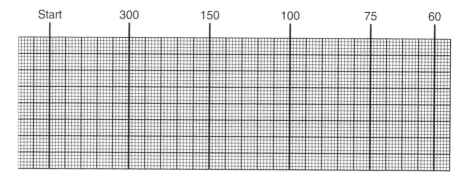

FIGURE 74•3 Measure rate.

➤ Look at the ECG paper and measure from one R wave to the next R wave.
  • First heavy black line to the next heavy black line (1/300 minute) = 300 beats/min
  • Then = 150 beats/min (2 heavy lines = 2/300 or 1/150)
  • Then = 100 beats/min (3 heavy lines = 3/300 or 1/100)
  • Then = 75 beats/min (4 heavy lines = 4/300 or 1/75)
  • Then = 60 beats/min (5 heavy lines = 5/300 or 1/60)
  • Then = 50 beats/min (6 heavy lines = 6/300 or 1/50)
➤ Within a 6-second strip, count cycles from R wave to R wave and multiply by 10 (the number of 6-second intervals in 1 minute = cycles/min).
  • Bradycardia (slow)—less than 60 cycles/min
  • Tachycardia (fast)—greater than 100 cycles/min
➤ Rhythm—The pattern of electrical conduction phenomena of the heart as the electrical current passes from the **sinoatrial node** (SA) through the AV node through the **bundle of His**, **bundle branches**, and the **Purkinje fibers**.
  ➤ Regular—distance between R waves is always equal.
    • Normal sinus rhythm (60 to 100 beats/min) (Fig. 74–4)
  ➤ Irregular—distance between R waves is not always equal.
    • AV blocks (Fig. 74–5)
      • First-degree AV block—P-R interval greater than 0.2 second on each cycle
      • Second-degree Wenckebach (type I)—P-R interval gets progressively longer until one P-R interval is finally dropped (not life-threatening)
      • Second-degree Mobitz II (type II)—a QRS complex is dropped with no lengthening of P-R interval (can lead to complete heart block)
      • Third-degree AV block (complete heart block)—none of the P-R intervals is related to a QRS complex

Equal distance between "QRS" complexes.

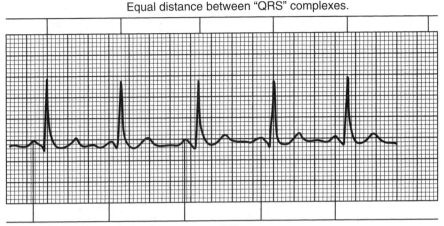

Equal distance between "P" waves.

FIGURE 74 • 4 Normal sinus rhythm.

- The rate lets you know the focus from which it originates.
- Ventricle focus is at a rate of 20 to 40 beats/min.
- A junctional focus is at a rate of 40 to 60 beats/min.
- Bundle-branch block (BBB) (Fig. 74–6)—usually the bundle branches are depolarized simultaneously.
  - A delay of electrical impulse to either the right or the left bundle branches results in one ventricular depolarization slightly later than the other.
  - On the ECG, a "Double-peaked" or "joined" widened QRS complex appears.
  - For a right BBB, check chest leads V_1 and V_2 for double-peaked QRS complexes.
  - For a left BBB, check chest leads V_5 and V_6 for double-peaked QRS complexes. These also are known as *hemiblocks* and commonly are associated with MI. MI is hard to diagnose, however, in the presence of a left BBB.
- Ectopic foci—stimulus from an ectopic focus (Fig. 74–7); results in premature beats (short beats) or escape beats (prolonged beats). Included are
  - Paroxysmal atrial tachycardia—150 to 250 beats/min
  - Supraventricular tachycardia—150 to 250 beats/min
  - Ventricular tachycardia—150 to 250 beats/min
  - Premature atrial contractions—early SA node contraction
  - Premature ventricular contractions (PVCs)—early ventricular firing
    - PVCs can be *unifocal* or *multifocal.*
    - A unifocal PVC comes from an abnormal focus in the *same place* in the ventricle *every* time and looks the same each time.

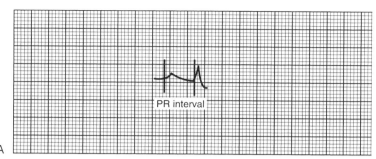

A

PR interval greater than 0.20 mm (5 small blocks)

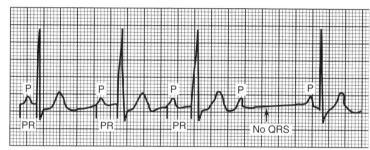

B

PR interval elongates and a QRS complex is dropped.

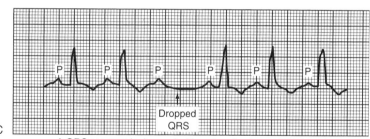

C

A QRS segment is dropped with no lengthening of PR intervals.

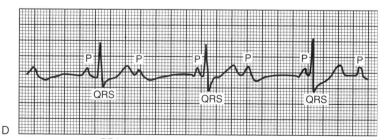

D

PR intervals are unrelated to QRS complexes.

FIGURE 74•5 AV blocks. (A) First-degree AV block, (B) second-degree Wenckebach (type I), (C) second-degree Mobitz II (type II), and (D) third-degree (complete heart block).

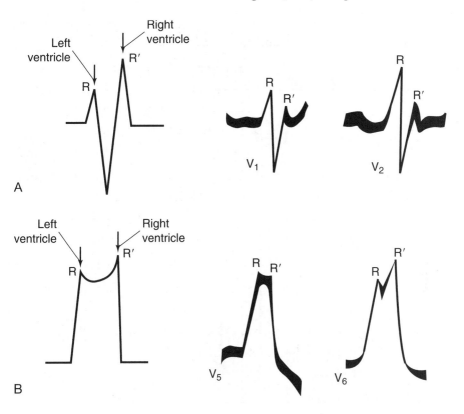

FIGURE 74 • 6 Bundle-branch blocks. (A) Right bundle-branch block and (B) left bundle-branch block.

- A multifocal PVC comes from *several* abnormal foci in the ventricles and looks different each time. A multifocal PVC is a much worse indicator of more serious heart disease is than a unifocal PVC.
- **Flutter**—250 to 300 beats/min
  - Flutter can be atrial or ventricular in origin.
  - A flutter has a regular single ectopic focus. It is sawtoothed in appearance.
- **Fibrillation**—350 to 450 beats/min
  - Fibrillation can be atrial or ventricular in origin.
  - A fibrillatory beat is irregular and comes from multiple foci. It is *irregular* in appearance and is an indicator of much worse heart disease.

➤ Axis (vector)—direction and magnitude of the electrical stimulus of depolarization starting at the AV node and continuing through the ventricles
  ➤ Axis is measured in degrees.

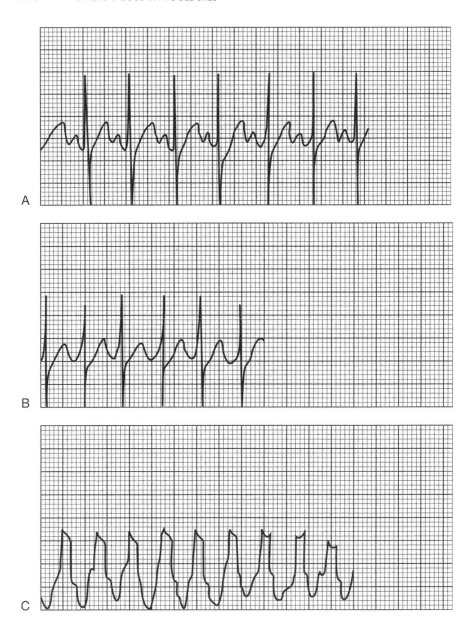

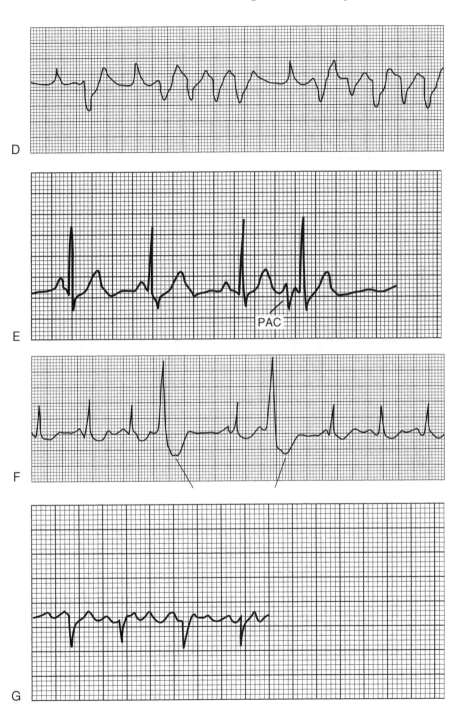

D

E

PAC

F

G

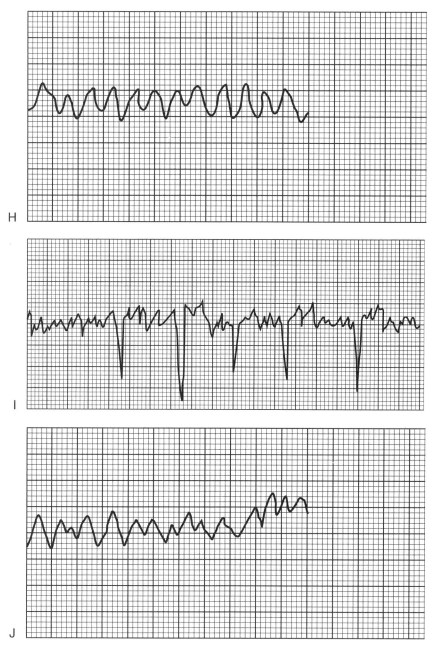

H

I

J

FIGURE 74 • 7 Ectopic foci. (A) Paroxysmal atrial tachycardia, 150 to 200 beats/min; (B) supraventricular tachycardia; (C) paroxysmal ventricular tachycardia; (D) runs of paroxysmal ventricular tachycardia; (E) premature atrial contraction; (F) premature ventricular contractions; (G) atrial flutter; (H) ventricular flutter; (I) atrial fibrillation; and (J) ventricular fibrillation.

➤ With a normal axis, the mean QRS (+0 to +90 degrees) **vector** points downward and toward the client's left side because that is the way the normal heart lies in the chest (Fig. 74–8). To measure axis, do the following
  • With the AV node as the center, imagine a circle around the heart measured in degrees positive (+) and negative (−).

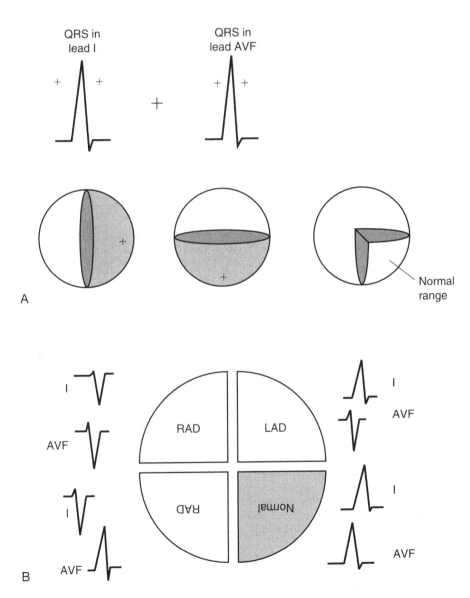

FIGURE 74 • 8 Check leads I and AVF to determine (A) normal axis or (B) axis deviation.

- Positive degrees are measured in the lower half of the heart.
- Negative degrees are measured in the top half of the heart.
- In lead I, measure the right and left spheres (halves) of axis (left is +, right is −).
  - A + deflection occurs when the stimulus is moving toward the left (left axis deviation).
  - A − deflection occurs when the electrical stimulus is moving toward the right (right axis deviation).
- aVF measures the upper and lower spheres (halves) of axis (upper is −, lower is +).
  - If the deflection is mainly +, the mean QRS vector is downward.
  - If the deflection is mainly −, the mean QRS vector is upward.
- Chest leads record axis on a horizontal plane.
  - They should be − in leads V_1 and V_2 and + in leads V_5 and V_6.
  - A progression from − in V_1 to + in V_6 is normal.
- Lead V_2, because of its position, projects through the anterior wall of the heart to the posterior wall of the heart and gives the best information on anterior and posterior wall MIs.

Things That Affect Axis

➤ Obesity—pushes the heart up, and the mean QRS vector is directed to the left of +0 degrees
➤ Infarction—no electrical stimulus goes through dead tissue, and the mean QRS vector *turns away* from the infarcted area of tissue
➤ Ventricular hypertrophy—has electrical activity, and the mean QRS vector *deviates* toward the enlarged ventricle
➤ Hypertrophy—increase in heart size or wall thickness because of an increased volume in the chambers of the heart (Fig. 74–9).
  ➤ Atrial hypertrophy
    - P wave depicts contraction of the atria.
    - Lead V_1 is placed directly over the atria (fourth intercostal space [ICS], right sternal border).
    - Hypertrophy of atria is shown as a diphasic wave (+ or − deflection) P wave in lead V_1.
    - If right atrial hypertrophy is present, the *beginning* portion of the diphasic wave is larger.
    - If left atrial hypertrophy is present, the *end* portion of the diphasic wave is larger.
  ➤ Ventricular hypertrophy—QRS wave depicts the contraction of the ventricles
    - Lead V_1 tracing is usually negative (small R wave and large S wave) because depolarization is *away* from the right side of the heart toward the thicker left side of the heart.
    - Hypertrophy of the ventricles is shown by the deflection of the QRS in lead V_1 (+ or −) (Fig. 74–10).
      - Right ventricular hypertrophy—V_1 has a + deflected QRS
        - The electrical stimulus is away from the left side toward the thicker right side.

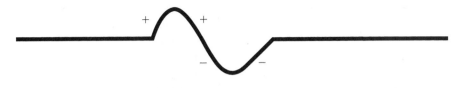

Diphasic P wave

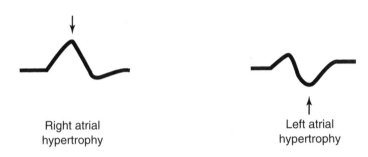

| Right atrial hypertrophy | Left atrial hypertrophy |

FIGURE 74 • 9 Atrial hypertrophy.

- Progression of V_1 to V_6 starts with large R waves in V_1 and ends with a small R wave in V_6.
- V_2 is directly over the right ventricle and is the best place to look for right ventricular *strain.*
- Left ventricular hypertrophy—more depolarization toward the left than usual
  - A *small R wave* and *deep S wave* in V_1.
  - Lead V_5 is directly over the left ventricle, so if the left ventricle is enlarged, V_5 has a more + deflection resulting in a *tall R wave.*
  - You must *add* the S wave in V_1 and the R wave in V_5 together in millimeters. If these add up to greater than 35 mm, left ventricular hypertrophy is present.
- T waves also indicate ventricular hypertrophy.
  - V_5 and V_6 are directly over the left ventricle and are the best place to look for left ventricular *strain.*
  - The wave is *inverted* and *asymmetric.*
- ➤ Hypoxia—occlusion of a coronary artery (by thrombus or arteriosclerotic plaques) producing lack of blood supply to the heart, resulting in decreased oxygenation to the cells
- ➤ Usually only the left ventricle suffers an MI.
- ➤ On the ECG, you can determine if the heart has suffered **ischemia,** *injury,* or *infarction.*

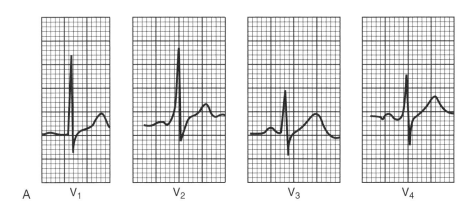

A   V₁   V₂   V₃   V₄

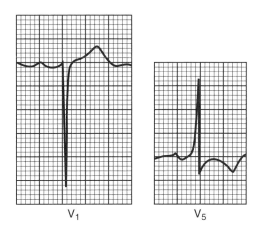

B   V₁   V₅

FIGURE 74 • 10 Ventricular hypertrophy. (A) Right ventricular hypertrophy; (B) left ventricular hypertrophy

- Ischemia (decreased blood supply)—"smiley" face (Fig. 74–11).
- Shown as a T-wave inversion and symmetry
  - In V_2 to V_6, this indicates pathology.
  - In limb leads, this is a normal variation.
- Injury (acuteness of infarct)—"frowny" face (Fig. 74–12).
  - Shown as elevated ST segment
  - Elevation of ST segment indicates *only* a small acute infarct, pericarditis, or ventricular aneurysm (T wave does *not* return to baseline).
  - Depressed ST segment may indicate a partial-thickness (subendocardial) infarct or digitalis effect.
- Infarction (Fig. 74–13)—not diagnosable if left BBB is present

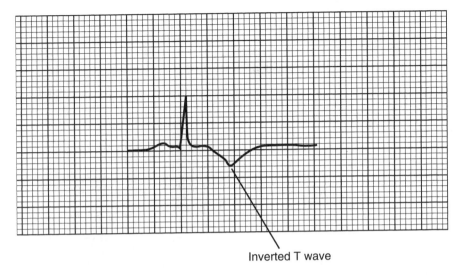

Inverted T wave

FIGURE 74 • 11 Myocardial ischemia.

- Check all leads for *significant Q waves.* Q waves that are significant are 0.04 second (1 small square) wide *or* 1/3 amplitude of the entire QRS complex.
- Q waves (first downward deflection of the QRS) are usually absent in the normal person.
- *Tiny Q waves are insignificant* in leads I, II, V₅, and V₆.

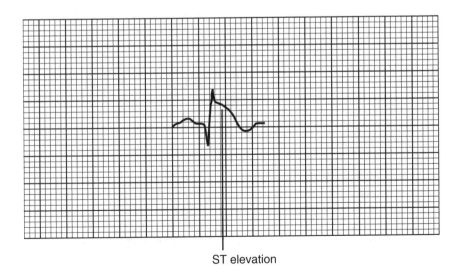

ST elevation

FIGURE 74 • 12 Myocardial injury.

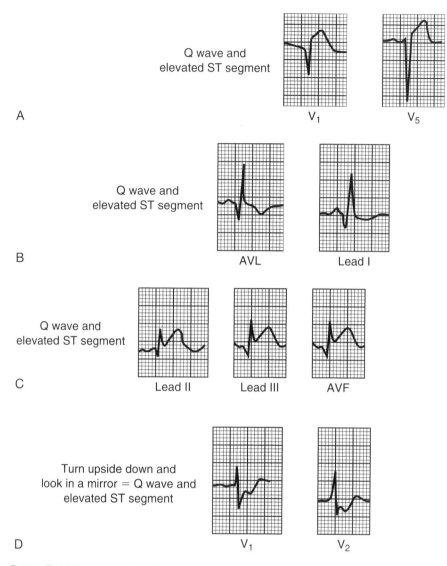

FIGURE 74•13 Myocardial infarction. (A) Anterior infarction, (B) lateral infarction, (C) inferior infarction, and (D) posterior infarction

- Anterior infarction (V_1 to V_4)
  - Check all chest leads (V_1 to V_4) for the presence of significant Q waves (0.04 second) and for elevated ST segment. Because all chest leads are anteriorly placed, it makes sense to check these leads.
- Lateral infarction (aVL, lead I)
  - Check aVL and lead I for significant Q waves and elevated ST segment.

- Inferior infarction (aVF, leads II and III)
  - Check aVF and leads II and III for significant Q waves or elevated or depressed ST segments.
- Posterior infarction (V_1 to V_2)
  - Opposite picture from anterior MI. There is a larger R wave and obviously depressed ST segment.
  - Do the mirror test. Turn the ECG upside down and look at it in a mirror. It should look like the classic acute infarct.

QUICK AND EASY INTERPRETATION

➤ Rate—300, 150, 100, 75, 60, 50
  ➤ If bradycardia, check 6-second strip and multiply by 10.
➤ Rhythm—regular or irregular? AV block or BBB?
➤ Axis—Right or left? Positive or negative? If present, think hypertrophy and infarction.
➤ Hypertrophy
  ➤ Atrial—V_1—diphasic P wave
    - Large *initial* positive deflection = right atrial hypertrophy
    - Large *ending* negative deflection = left atrial hypertrophy
  ➤ Ventricular
    - V_1—positive deflection of QRS = right ventricular hypertrophy
    - V_2—inverted and asymmetric T = right ventricular hypertrophy
    - Check V_1—if deep S wave, measure
    - Check V_5—if large R wave, measure
    - Add V_1 and V_5 together; if greater than 35 mm = left ventricular hypertrophy
    - Check V_5 and V_6—if inverted and asymmetric T wave = left ventricular hypertrophy
➤ Hypoxia
  ➤ Ischemia—smiley face—T wave inverted and symmetric in V_1 to V_6 only
  ➤ Injury—frowny face—ST segment elevated = acute full-thickness MI
    - Depressed ST segment = partial-thickness MI
  ➤ Infarction
    - Q wave present
    - ST elevation
      - Anterior MI—Q in V_1 to V_4 and ST wave elevation
      - Lateral MI—aVL and lead I—Q wave and ST wave elevation
      - Inferior MI—aVF, leads II and III—Q wave and ST wave elevation
      - Posterior MI—opposite of anterior MI; larger R wave with ST wave depression

OTHER HEART PROBLEMS

See Figures 74–14 and 74–15.
➤ Digitalis effect—downsloping QT segment
➤ Digitalis toxicity—PVCs (bigeminy or trigeminy), ventricular tachycardia, ventricular fibrillation, atrial fibrillation
➤ Emphysema—low voltage in leads I, II, and III and right axis deviation (lead I negative, aVF positive)

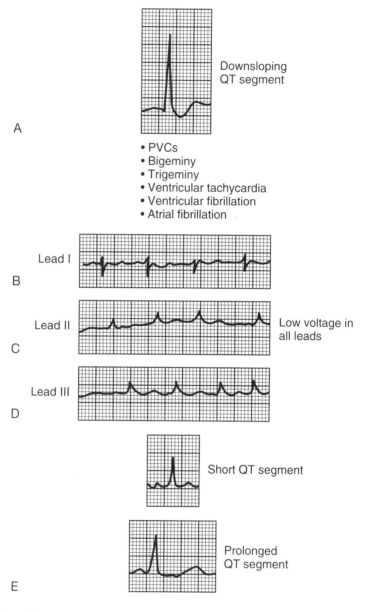

FIGURE 74 • 14 Other heart problems. (A) Digitalis effect, (B) digitalis toxicity, (C) emphysema, (D) hypercalcemia, and (E) hypocalcemia.

➤ Hypercalcemia—short QT segment
➤ Hypocalcemia—long QT segment
➤ Hyperkalemia—peaked T wave, flattened P wave, widened QRS

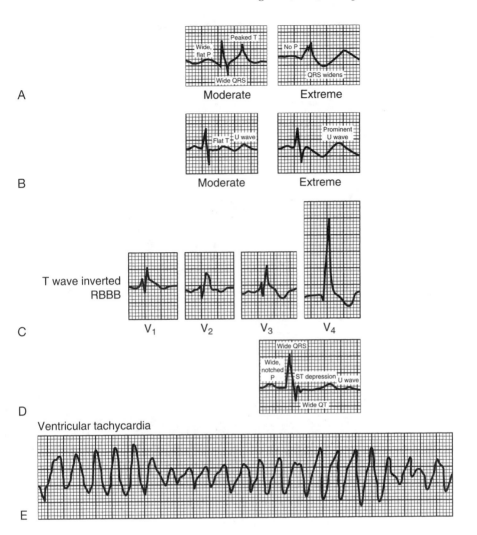

FIGURE 74 • 15 Other heart problems. (A) Hyperkalemia, (B) hypokalemia, (C) pulmonary embolus, (D) quinidine effect, and (E) quinidine toxicity.

➤ Hypokalemia
  ➤ Moderate—flat T wave
  ➤ Extreme—prominent U wave (wave sometimes appearing immediately after the T wave)
➤ Pulmonary embolus
  ➤ Large S wave in lead I
  ➤ ST segment depression in lead II
  ➤ Large Q wave in lead III with T wave inversion
  ➤ Right BBB and T wave inversion in V_1 to V_4

➤ Quinidine effect—notched P wave, widened QRS, ST segment depressed, prolonged QT segment, U waves
➤ Quinidine toxicity—ventricular tachycardia

BIBLIOGRAPHY

Dubin, D. (1994) (4th ed.). *Rapid interpretation of EKGs.* Tampa: Cover Publishing.
Grauer, K. (1991). *ECG interpretation.* St. Louis: Mosby.
Thaler, M.S. (1995) (2nd ed.). *The only EKG book you'll ever need.* Philadelphia: Lippincott.

75

ELECTROCARDIOGRAM (ECG) LEAD PLACEMENT

MARGARET R. COLYAR

CPT Code	
93000	ECG, routine; with at least 12 leads; with interpretation and report
93005	ECG tracing only; with interpretation and report
93010	ECG interpretation and report only

To ensure an accurate ECG, correct lead placement is vital. Leads that are misplaced can cause potentially dangerous interpretation errors.

OVERVIEW

➤ Incidence unknown
➤ Common errors include
  ➤ Placement of leads in wrong anatomic locations
    • Switching one lead with another lead in a comparable area
    • Inaccurate positioning, especially precordial, can create the impression of mirror-image dextrocardia or possible lateral **MI**.
  ➤ Exchange of two or more precordial leads can produce misleading patterns.
  ➤ Exchange of right and left leg leads—no significant change

> Exchange of left leg and left arm leads—insignificant Q wave in lead III
> Exchange of left arm and right leg leads—low voltage in lead III
> Leg leads placed on abdomen or arm leads placed on upper chest— distortion of pattern
> Exchange of right and left *arm* leads—misinterpretation of pattern— lateral MI
> Exchange of right arm and right or left leg leads—misinterpretation of pattern—inferior wall MI or previous MI, pericardial effusion, emphysema, or thyroid problem

RATIONALE

> To ensure satisfactory ECG tracings
> To promote pertinent ECG readings

INDICATIONS

> Chest pain
> Rule out cardiac involvement

CONTRAINDICATIONS

> None

PROCEDURE
ECG Lead Placement
Equipment

> ECG machine with limb leads, chest leads, and cable
> ECG paper
> Electrodes
> Grounded safe electrical outlet

Procedure

> Position the client supine.
> Plug in machine.
> Enter client identification data into the machine, if required.
> Set speed at 25 mm/sec and size sensitivity at 10 mm/sec.
> Cleanse skin with alcohol if dirty or oily.
> Apply electrodes in proper configuration.
> Limb leads (Fig. 75–1)
  • Legs—distal third of lower leg on anterior medial surface
  • Arms—volar surface of distal third of forearms
> Chest leads (Fig. 75–2)
  • V_1—fourth ICS right sternal border
  • V_2—fourth ICS left sternal border
  • V_3—halfway between V_2 and V_4

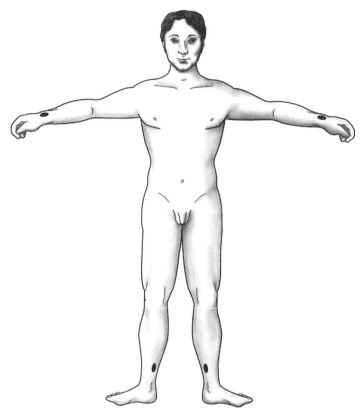

FIGURE 75 • 1 Limb lead placement.

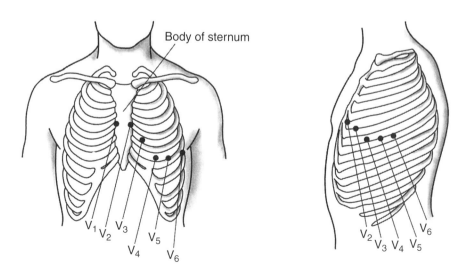

FIGURE 75 • 2 Chest lead placement.

- V_4—fifth ICS midclavicular line
- V_5—anterior axillary line lateral to V_4
- V_6—midaxillary line lateral to V_5

➤ Attach cable to the electrodes.
➤ Push the record button.
➤ If an arrhythmia is seen, obtain a rhythm strip (long lead II).
➤ Remove the electrodes and cleanse the skin if needed.

Client Instructions

➤ Lie still while the ECG machine is running.
➤ There will be no electrical shock.

B I B L I O G R A P H Y

Edmunds, M.W., and Mayhew, M.S. (1996). *Procedures for primary care practitioners*. St. Louis: Mosby.

Peberdy, M.A., and Ornato, J.P. (1994). ECG leads: misplacement and misdiagnosis. *Emerg Med*, Oct., 37–38.

HOLTER MONITOR APPLICATION
CONTINUOUS 24-HOUR AMBULATORY CARDIAC MONITORING

76

MARGARET R. COLYAR

CPT Code

93230–93237   ECG monitoring for 24 hours

A Holter monitor is a portable ECG machine with memory. A Holter monitor oversees cardiac activity for 24 hours, usually to detect and evaluate cardiac disease, drug effects, and pacemakers. During the 24-hour period, the heart has approximately 100,000 cardiac cycles.

OVERVIEW

- ➤ Incidence unknown
- ➤ Used to detect and evaluate
  - ➤ Arrhythmias
  - ➤ Chest pain
  - ➤ Effect of antiarrhythmic drug therapy
  - ➤ Client status after an acute MI
  - ➤ Client status after the implantation of a pacemaker

RATIONALE

- ➤ To detect and evaluate cardiac disease, drug effects, and operation of pacemakers

INDICATIONS

- ➤ MI
- ➤ Pacemaker
- ➤ Chest pain
- ➤ Cardiac symptoms
- ➤ Unexplained fainting

CONTRAINDICATIONS

- ➤ None

PROCEDURE

Holter Monitoring

Equipment

- ➤ Monitor with new battery
- ➤ Case with strap
- ➤ Cassette tape
- ➤ Electrodes
- ➤ Electrode gel
- ➤ Cable and lead wires
- ➤ Alcohol or **acetone**
- ➤ 4 × 4 gauze—nonsterile
- ➤ Disposable razor
- ➤ Tape
- ➤ Diary

Procedure

- ➤ Position the client in a seated, upright position.
- ➤ Shave the electrode-placement sites.
- ➤ Cleanse the electrode sites with alcohol or acetone to remove body oils.
- ➤ Apply electrodes.
  - ➤ Remove paper backing.
  - ➤ Press firmly in position.
  - ➤ Attach the cables to the electrodes.

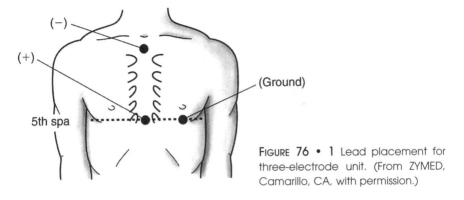

FIGURE 76 • 1 Lead placement for three-electrode unit. (From ZYMED, Camarillo, CA, with permission.)

➤ Attach the cables to the monitor.
➤ Place the monitor strap around the client's neck.
➤ Place the monitor in the monitor case.
➤ Run the monitor cables through the front of the client's shirt or blouse and button.

LEAD PLACEMENT FOR THREE-ELECTRODE UNIT

See Figure 76–1
➤ Place over bone, not ICSs; this prevents distortion caused by muscle movement.
➤ Positive electrode—Place over the fifth rib left midclavicular line.
➤ Negative electrode—Place over the manubrium.
➤ Ground wire—Place over the fifth right midclavicular line.

LEAD PLACEMENT FOR FIVE-EECTRODE UNIT

See Figure 76–2
➤ Place over bone, not ICSs; this prevents distortion caused by muscle movement.
➤ Positive electrodes—Place over the sternum at the fifth ICS and the left anterior axillary line at the fifth ICS.

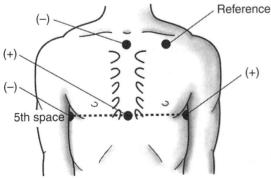

FIGURE 76 • 2 Lead placement for five-electrode unit. (From ZYMED, Camarillo, CA, with permission.)

➤ Negative electrodes—Place over right anterior axillary line at the fifth ICS and the top of the sternum below the sternal notch.
➤ Ground wire—Place over the left midclavicular line at the first ICS.

DIARY

Log all daily activities (Fig. 76–3). Compare with the Holter recording to determine a correlation between the client's symptoms and cardiac arrhythmias.

Time	Activity	Symptoms
9 AM	Watching TV	
11:30	Eating lunch	Short of breath
1 PM	Reading	
2 PM	Taking a walk	Dizzy, Short of breath
3:30	Went to pick up children	Dizzy, Chest pain, Sweaty
5 PM	Eating supper	Short of breath
7 PM	Watching TV	
9:30	To bed	Weak
6 AM	Getting ready for work	Short of breath, Chest pain
7 AM	At computer at work	Dizzy, weak

FIGURE 76 • 3 Example of a daily diary.

➤ Fill the diary with time and activity whenever you change activity, such as
  ➤ Stair climbing
  ➤ Running
  ➤ Walking
  ➤ Sleeping
  ➤ Elimination
  ➤ Intercourse
  ➤ Emotional upset
  ➤ Physical symptoms such as
    • Dizziness
    • Palpitations
    • Chest pain
    • Any pain
    • Fatigue
    • Shortness of breath
  ➤ Ingestion of medications
  ➤ Eating

Client Instructions

➤ Wear loose-fitting clothes.
➤ Wear a watch so that you can complete accurately the activity and symptom diary.
➤ You may take a sponge bath, but avoid wetting the equipment and dislodging the electrodes. If the electrodes become dislodged, do the following
  ➤ Partially dislodged—Depress the center to reattach.
  ➤ Fully dislodged—Return to the office for lead placement.
➤ Avoid magnets, metal detectors (e.g., at airports), high-voltage areas, and electric blankets.

BIBLIOGRAPHY

Grauer, K. (1994). Holter monitoring. In Pfenninger, J.L., and Fowler, G.C. (eds.). *Procedures for primary care physicians*. St. Louis: Mosby, pp. 378–407.

Grauer, K., and Leytem, B. (1992). A systemic approach to Holter monitor interpretation. *Am Fam Physician*, 45, 1641–1645.

Thaler, M.S. (1995). *The only EKG book you'll ever need*. Philadelphia: Lippincott.

Zymed, Inc. (1997). *Automatic 12-lead data from Holter and telemetry patients*. Camarillo, CA: Author.

77 ARTERIAL PUNCTURE

MARGARET R. COLYAR

CPT Code

82803   Gases, blood, any combination of pH, P_{CO_2}, P_{O_2}, CO_2, HCO_3 (including calculated O_2 saturation)

Arterial puncture is performed to determine the client's acid-base balance, oxygenation, and ventilation. Arterial blood gases (ABGs) are a mixture of measured and calculated values. The pH, P_{O_2}, P_{CO_2}, and HCO_3 measurements are used to interpret the meaning of the ABGs. Analysis of ABGs is usually a two-step process. First, the acid-base balance is determined. Second, the oxygenation status is determined. Normal ABG values are given in Table 77–1. Abnormal ABG values with interpretation are given in Table 77–2.

OVERVIEW

➤ Incidence unknown
➤ Site selection (Fig. 77–1)
  ➤ First choice—radial artery
    • Less chance of hematoma because of the ease of compression over bones and ligaments of wrist.
    • Do **Allen's test** to check for collateral circulation through the ulnar artery before the stick (Fig. 77–2).
  ➤ Second choice—brachial artery
    • Larger artery but deeper and close to a vein and nerve
  ➤ Third choice—femoral artery
    • Large artery
    • Easily palpated and punctured but poor collateral circulation
    • Increased risk of infection because of the location of the site
    • Palpate just below inguinal ligament
    • From lateral to medial, structures are
      • Nerve
      • Artery
      • Vein

TABLE 77 •1   NORMAL VALUES FOR ARTERIAL BLOOD GASES

pH	P_{CO_2}	HCO_3	P_{O_2}
7.35–7.45	35–45 mm Hg	24–28 mEq/L	75–100 mm Hg

TABLE 77•2 ABNORMAL (ARTERIAL BLOOD GAS) VALUES
WITH INTERPRETATION

pH	PCO₂	HCO₃	INTERPRETATION
<7.35	>45	Normal	Respiratory acidosis
<7.35	>45	>28	Respiratory acidosis with metabolic compensation
>7.45	<35	Normal	Respiratory alkalosis
>7.45	<35	<24	Respiratory alkalosis with metabolic compensation
<7.35	Normal	<24	Metabolic acidosis
<7.35	<35	<24	Metabolic acidosis with respiratory compensation
>7.45	Normal	>28	Metabolic alkalosis
>7.45	>45	>28	Metabolic alkalosis with respiratory compensation

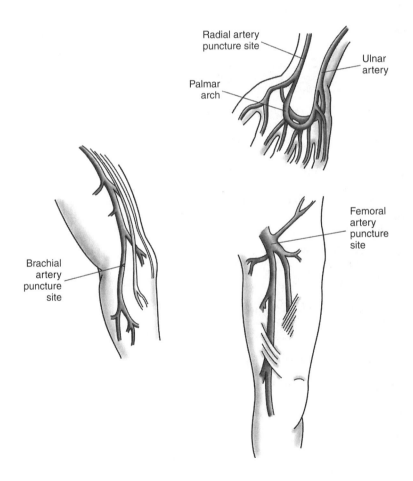

FIGURE 77 • 1 Site selection for arterial puncture.

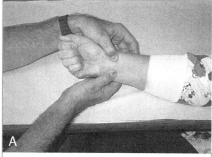
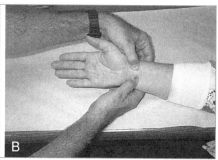
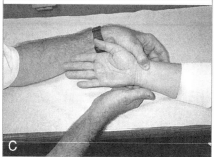

FIGURE 77 • 2 Check for collateral circulation using the Allen's test. The client makes a fist while the radial and ulnar arteries are occluded. *(A)* The thenar surface of the palm becomes pale. *(B)* The client opens the palm and the pallor remains while the arteries are occluded. *(C)* When the ulnar occlusion is removed, the palm should return to pink.

- Empty space
- Lymphatics

RATIONALE

➤ To determine acid-base balance, oxygenation, and ventilation

INDICATIONS

➤ Respiratory disorder
➤ Cardiac failure
➤ Renal disease
➤ Drug overdose
➤ Uncontrolled diabetes mellitus
➤ Metabolic disorder

CONTRAINDICATIONS

➤ No collateral circulation

PROCEDURE

Arterial Puncture

Equipment

➤ Gloves—nonsterile
➤ Syringe—3 to 5 mL

➤ 23- to 25-gauge, 1-inch needle
➤ Heparin (1000 U/mL), 1 mL
➤ Alcohol swabs
➤ Povidone-iodine (Betadine) swabs
➤ Cup of ice
➤ Small block of rubber or latex
➤ 2 × 2 gauze
➤ Tape

Procedure

➤ Select the site.
➤ Position the client with the site easily accessible. If using the radial artery, the wrist should be hyperextended.
➤ Put on gloves.
➤ Draw up 1 mL of 1:1000 heparin into the syringe.
  ➣ Pull the plunger all the way back.
  ➣ Expel all the heparin. The syringe is now coated with heparin.
➤ Palpate the artery proximally and distally (Fig. 77–3).
➤ Trap the artery between two fingers placed on each side.
➤ Cleanse the site with alcohol.
➤ Apply povidone-iodine to the area in a circular motion, starting where you plan to puncture and working outward.
➤ Hold the syringe like a pencil, with the bevel up.
➤ Using a 90-degree angle, insert the needle.
➤ The syringe usually fills spontaneously. If it does not fill spontaneously, aspirate gently.
  ➣ If you do not get blood, pull back the needle without coming out of the skin and redirect toward the artery.
➤ When the specimen is obtained, withdraw the needle.
  ➣ Apply firm pressure to the site for 5 minutes; apply pressure for 10 minutes if the client is on anticoagulants.
  ➣ Expel the air from the syringe.
  ➣ Rotate the syringe to mix the contents.

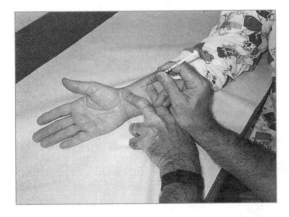

FIGURE 77 • 3 Trap the artery between two fingers. After preparing the site, insert the needle at a 90-degree angle into the artery.

➤ Place the needle tip into a rubber block.
➤ Place the syringe into a cup of ice.
➤ Check the site for bleeding.
➤ Cleanse the site with alcohol, and apply a 2 × 2 pressure dressing.

Client Instructions

➤ Keep pressure dressing in place for 30 minutes, then remove.
➤ Observe for signs and symptoms of infection, such as
  ➤ Increase in pain after 24 hours
  ➤ Increase in temperature
  ➤ Redness or swelling
  ➤ Yellow or greenish drainage
  ➤ Foul odor
➤ If any signs or symptoms of infection are found, return to the office.

B I B L I O G R A P H Y

Gomella, L.G. (1993). *Clinician's pocket reference.* Norwalk, CT: Appleton & Lange.
McCall, R.E., and Tankersley, C.M. (1993). *Phlebotomy essentials.* Philadelphia: Lippincott.
Swartz, G.R. (1992). *Principles and practices of emergency medicine.* St. Louis: Mosby.

78

BLOOD CULTURE SPECIMEN COLLECTION

MARGARET R. COLYAR

CPT Code
36415   Blood specimen collection
87040   Blood culture collection

Blood culture specimen collection requires a precise specimen collection procedure to obtain, store, and transport correctly. Culture medium is inoculated with a blood sample and incubated for isolation and identification of pathogens. Many laboratories have their own policy for blood culture specimen collection. Check with the laboratory to determine any special requirements.

TABLE 78•1 TYPES OF BLOOD CULTURES

Aerobic
Anaerobic
Fungal
Mycobacterial
Viral

OVERVIEW

➤ Incidence unknown
➤ Identification of approximately 70% of pathogens within 24 hours
➤ Identification of approximately 90% of pathogens with 72 hours
➤ Sample collection
  ➣ Types of blood cultures (Table 78–1)
  ➣ Number and timing of blood cultures (Table 78–2)
    • Microorganisms enter bloodstream 30 to 90 minutes before fever spikes.
  ➣ Amount of blood needed (Table 78–3)
➤ Do *not* use vacutainer needle to draw cultures.
➤ Do *not* change needle between blood draw and transfer to culture medium (chance of contamination). Some laboratories require change of needle at this step.

RATIONALE

➤ To confirm bacteremia or septicemia
➤ To identify causative organisms

INDICATIONS

➤ Fever/chills
➤ Sepsis
➤ Prostration
➤ Pain/headache
➤ Nausea/vomiting

TABLE 78•2 BLOOD CULTURES—NUMBER AND TIMINIG

DISEASE PROCESS	NUMBER/TIMING
Acute sepsis	2 or 3 sets from separate sites
Endocarditis	
Acute	3 sets from 3 separate sites over 1–2 hr
Subacute	3 sets on day 1 (15 min apart)
Fever of unknown origin	2 separate sets 1 hr apart. If negative, redraw in 36 hr
On antimicrobial treatment for 1–2 wk	2 separate sets on 3 successive days

TABLE 78•3 BLOOD CULTURES—AMOUNT OF BLOOD TO OBTAIN

AGE	AMOUNT OF BLOOD
Neonate	1 mL
Small child	4 mL
Adults	Bacterial—20 mL
	Fungal—30 mL

➤ Diarrhea—unexplained
➤ Signs of shock—drop in blood pressure, increased respirations, tachycardia
➤ Coma
➤ Mental confusion/anxiety
➤ Bacterial pneumonia
➤ Infectious endocarditis

CONTRAINDICATIONS

➤ Surveillance of infection before the clinical suspicion of infection exists

PROCEDURE

Blood Culture Specimen Collection

Equipment

➤ 2 innoculated culture media—in bottles (Fig. 78–1)
➤ 3 alcohol swabs
➤ 3 povidone-iodine swabs
➤ Gloves—nonsterile
➤ Tourniquet
➤ Syringes—2 to 3 each—20 mL
➤ Needles—20-gauge
➤ 2 × 2 gauze or cotton balls
➤ 2 adhesive bandages (Band-Aids) or tape
➤ 1 4 × 4 gauze

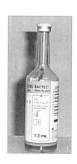

FIGURE 78 • 1 Blood culture medium bottle.

Procedure

➤ Put on gloves.
➤ Remove outer cap from blood culture medium bottles.
➤ Cleanse top of bottles with alcohol.
➤ Vigorously cleanse site with alcohol swab for 1 minute.
➤ Allow to air dry.
➤ Cleanse site with 10% iodine/povidone-iodine swab in circular motion from center outward in concentric circles.
➤ Let dry for 1 minute.
➤ Cleanse top of culture medium bottles with povidone-iodine.
➤ Apply tourniquet to client's arm.
➤ Do *not* palpate vein after prepared.
➤ Draw blood specimen.
➤ Remove the tourniquet from the arm.
➤ Remove the needle from the arm.
➤ Apply pressure to the puncture site with a cotton ball or 2 × 2 gauze.
  ➤ Keep pressure to site for 1 minute (if client is on anticoagulant therapy, apply pressure to 3 to 5 minutes).
  ➤ Wipe residual povidone-iodine from site with alcohol prep pads.
➤ Apply a Band-Aid or tape to secure.
➤ Inject appropriate amount of blood in each of two inoculated culture medium bottles.
➤ Invert bottles four to five times.
➤ Deposit the needles in a puncture-proof container.
➤ Label the culture medium bottles with the appropriate information (i.e., client's name, date, time, ID number, and your initials).
➤ Transport to the laboratory.
  ➤ Do not refrigerate.

Client Instructions

➤ Band-Aid may be removed in 15 minutes.
➤ Do not rub the site because rubbing increases risk of oozing and results in a bruised appearance.

BIBLIOGRAPHY
Colyar, M.R. (in press). *Well child assessment for health care providers.* Philadelphia: F.A. Davis.
Springhouse (2000). Diagnostics, nurse's reference library. Springhouse, PA: Author.
http://www.ehendrick.org/healthy/ (2002).
http://www.internalmed.wustl.edu (2002).
http://researchpath.hitchcock.org (2002).
http://www.uams.edu/nursing manual/procedures/procedure34.htm (2002).
http://www.uphs.upenn.edu/bug drug/antibiotic manual/ (2002).

79

Capillary Blood Collection— Heel/Finger Stick

MARGARET R. COLYAR

CPT Code

36415   Routine venipuncture of finger, heel, or ear stick for collection of specimens

Capillary blood collection is a method used to obtain blood specimens from the finger, heel, or in some cases the ear. This procedure is used when only a few drops of blood are required for performance of the test; when venous access fails; or when blood is required from small children, infants, or neonates.

OVERVIEW

➤ Incidence unknown
➤ Heel stick performed frequently on neonates and young infants
➤ Finger stick performed frequently on older children, adolescents, and adults
➤ General principles
  ➤ Collect enough blood to perform the required test.
  ➤ Collect specimen in proper container.
    • Capillary tube
    • Filter testing paper
  ➤ Minimize discomfort.
    • Side of fingertip
  ➤ Maintain sterile technique.

RATIONALE

➤ To obtain information about biochemical and biophysical status of the human organism

INDICATIONS

➤ Specific testing ordered to determine biochemical and biophysical information

CONTRAINDICATIONS

➤ Necrosis at the site
➤ Poor circulation at the site

PROCEDURE

Capillary Blood Collection—Heel/Finger Stick

Equipment

➤ Capillary specimen tube or filter paper for required test
➤ Lancet—2.4 mm or smaller
➤ Alcohol swabs
➤ Povidone-iodine swabs
➤ Cotton balls or 2 × 2 gauze
➤ Band-Aids
➤ Gloves—nonsterile
➤ Puncture-resistant sharps box container (biohazard approval and markings)

Procedure

See Figure 79–1
➤ Warm heel or finger to increase blood flow.
➤ Cleanse area with alcohol.

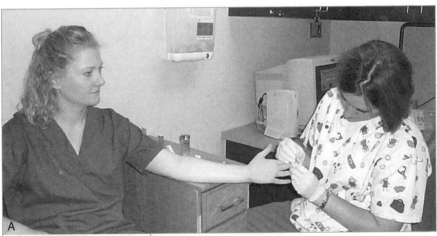

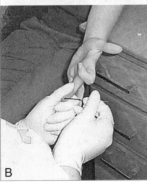

FIGURE 79 • 1 Capillary blood collection—finger stick on an adult.

➤ Dry with sterile gauze or cotton ball.
➤ Don gloves.
➤ Using a 2.4 mm or smaller lancet, perform a swift, clean puncture on plantar surface of heel or side of distal finger tip.
➤ Wipe away first drop of blood.
➤ Allow large blood drop to form.
➤ Gently milk the heel or finger and use gravity to produce enough blood for the test.
  ➤ Capillary tube—Fill tube to specified line.
  ➤ Filter paper—Completely cover the required space with blood.
➤ Cover the puncture site with a Band-Aid.
➤ Send specimen to laboratory for evaluation.
  ➤ Filter test paper
    • Dry the specimen in a horizontal position and mail within 24 hours.
    • Do not transport in plastic bag due to condensation.

Client Instructions

➤ Keep site clean and dry until healed.
➤ If bleeding reoccurs, apply a pressure dressing.
➤ Monitor for signs of infections (red streaks, yellow-green drainage).

BIBLIOGRAPHY
Edmunds, M.W., and Mayhew, M.S. (1996). Procedures for primary care practitioners. St. Louis: Mosby.
McCall, R.E., and Tankersley, C.M. (1997). Phlebotomy essentials. Philadelphia: Lippincott.
http://www.upstate.edu. (2002).

CENTRAL VENOUS CATHETER ACCESS— PORTACATH

80

GEETA MAHARAJ

CPT Code

36540   Collection of blood specimen from
90780   Intravenous infusion for therapy/diagnosis

Portacaths (ports) or Mediports are central vascular access devices, fully implanted under the skin usually on the patient's chest under general anesthesia. Ports consist of a metal or plastic housing attached to a silicone catheter with a self-sealing silicone gel inside the housing. The tip of the catheter is inserted in the subclavian vein and advanced to the superior vena cava.

OVERVIEW

➤ Incidence unknown
➤ When accessing, using, and maintaining the port, the risk of life-threatening complications, such as infection, makes it important to use correct and sterile technique.
➤ Advantages of the portacath include
  ➤ Nothing external when the port is not in use
  ➤ Little maintenance when the port is not accessed
  ➤ Quick needle-stick venous access versus repeated venipunctures
  ➤ Irritating medicines infused without discomfort into larger veins due to dilution by rapid blood flow
➤ Disadvantages of the portacath include
  ➤ Surgical implantation needed
  ➤ Painful access unless topical anesthetic cream used
  ➤ Frequent access may lead to increased infection risk
  ➤ Catheter thrombosis
  ➤ Mechanical problems, such as leaking around the diaphragm
➤ To be used for continuous infusions, bolus injections, cyclic therapies such as chemotherapy, hypertransfusion with blood products for patients with hemoglobinopathies, and primary/secondary prophylaxis in children with hemophilia

RATIONALE

➤ To allow irritating medicines to be infused without discomfort
➤ To provide easy venous access for adults and children with chronic problems who need continuous infusion, bolus injections, cyclic therapies, hypertransfusion, or primary/secondary prophylaxis

INDICATIONS

➤ Cancer
➤ Hemophilia
➤ Sickle cell disease
➤ Cystic fibrosis
➤ Other chronic illness with poor intravenous access
➤ Infections requiring long-term antibiotics

CONTRAINDICATIONS

➤ Redness, swelling, or tenderness over or around the site of the port
➤ Unable to get a free-flowing blood return from the port
➤ Pain or a stinging sensation during infusion

PROCEDURE

Central Venous Access (Portacath)

Equipment

➤ Topical anesthetic cream (Emla)
➤ Tegaderm to cover (Emla)
➤ Alcohol wipes
➤ Povidone-iodine wipes
➤ Gloves—sterile
➤ Huber noncoring needle
➤ Semipermeable transparent dressing to cover Huber needle
➤ 2 × 2 sterile gauze
➤ 0.9% normal saline—10 mL
➤ Syringe—10 mL
➤ Heparin 100 U/mL or 10 U/mL/kg

Procedure

➤ Palpate upper chest to locate port.
➤ Observe site for redness, swelling, or tenderness.
➤ To numb the skin, apply Emla cream over port and cover with Tegaderm. Leave Emla on for 30 minutes.
➤ Remove Tegaderm and wipe off anesthetic cream.
➤ Set up sterile field.
➤ Put on sterile gloves.
➤ Do not touch anything outside the field until the procedure is done.
➤ Using sterile technique, cleanse the area over the port with alcohol, then povidone-iodine.
  ➤ Start cleansing in the center of the port, and wipe outward in a circular pattern with a 2-inch radius.
➤ Leave povidone-iodine to dry for 30 seconds.
➤ Using your nondominant hand, locate the edge of the port housing, and stabilize with the thumb and index finger.
➤ Insert the Huber needle through the skin and silicone gel until the port's rigid housing is felt (Fig. 80–1).
➤ Aspirate for blood return, to confirm the needle is in the port.
➤ Flush with 10 mL of 0.9% saline.
➤ Place sterile gauze under the wings of the Huber needle.
➤ Cover Huber needle with semipermeable transparent dressing.
➤ Start infusion.
➤ Change Huber needle and transparent dressing every 7 days using sterile technique.
➤ Change administration set using sterile technique every 72 hours if medications or fluids infusing and every 24 hours if total parental nutrition or blood products are infusing.
➤ To discontinue the Huber needle, first flush with 20 mL of 0.9% saline and 5 mL of heparin. Then remove the transparent dressing and needle, and cover with sterile gauze and tape.

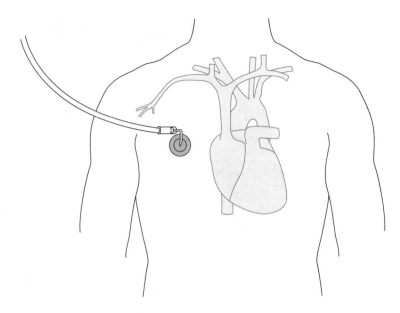

FIGURE 80 • 1 Positioning of Huber needle.

➤ Heparin lock (Heplock) the central venous access port if it is not being used for infusion using sterile technique.
➤ When port is accessed and not being used for infusion, flush daily with 5 mL of heparin (patients weighing more than 10 kg, use 100 U/mL of heparin; patients weighing less than 10 kg, use 10 U/mL of heparin).

Client Instructions

➤ After portacath needle is removed, sterile gauze is taped to cover the portacath.
  ➤ Gauze and tape should be removed by the next day.
➤ No dressing is needed when the port is not accessed.
➤ If the access site becomes red, becomes painful, or has yellow-green drainage, contact your health-care provider immediately.

B IBLIOGRAPHY

Intravenous therapy (2002). Available at: www.barttersite.com/port.
Bollard, C.M., et al (2000). The use of central venous catheters (portacaths) in children with hemophilia. *Hemophilia*, 6(2), 66–70.
Masoorli, S., and Angeles, T. (2002). Getting a line on central vascular access devices. *Nursing*, 32(4), 36–43.

81

Unna's Boot Application

MARGARET R. COLYAR

CPT Code
29580   Unna's paste boot application
29405   Ankle immobilization

The Unna's boot is a compression paste and dressing bandage used mainly for treatment of ulcers arising from venous insufficiency. The Unna's boot is a moist dressing that works to decrease venous hypertension and so diminish the movement of fluids into the interstitium. Moist wound healing prevents the release of moisture, allowing higher collagen production, less **eschar** formation (eschar can diminish wound healing), and an increased rate of **epithelialization**.

OVERVIEW

➤ Incidence is unknown.
➤ Venous ulcers constitute 67% to 90% of all leg ulcers (usually elderly women).
➤ The Unna's boot is used to
  ➤ Decrease pain
  ➤ Assist venous return
  ➤ Decrease superficial venous distention
➤ Venous insufficiency symptoms include
  ➤ Pitting edema in lower legs that responds poorly to diuretics
  ➤ Tenderness
  ➤ Hemosiderin—reddish brown discoloration of lower calf
  ➤ Scaling
  ➤ **Pruritus**
  ➤ **Erythema**
➤ Venous ulceration usually occurs at the medial aspect of the lower leg, especially at the medial malleolus (Fig. 81–1).

RATIONALE

➤ To increase wound healing in patients with venous insufficiency and venous stasis ulcers
➤ To promote ankle stabilization

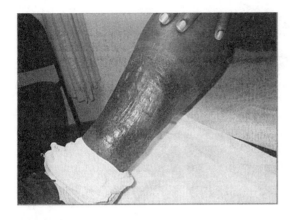

FIGURE 81 • 1 Venous ulceration on the medial aspect of the lower leg.

INDICATIONS

➤ Venous ulcers
➤ Ankle sprain with severe swelling

CONTRAINDICATIONS

➤ Acute pulmonary edema
➤ Cellulitis
➤ Deep vein thrombosis
➤ Arterial insufficiency
➤ Infected venous ulcers
➤ Phlebitis

PROCEDURE

Unna's Boot Application

Equipment

➤ Nonadherent wound dressing (e.g., Telfa)
➤ Mineral oil
➤ Paste bandage—impregnated with calamine, gelatin, and zinc oxide
➤ Soft roll, Kling, or Kerlex
➤ Elastic wrap (e.g., Ace wrap)
➤ Gloves—nonsterile
➤ Tape or metal fasteners

Procedure

➤ Position the client with the affected leg elevated above the heart and foot flexed at a right angle, promoting venous return and good ankle alignment.
➤ Apply a nonadherent dressing over any skin lesions.
➤ Moisturize the rest of the leg with mineral oil to decrease pruritus.
    ➤ Do *not* put mineral oil on any skin lesions.

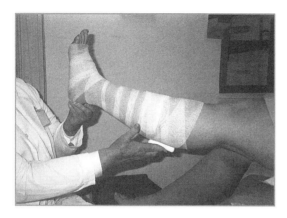

FIGURE 81 • 2 Wrap the paste bandage in an overlapping method to just below the knee.

➤ Starting at the base of the toes, wrap the paste bandage snugly in an overlapping method to just below the knee.
  ➤ Smooth out any wrinkles.
  ➤ Each layer should overlap the previous wrap by 50% (Fig. 81–2).
➤ Wrap Kerlex, Kling, or soft roll in the same fashion over the paste bandage (Fig. 81–3).
➤ Cover with the elastic bandage. Start at the toes and work up until all the previous bandage is covered (Fig. 81–4).
➤ Secure with metal clips or tape.
➤ Keep in place 3 to 14 days. Seven days is the average.
  ➤ The length of time the Unna's boot bandage stays on depends on the amount of exudate from the venous ulcer.

Client Instructions

➤ To decrease swelling and pain, elevate the foot above the heart as much as possible during the day and at bedtime.

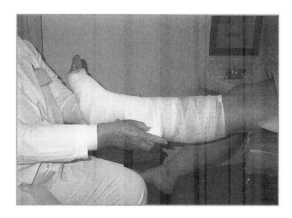

FIGURE 81 • 3 Wrap Kerlex, Kling, or soft roll in an overlapping method over the paste bandage.

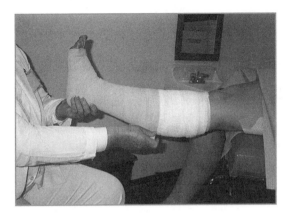

FIGURE 81 • 4 Cover the second layer with an elastic bandage in an overlapping method. Secure with metal clips or tape.

➤ Do *not* get the Unna's boot bandage wet.
  ➤ Wrap the Unna's boot in plastic before bathing and wrap with an elastic bandage up to the knee to prevent seepage of water.
➤ Check circulatory status frequently.
  ➤ Check for change in color of the toes, numbness, swelling, and pain.
  ➤ Report any changes to the practitioner immediately.
➤ Report any odor, drainage, or increase in itching to the practitioner.
➤ Do *not* scratch under the Unna's boot because this may cause wounds.

BIBLIOGRAPHY

Barr, D.M. (1996). The Unna's boot as a treatment for venous ulcers. *Nurse Practitioner,* 21(7), 55–75.

Rubin, J.R., et al (1990). Unna's boot vs. polyurethane foam dressings for the treatment of venous ulceration: a randomized prospective study. *Arch Surg,* 125(4), 489–490.

82 VENIPUNCTURE

CYNTHIA R. EHRHARDT

CPT Code

36415   Routine venipuncture or finger, heel, or ear stick for collection of specimens

Venipuncture is a method used to obtain blood specimens from a vein.

OVERVIEW

➤ Incidence unknown
➤ General principles
  ➤ Collect enough of blood specimen to perform the required test.
  ➤ Collect specimen in proper container.
  ➤ Minimize discomfort as much as possible.
  ➤ Minimize inconvenience to client as much as possible.
  ➤ Know proper techniques to obtain specimen.
  ➤ Maintain sterile technique when drawing blood specimen.
  ➤ Be aware of state law for informed consent in obtaining blood specimens (i.e., alcohol, human immunodeficiency virus, drug screening).
  ➤ Know specific requirements for informed consent (i.e., chain-of-command documentation).

RATIONALE

➤ To obtain information about biochemical and biophysical status of the human organism

INDICATIONS

➤ Need to obtain biochemical and biophysical information concerning the physiology of a client

CONTRAINDICATIONS

➤ Inability to stabilize the vein site as required for successful blood drawing

PROCEDURE

Venipuncture

Equipment

➤ Blood specimen tube (Table 82–1)
➤ Plastic needle holder
➤ Needles for plastic needle holder (16-, 18-, 21-gauge)
➤ Vacuum butterfly adapters
➤ Alcohol swabs
➤ Povidone-iodine swabs
➤ Cotton balls
➤ Adhesive tape
➤ Band-Aids
➤ Timer
➤ Blood specimen stacking tray
➤ Centrifuge
➤ Blood collection tray
➤ Transport container
➤ Labels
➤ Laboratory order sheets
➤ Gloves—nonsterile

TABLE 82•1 COLOR OF BLOOD SPECIMEN TUBES AND COMMON USES

Color of Specimen Container	Use
Red (no coagulation chemicals)	Depakene, digoxin, phenytoin (Dilantin) levels
Speckled or marbled (serum separator)	Chemistry profiles, *Helicobacter pylori* titer, lipid survey, thyroid profile
Purple (EDTA)	Complete blood count, alcohol level, hemoglobin and hematocrit measurements, sedimentation rate
Blue (citrate)	Partial thromboplastin time (INR)
Green (heparin)*	Ammonia, troponin levels
Gray (fluoride-oxalate)	Glucose, lactic acid levels

Note: A catalog of laboratory tests usually is provided by the laboratory facility to assist in choosing the appropriate blood specimen tube for the test ordered.

* Not commonly used.

➤ 2 × 2 gauze
➤ Indelible marking pen
➤ Needle holders
➤ Tourniquets
➤ Puncture-resistant sharps box container (biohazard approval and markings)

Procedure

➤ Equipment preparation
  ➣ Determine the type of needle or butterfly infusion needle required.
  ➣ Attach the unused needle to the plastic needle holder.
  ➣ Select the appropriate blood specimen tube for test.
  ➣ Determine whether the blood sample will need special preparation after collection. Refer to the laboratory catalog of tests provided in your laboratory.
➤ Position the client in comfortable position.
➤ Position yourself in a comfortable position with all required equipment within reach.
➤ Site location
  ➣ Usually the median vein of the antecubital space of the arms is the best site in adults and children older than age 1 year (Fig. 82–1).
  ➣ Avoid thrombosed veins.
  ➣ If no viable antecubital veins, inspect sites distally.
  ➣ Choose a distal site before a proximal site.
➤ Put on gloves.
➤ Cleanse the site with antiseptic (povidone-iodine or alcohol prep pads) in a circular pattern beginning at the center and expanding outward.
  ➣ *Alcohol is avoided in cases in which drug and alcohol levels are to be measured. (This should be documented on the record.)*

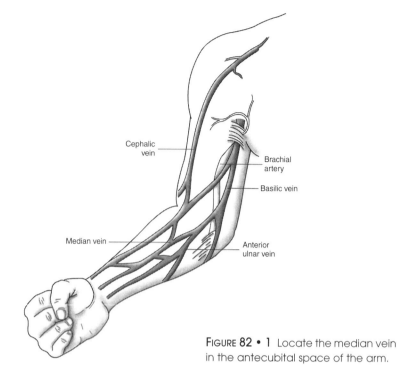

Cephalic vein

Brachial artery

Basilic vein

Median vein

Anterior ulnar vein

FIGURE 82 • 1 Locate the median vein in the antecubital space of the arm.

➤ Apply a tourniquet approximately 4 to 6 inches above the vein selected firmly enough to obstruct venous flow without obstruction to arterial flow.
➤ Do not leave the tourniquet on longer than 1 minute.
➤ When a suitable vein is located, have the client make a fist.
➤ Palpate the vein. It should be an elastic sensation without pulsation.
➤ Uncap the needle.
➤ Stabilize the site.
➤ Insert the needle bevel side up at a 15-degree angle (Fig. 82–2) in line with the vein in a smooth, clean motion.
➤ When the needle penetrates the vein, a "give" will be felt.
➤ Decrease the angle and slowly insert the needle approximately 1/8 inch more or until the blood flow is adequate.
  ➤ Push blood specimen tube onto the needle.
➤ Allow the blood to flow until the tube is filled.
➤ Pull back on the blood specimen tube to dislodge it from the needle in the plastic needle holder. This releases the pressure.
➤ Release the tourniquet.
➤ Remove the needle.
➤ Apply pressure to the puncture site with a cotton ball in a smooth motion.
  ➤ *Great care should be taken during this part of the procedure because this has the highest incidence of accidental needle sticks.*

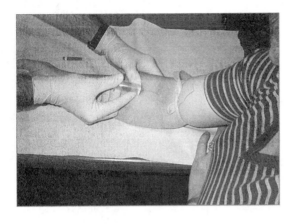

FIGUER 82 • 2 Insert the needle bevel up at a 15-degree angle in line with the vein.

➤ Have the client apply pressure to the site.
  ➤ Keep pressure to site for 1 minute (if client is on anticoagulant therapy, apply pressure for 3 to 5 minutes).
➤ Deposit the needle in a puncture-proof container.
➤ Apply a Band-Aid or cover the cotton ball with tape at the venipuncture site.
➤ Label the specimen with the appropriate information (i.e., client's name, date, time, ID number, and your initials).
➤ If the specimen tube containing blood needs to be centrifuged, consult the laboratory manual for time duration.
➤ Fill out the appropriate laboratory form, and specify what test is to be done.
➤ On completion, package as directed by the laboratory for transport.

Client Instructions

➤ You may remove the Band-Aid in 15 minutes.
➤ Do not rub site because rubbing increases risk of oozing and results in a bruised appearance.

BIBLIOGRAPHY
American College of American Pathologists. (1992) (5th ed.). *So you're going to collect a blood specimen: an introduction to phlebotomy.* Washington, DC: Author.
McCall, R.E., and Tankersley, C.M. (1993). *Phlebotomy essentials.* Philadelphia: Lippincott.

Respiratory Procedures

AEROSOL/INHALATION ADMINISTRATION (NEBULIZER)

83

CYNTHIA R. EHRHARDT

CPT Code
94664   Aerosol inhalation—initial
94665   Aerosol inhalation—subsequent

Inhalation via aerosol administration of medication is used commonly in medical conditions of airflow obstruction, such as bronchospasm and airway hyperresponsiveness. This is considered an effective method of medication administration of drug therapy for the treatment of bronchioli pathway disorders with fewer side effects. Aerosol inhalation is extremely effective in the administration of medication in children younger than age 5 years. Fewer drug interactions and side effects have been associated with aerosol administration. Aerosol inhalation may be used as an episodic or long-term therapy.

OVERVIEW

➤ Incidence
   ➤ Usage in episodic illnesses is unknown.
   ➤ Use in chronic obstructive disorders, such as asthma and chronic pulmonary obstructive disease, is estimated at 5 million individuals.

RATIONALE

➤ To facilitate oxygenation in diseases affecting airflow

INDICATIONS

➤ Presence of medical conditions associated with bronchospasm (airflow obstruction) and hyperresponsiveness that result in compromise of the client's health status

CONTRAINDICATIONS

➤ None

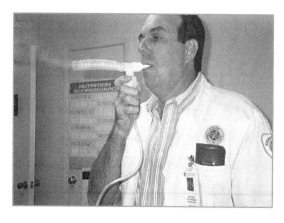

FIGURE 83 • 1 Aerosol or inhalation administration.

PROCEDURE

Aerosol/Inhalation Administration

See Figure 83–1.

Equipment

➤ Pulse oximeter
➤ Peak flowmeter
➤ Oxygen with tubing and nebulizer mask
➤ Aerosol administration kit
➤ Air compressor (such as Pulmo-aide or Invacare Passport)
➤ 0.9% sodium chloride—3 mL
➤ Medication (commonly used) (Table 83–1)

Procedure

➤ Position the client in a comfortable upright position.
➤ Apply the pulse oximeter, and monitor continuously throughout the procedure.
➤ Perform a peak flow reading and record (see Chapter 84).
➤ Plug the air compressor in, and open the aerosol administration kit.
➤ Insert the aerosol medication into the aerosol administration kit at an appropriate dosage and mixture.
➤ Determine the best method of administration (mask versus mouthpiece). This depends on the age of the client and ability to handle the mouthpiece versus the mask.
➤ Turn on the machine; a fine mist should form.
➤ Instruct the client to breathe in until the mist disappears, then slowly exhale.
   ➤ Slow inhalation and exhalation should allow effective administration of medication with fewer side effects.
   ➤ Continue the treatment until all the medication is depleted. This is indicated by no further production of aerosol mist.
   ➤ Perform post-treatment peak flow and record.

TABLE 83•1 MEDICATIONS COMMONLY USED IN AEROSOL INHALATION
ADMINISTRATION

β₂-Agonists—Short-acting Bronchodilators
➤ Albuterol 2.5 mg/mL
  ➤ Dosage: 0.2–0.3 mg/3 mL 0.9% sodium chloride every 4 hr
  ➤ Precautions with children less than 2 years of age and pre-existing cardiac conditions

Anti-inflammatories
➤ Corticosteroids
  ➤ Methylprednisolone (Decadron) 0.5 mg
    • 1 mg mixed in 3 mL 0.9% sodium chloride with or without administration of albuterol
    • One-time dosage administration
    • Rapid and direct administration of corticosteroids to the lining of the bronchioles
  ➤ Cromoglycates:
    ➤ Cromolyn sodium—20 mg per 2-mL ampule
    • Dosage: 1 ampule every 6 hr
    • May be mixed with albuterol and administered simultaneously
    • Slow onset of action; may be several days before significant reduction of airway obstruction occurs

Anticholinergics (Rarely used)
➤ Atropine 0.1 mg/mL
  ➤ Rarely used because of potential side effects
  ➤ Use only when reduction in bronchospasm has not occurred with conventional therapy and potential life-threatening situation is occurring

Client Instructions

➤ Perform home treatments four times a day using medications ordered. Do not perform treatments more than four times a day unless instructed by a health-care provider.
➤ Breathe slowly in and out to maximize the effectiveness of medication.
➤ Side effects of the medication may include
  ➤ Nervousness or jittery feeling
  ➤ Fast heart rate or palpitations
➤ *Seek emergency treatment if any of the following occur*
  ➤ Nasal flaring
  ➤ Intercostal retractions
  ➤ Blueness of fingertips, nail beds, or around the mouth

BIBLIOGRAPHY
American Medical Association (1996). *Physicians' current procedural terminology*. Chicago: Author.
Busse, W., and Holgate, S. (eds.). (1995). *Asthma and rhinitis*. Cambridge, MA: Blackwell.
Invacare (1996). *Operator's manual for passport nebulizer*. Elyria, OH: Author.
Katzung, B. (ed.). (1989). *Basic and clinical pharmacology*. Norwalk, CT: Appleton & Lange.
Pulmo-aide. (1994). *Operator's manual for Pulmo-aide nebulizer*. Somerset, PA: Author.

Summer, W., et al (1989). Aerosol bronchodilator delivery methods. *Arch Intern Med*, 149(7), 618–623.

United States Department of Health and Human Services, National Institutes of Health (1992). *International consensus report on the diagnosis and management of asthma*. Washington, DC: Author.

84 PEAK FLOWMETER

Cynthia R. Ehrhardt

CPT Code

94160   Vital capacity screening tests; total capacity, with timed forced expiratory volume (state duration), and peak flow rate

The peak flowmeter is a handheld device that provides an objective assessment of dynamic pulmonary function and response to clinical therapy of pulmonary diseases. This is particularly beneficial for asthmatics because it has been shown that regular monitoring has reduced the frequency, duration, and severity of attacks. Peak flowmeters are relatively inexpensive and easily transported apparatus. The result of the peak flowmeter evaluation is expressed as the peak flow rate.

OVERVIEW

➤ Incidence unknown
➤ Limitations of the peak flowmeter
  ➤ Poor user skills
  ➤ Lack of motivation and individual effort
  ➤ Younger than age 5 years
➤ The normal predicted average peak expiratory flow for males and females is shown in Table 84–1.
➤ The normal predicted average peak expiratory flow for children and adolescents is shown in Table 84–2.

RATIONALE

➤ Allows asthmatics to self-monitor their respiratory status objectively
➤ Permits clinicians treating asthmatics to intervene earlier in therapy
➤ Reduces the frequency of emergency department visits and/or hospitalizations

TABLE 84•1 NORMAL PREDICTED AVERAGE PEAK EXPIRATORY FLOW RATE—ADULTS*

AGE (YEARS)	MALE HEIGHT (INCHES)					FEMALE HEIGHT (INCHES)				
	60	65	70	75	80	55	60	65	70	75
20	554	602	649	693	740	390	423	460	496	529
25	543	590	636	679	725	385	418	454	490	523
30	532	577	622	664	710	380	413	448	483	516
35	521	565	609	651	695	375	408	442	476	509
40	509	552	596	636	680	370	402	436	470	502
45	498	540	583	622	665	365	397	430	464	495
50	486	527	569	607	649	360	391	424	457	488
55	475	515	556	593	634	355	386	418	451	482
60	463	502	542	578	618	350	380	412	445	475
65	452	490	529	564	603	345	375	406	439	468
70	440	477	515	550	587	340	369	400	432	461

*This table shows values at sea level; these are considered averages and may vary widely from individual to individual.

INDICATIONS

➤ Asthma
➤ Monitor respiratory status

CONTRAINDICATIONS

➤ None

TABLE 84•2 NORMAL PREDICTED AVERAGE PEAK EXPIRATORY FLOW RATE (PFR)—CHILDREN AND ADOLESCENTS*

		Male and Female Heights			
HEIGHT (INCHES)	AVERAGE PFR	HEIGHT (INCHES)	AVERAGE PFR	HEIGHT (INCHES)	AVERAGE PFR
43	147	51	254	59	360
44	160	52	267	60	373
45	173	53	280	61	387
46	187	54	293	62	400
47	200	55	307	63	413
48	214	56	320	64	427
49	227	57	334	65	440
50	240	58	347	66	454

*This table shows values at sea level; these are considered averages and may vary widely from individual to individual.

PROCEDURE

Peak Flowmeter

Equipment

➤ Peak flowmeter (Fig. 84–1)
➤ Mouthpiece

Procedure

➤ Place the appropriate-size mouthpiece over the peak flowmeter.
➤ Check that the indicator is at the bottom of the chamber.
➤ Hold the peak flowmeter in the proper direction (as recommended by the manufacturer).
➤ Ask the client to take as deep a breath as possible.
➤ Ask the client to seal his or her lips over the mouthpiece and blow out as quickly as possible (like blowing candles out) (Fig. 84–2).
➤ Note the reading on the dial.
➤ Repeat the procedure three times, and record the highest reading.

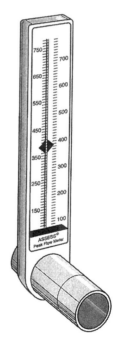

FIGURE **84** • 1 Peak flowmeter. (Courtesy of Healthscan Products, Inc., Cedar Grove, NJ.)

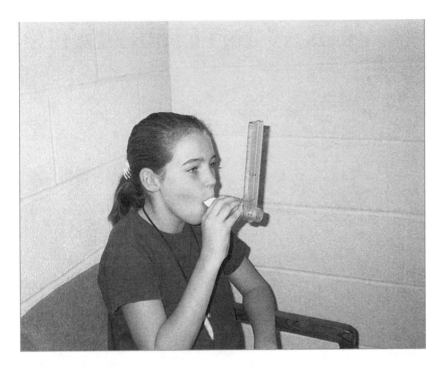

FIGURE 84 • 2 Seal lips over the mouthpiece, and blow out as quickly as possible.

B I B L I O G R A P H Y

Fisons Pharmaceuticals. (1995). *Handout: using a peak flow meter.* St. Louis: Mosby.

Johnson, K. (1993) (13th ed.). *The Johns Hopkins Hospital: the Harriet Lane handbook.* St. Louis: Mosby.

National Asthma Education Program, Expert Panel Report. (1991). National Heart, Lung, and Blood Institute: guidelines for the diagnosis and management of asthma. *J Allergy Clin Immunol,* 88, 477–492.

Polgar, G., and Promadhat, V. (1971). *Pulmonary function testing in children: techniques and standards.* Philadelphia: Saunders.

Habiff, T. (1996) (3rd ed.). *Clinical dermatology: a color guide to diagnosis and therapy.* St. Louis: Mosby.

Murtagh, J. (1995) (2nd ed.). *Practice tips.* New York: McGraw-Hill.

Pfenninger, J.L., and Fowler, G.C. (1994). *Procedures of primary care physicians.* St. Louis: Mosby.

85

X-RAY INTERPRETATION —CHEST

CYNTHIA R. EHRHARDT

CPT Code
Usually included as part of the office visit charge. Actual x-ray films are billed according to the views taken.

A chest x-ray (radiograph) is considered the best radiologic screening and diagnostic tool of most lung disease because of its ability to generate high spatial resolution and to visualize various densities within the thoracic cavity.

OVERVIEW
➤ Incidence unknown
➤ General principles
  ➤ Adequate knowledge of anatomy and physiology is necessary for proper interpretation of the chest film.
  ➤ Use an orderly and systematic approach to interpret the chest film.
  ➤ Order posteroanterior and lateral views. When a portable chest x-ray is taken, you get an anteroposterior view, which makes the heart look artificially large.
➤ Order an expiratory view if a pneumothorax is suspected.

RATIONALE
➤ To diagnose diseases and disorders of the chest

INDICATIONS
➤ Trauma to the chest area
➤ Chronic cough
➤ Chest pain
➤ Suspicion of lung infection
➤ Suspicion of lung carcinoma

CONTRAINDICATION
➤ Pregnancy (unless shielded)

PROCEDURE

X-ray Interpretation—Chest

Equipment

➤ X-ray view box with proper illumination for films
➤ Storage cover for films
➤ Folder storage to prevent bending of films

Procedure

➤ Place the posteroanterior and lateral views on the view box with adequate illumination.
➤ Inspect for the presence of any foreign bodies in the thoracic cavity.
➤ Systematically inspect the skeletal system of the thoracic region
  ➤ Identify anatomic skeletal landmarks within the thoracic cavity and occurrence of any aberration (Figs. 85–1 and 85–2).
  ➤ Identify any demineralization in the skeleton structure.
  ➤ Determine the lack of continuity and symmetry of skeletal structure (including clavicles, scapulae, humeri, and sternum).
  ➤ Note the appearance of the ribs, beginning with identification of the posterior segments of the first rib on the right and proceeding through the 12th rib. Repeat this process on the opposite side of the thoracic cavity.
  ➤ Note any widening of the rib spaces.

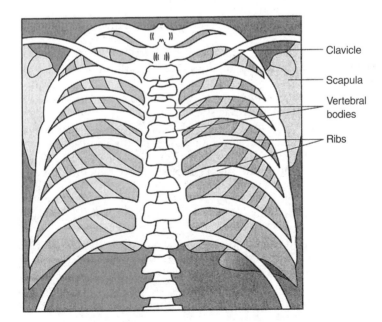

FIGURE 85 • 1 Anatomic skeletal landmarks as seen on the posteroanterior view of the chest.

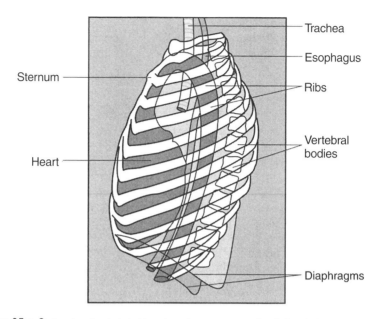

Trachea

Esophagus

Sternum

Ribs

Vertebral bodies

Heart

Diaphragms

FIGURE 85 • 2 Anatomic skeletal landmarks as seen on the lateral view of the chest.

➤ Systematically inspect for the presence of soft tissue masses.
  ➤ Note the contour of the neck.
  ➤ Look for asymmetry and shadow density changes in
    • Breast shadows
    • Hepatic and splenic shadows
  ➤ Check for the presence of a gas bubble in the stomach shadow (Fig. 85–3).
  ➤ Note any evidence of changes in or shifting of the mediastinal shadows.
➤ Systematically inspect cardiac system.
  ➤ Note the shape of the cardiac silhouette, which is easily visible.
  ➤ Measure the intrathoracic diameter. Note the width of inside of the rib cage at level of the diaphragm's right side plus the left side.
  ➤ Divide the width of the rib cage by one half. This should equal the cardiac size. Normal cardiac size is less than half the thoracic size (Fig. 85–4).
  ➤ Note the clarity of the cardiac borders. The cardiac borders should be well defined.
  ➤ Note increased calcification of silhouette of the heart.
  ➤ Calcifications within the silhouette represent the valvular structures of the heart (Fig. 85–5).
➤ Systematically inspect the presentation of the vascular system.
  ➤ Note any anatomic shift or calcifications in the pulmonary arteries and aorta.
    • The main pulmonary arterial branches should be equal in size, shape, and contour.

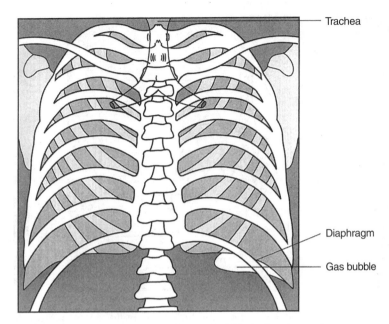

FIGURE 85 • 3 Check for the presence of a gas bubble in the stomach.

PA view

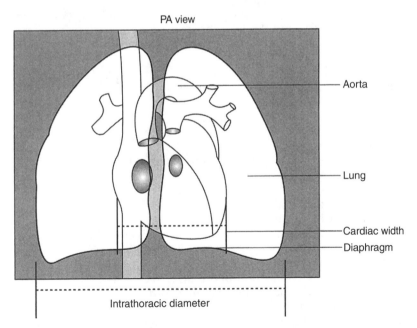

FIGURE 85 • 4 Inspect the cardiac system. Measure the intrathoracic diameter. Divide the intrathoracic diameter by 2. Measure the cardiac width. Normal cardiac size is less than half the intrathoracic diameter.

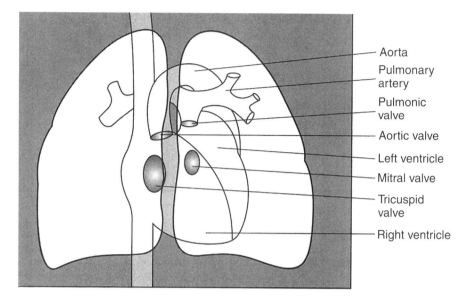

Aorta

Pulmonary artery

Pulmonic valve

Aortic valve

Left ventricle

Mitral valve

Tricuspid valve

Right ventricle

FIGURE 85 • 5 Calcifications within the cardiac silhouette represent the valves of the heart.

➤ Inspect the size and shape of thoracic aorta.
➤ Locate the base of aorta as it extends from cardiac silhouette.
➤ Note the presence of
  • Aortic dilatation
  • Straightening or coarctation of the aortic arch
  • Aortic calcifications
➤ Systematically inspect the diaphragm
  ➤ Note the presence or absence of flattening.
  ➤ Note the integrity and symmetry of the anatomic location.
  ➤ Note the absence or presence of ipsilateral hemidiaphragm.
➤ Systematically inspect the lung silhouette.
  ➤ Check for
  • Cohesiveness to the pleural borders.
  • Lucency of air within the lungs.
  • Presence of pleural lines within the confines of the ribs.
  • Calcifications or densities within the lung field.
  • Accentuated areas of white within the pulmonary black background. This represents pleural thickening or pleural fluid and can prevent clear demarcation of the anatomic borders.
  • Blunting of the costophrenic borders.
➤ Some common abnormalities include
  ➤ Abscesses, fungus, and lymphomas
  • Appearance of "balls" in the chest
  • Diaphragm may be pulled up

➤ Cystic fibrosis
  • Low, flat diaphragm
  • Small heart
  • Large lungs
➤ Pneumonia
  • More white and less black in whichever lobe is affected (Fig. 85–6).
➤ Pneumothorax
  • Lobe of lung is decreased in size or absent
➤ Sarcoidosis
  • Masses in hylar area
➤ Tuberculosis
  • Infiltrates and ball-like scarring in apices

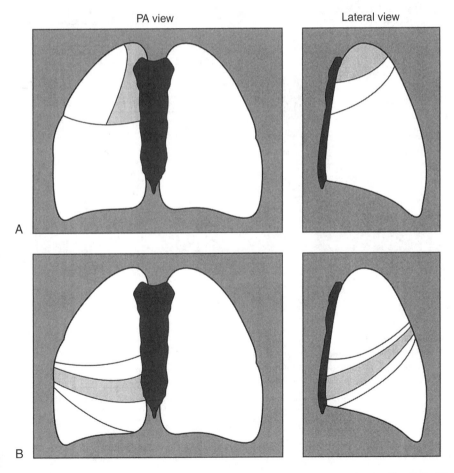

FIGURE 85 • 6 Pneumonia—more white and less black in whichever lobe is affected. (A) Right upper lobe pneumonia; (B) right middle lobe pneumonia; (C) right lower lobe pneumonia; and (D) left upper lobe pneumonia.

PA view   Lateral view

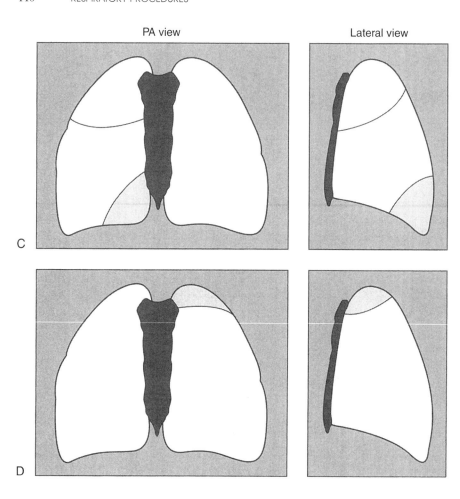

C

D

FIGURE 85 • 6 *(Continued)*

BIBLIOGRAPHY

Hurst, W. (1995). *Cardiac puzzles.* St. Louis: Mosby.

Scialabba, F., and Salvatore, D. (1990). Saccular aneurysms of thoracic aorta. *Am Fam Physician,* 42(5), 1475–1478.

Spilane, R., et al (1994). Radiographic aspects of pneumothorax. *Am Fam Physician,* 51(2), 459–464.

Stimac, G. (1992). *Introduction to diagnostic imaging.* Philadelphia: Saunders.

Vine, D. (1990). Congestive heart failure. *Am Fam Physician,* 42(3), 739.

Wilson, J. (ed.). (1991) (12th ed.). *Harrison's principles of internal medicine.* New York: McGraw-Hill.

CHEST TUBES
FOR EMERGENCY
86 TRANSPORT

MARGARET R. COLYAR

CPT Code
32020   Chest tubes (thoracotomy)

The Heimlich valve, a plastic portable one-way valve used for chest drainage, allows evacuation of the lung during coughing and breathing, while preventing return of secretions to the lung. It was introduced in the late 1960s to drain the pleural space, avoiding the need for an underwater seal during wartime. Insertion of a portable one-way chest tube is an important procedure for managing life-threatening respiratory situations and to stabilize the patient for emergency transport.

OVERVIEW

➤ Allows freedom of movement
➤ Used to drain blood, fluid, or air from the space between inner and outer linings of the lung
➤ Placement for different types of chest trauma (Table 86–1)

RATIONALE

➤ To relieve pain due to pressure exerted by excess fluid in the chest cavity
➤ To drain excess air and fluid from the chest cavity
➤ To prevent collapse of the lung caused by increased pressure
➤ To allow lungs to reinflate

TABLE 86•1 PLACEMENT OF CHEST TUBES

TYPE OF CHEST TRAUMA	PLACEMENT OF CHEST TUBES
Hemothorax	4th–5th intercostal spaces midaxillary line
Pneumothorax	2nd–3rd intercostal spaces anterior chest at midclavicular line

441

INDICATIONS

➤ Pleural effusion
➤ Empyema
➤ Spontaneous pneumothorax
➤ Sucking chest wound from penetrating trauma
➤ Hemothorax

CONTRAINDICATIONS

➤ Clinically stable patients with a small pneumothorax

☑ *Informed consent required*
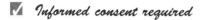

PROCEDURE

Chest Tube Insertion for Emergency Transport

Equipment

➤ Heimlich valve (Fig. 86–1)
➤ Vented drainage bag—urinary or ostomy bag
➤ Mask
➤ Scalpel
➤ Kelly clamp—2 rubber-tipped
➤ Forceps—sterile
➤ Syringe—10 mL
➤ Needle—22-gauge, 1-inch
➤ Local anesthetic—10 mL
➤ Tape—2-inch cloth/elastic
➤ Scissors
➤ Gloves—nonsterile
➤ Gloves—sterile
➤ Povidone-iodine (Betadine)
➤ Drape—fenestrated
➤ Alcohol swabs
➤ 4 × 4 gauze—sterile
➤ Vaseline gauze or clear plastic that clings (i.e., Saran Wrap)
➤ Suture—large filament—optional

Procedure

➤ Position client according to type of chest tube placement needed (Table
86–2; Fig. 86–2).

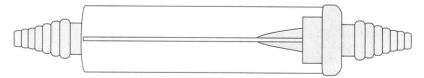

Figure 86 • 1 Heimlich valve.

TABLE 86•2 POSITIONING OF CLIENT FOR CHEST TUBE PLACEMENT

TYPE OF CHEST TRAUMA	POSITION FOR CHEST TUBE PLACEMENT
Hemothorax	Orthopneic
Pneumothorax	Supine, high Fowler's, semi-Fowler's

➤ Put on nonsterile gloves.
➤ Place rubber-tipped Kelly clamps in opposite directions on proximal end of the urinary/ostomy bag tube.
➤ Attach the urinary/ostomy bag tube to blue end of the Heimlich valve.
➤ Attach the Heimlich valve connecting tube to other end of Heimlich valve.
➤ Tape connection site at both ends of the valve.
➤ Cleanse site with povidone-iodine starting at insertion site in concentric circles three times in outward motion.

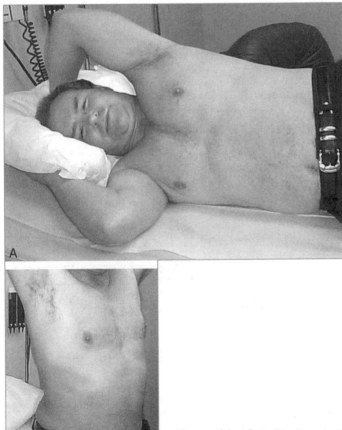

Figure 86 • 2 Positioning of client for chest tube placement. *(A)* Supine; *(B)* orthopneic.

➤ Administer local anesthetic to skin between ribs identified as insertion site.
➤ Drape the chest tube insertion site.
➤ Remove nonsterile gloves and put on sterile gloves.
➤ Palpate intercostal space.
➤ Stabilize surrounding tissue with nondominant hand.
➤ Make a small incision where the catheter is to be inserted.
➤ Insert catheter through the skin, intercostal space, and parietal pleura and into pleural space. A "pop" may be heard or felt.
➤ Remove the inner blunt-tip obturator and advance the catheter.
➤ Attach the radiopaque catheter to the Heimlich valve connecting tube.
➤ Suture tube to skin or tape securely.
➤ Place Vaseline gauze or cling-film over chest tube insertion site.
➤ Apply sterile 4 × 4 gauze on top of Vaseline gauze.
➤ Tape with 2-inch cloth or elastic tape making an occlusive dressing.
➤ If available, obtain chest radiograph to ensure proper placement.

Client Instructions

➤ Transport to emergency department.
➤ Chest tube is removed when lung has reinflated.

BIBLIOGRAPHY
American College of Chest Physicians (2002). *Consensus panel on the management of spontaneous pneumothorax: management of spontaneous pneumothorax: quick reference guide.* Available at: www.chestnet.org/education/physician/statements,pneumothorax/.
Baumann, M.H. (2002). *Management of spontaneous pneumothorax.* Available at: www.chestnet.org.
Chest tubes. Available at: http://medicine.creighton.edu.
Heimlich, H.J. (1968). Valve drainage of the pleural cavity. *Dis Chest,* 53, 282–286.
Procedure for proper usage of the Heimlich valve. Available at: www.uams.edu.

FLAIL CHEST STABILIZATION
WITH OR WITHOUT OPEN CHEST WOUND

87

CYNTHIA R. EHRHARDT

CPT Code
None specific

Flail chest is the consequence of blunt or penetrating (open chest wound) trauma in which there are multiple fractures to the ribs (usually more than three consecutive ribs on the same side) resulting in instability to the chest wall. Flail chest with or without open chest wounds is a potentially life-threatening situation. In an ambulatory setting, the focus is on stabilizing the injury, providing adequate ventilation, and transporting to an appropriately equipped emergency department.

OVERVIEW

➤ Incidence
  ➤ Accounts for 25% to 30% of the 45,000 automobile deaths in the United States each year
  ➤ Three times as likely to occur in individuals not wearing seat belts
➤ Complications
  ➤ Pneumothorax
  ➤ Hemothorax
  ➤ Hemopneumothorax
  ➤ Cardiac contusions, including cardiac tamponade and thoracic aortic trauma
  ➤ Cardiac arrhythmias
  ➤ Systemic/cardiogenic shock
  ➤ Death
➤ General principles
  ➤ Activate emergency medical system (EMS).
  ➤ Maintain ABCs (airway, breathing, circulation) of basic life support.
  ➤ Apply oxygen in as high a concentration as possible.
  ➤ Establish monitoring with pulse oximetry and cardiac monitoring.
  ➤ Seal as quickly as possible if an open chest wound.
  ➤ Establish intravenous lines (two) as quickly as permitted.
  ➤ Treat for cardiogenic shock.
  ➤ Transport as quickly as possible.
➤ Physical examination
  ➤ Observe for signs and symptoms of systemic cardiogenic shock.
  ➤ Inspection
    • Presence or absence of chest wall motion
    • Paradoxical chest wall motion
    • Presence or absence of air-movement noise
    • Cyanosis of the face and neck
    • Subcutaneous emphysema (**crepitus** skin)
    • Excessive abdominal muscular movement
  ➤ Palpation
    • Crepitus anywhere in the chest wall region with particular attention at the location of blunt trauma
    • Palpable rib or sternal fractures
    • Movable sternum
    • Decrease in intensity of point of maximal impulse, which can be associated with cardiac tamponade, or shift in point of maximal impulse if mediastinal shift occurs and congestive heart failure can be excluded

➤ Percussion
  • Dullness suggests **hemothorax** or pneumothorax
  • Hyperresonance suggests pneumothorax
➤ Auscultation
  • Unilateral decreased breath sounds

HEALTH PROMOTION/PREVENTION

➤ Prevention is focused on eliminating situations that can result in the incidence of blunt trauma and penetration wounds. This includes
  ➤ Properly worn seat belts in automobiles with or without airbags
  ➤ Gun and hunting safety
  ➤ High-rise safety (ladders and roofs)
  ➤ Protection against and avoidance of situations that produce projectile objects

OPTIONS

➤ *Method 1*—flail chest stabilization without open chest wound
➤ *Method 2*—flail chest stabilization with open chest wound

RATIONALE

➤ To prevent life-threatening complications

INDICATIONS

➤ Blunt trauma
➤ Penetrating chest wound
➤ Rib injuries

CONTRAINDICATIONS

➤ None

PROCEDURE

Flail Chest Stabilization

Equipment

➤ Pulse oximeter
➤ Oxygen with nasal cannula, mask, or rebreather mask
➤ Cardiac monitoring if available
➤ Intravenous solution kits of Ringer's lactate or 0.9% sodium chloride
➤ Large-bore intravenous catheters (16- to 18-gauge for adults; 18- to 21-gauge for children)
➤ 0.9% sodium chloride irrigation solution—500 mL—sterile
➤ Abdominal dressings (6 inch × 12 inch or larger)—sterile
➤ Gloves—sterile
➤ 4 × 4 gauze—sterile
➤ Occlusive dressing (petroleum or polytetrafluoroethylene [Teflon] base)—sterile

➤ 4-0 Ethicon suture material
➤ Adhesive tape rolls (1-, 2-, 4-, or 6-inch)
➤ Pillow or sandbag
➤ Sterile dressing or suture tray including
  ➤ Straight and curved **hemostats**
  ➤ Needle holder
  ➤ **Forceps** with teeth
  ➤ Iris scissors
  ➤ Emesis basin
  ➤ Sterile towels (fenestrated and nonfenestrated)
➤ 1% or 2% lidocaine without epinephrine
➤ 5-mL syringe—sterile
➤ 22-gauge, $1^1/_2$-inch needle—sterile
➤ Intubation tray—optional

Procedure

METHOD 1—FLAIL CHEST STABILIZATION WITHOUT OPEN CHEST WOUND

➤ Activate the EMS system.
➤ Maintain ABCs of basic life support.
➤ Apply oxygen in as high a concentration as possible.
➤ Establish monitoring with pulse oximetry and cardiac monitoring.
➤ Locate the edges of the flail section with gentle palpation.
➤ When located, establish that there is no evidence of open chest injury.
➤ Apply a thick dressing of at least 3 inches over the site. A small pillow or small sandbag (5 lb or less) can be used.
➤ Use large strips of tape across the dressing or pad to secure (Fig. 87–1)
➤ Ensure that the tape tension causes the dressing to support the flail region.
  ➤ Strips of cloth may be used to anchor if tape is not available.
➤ Initiate two intravenous sites and run intravenous solution (if stable) to keep patent.
➤ *Monitor and transport to the nearest emergency department equipped to handle the potential secondary complications that can occur with flail chest.*

METHOD 2—FLAIL CHEST STABILIZATION WITH OPEN CHEST WOUND

➤ Activate the EMS system.
➤ Maintain ABCs of basic life support.
➤ Apply oxygen in as high a concentration as possible.
➤ Establish monitoring with pulse oximetry and cardiac monitoring.
➤ With gentle palpation, locate the edges of the flail section.
➤ Note the presence or absence of sucking sound of air movement each time the individual inhales.
➤ Locate the open chest wound.
➤ Put on gloves.
➤ Seal the open chest wound as quickly as possible.
  ➤ Clean the area around the wound with sterile 0.9% sodium chloride, ensuring that none of the solution enters the wound.

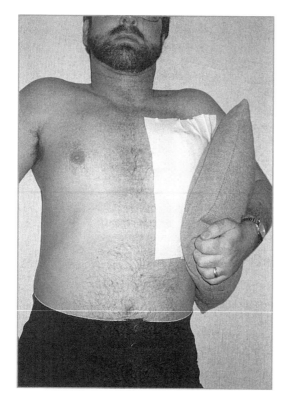

Figure 87 • 1 Secure the dressing with tape, and stabilize with a pillow or sandbag.

- ➤ Dry with sterile 4 × 4 gauze.
- ➤ Apply petroleum-impregnated dressing or occlusive dressing over the open wound and extending 2 to 3 inches beyond the site.
- ➤ Anchor securely with tape, then proceed with method 1—flail chest stabilization without chest wound dressing.
- ➤ If wound is gaping, or dressing does not hold well, apply temporary sutures (see Chapter 22) to the wound, then reapply the occlusive dressing.
- ➤ *Monitor and transport to the nearest emergency department equipped to handle the potential secondary complications that can occur with flail chest.*

Client Instructions

➤ Transport to appropriately staffed emergency department.

BIBLIOGRAPHY

American Medical Association (1996). *Physicians' current procedural terminology.* Chicago: Author.

Grant, H., et al (1986) (4th ed.). *Emergency care.* Englewood Cliffs, NJ: Prentice-Hall.

Peterson, T., and Royer, K. (1991). Motor vehicle crash injuries: mechanisms and prevention. *Am Fam Physician,* 44(4), 804–810.

Rosen, P., et al (1992) (3rd ed.). *Emergency medicine: concepts and clinical practice.* St. Louis: Mosby.

Thelan, L., et al (1994) (2nd ed.). *Critical care nursing.* St. Louis: Mosby.

88

STAB/PENETRATING WOUND STABILIZATION

CYNTHIA R. EHRHARDT • MARGARET R. COLYAR

CPT Code

20100 Exploration—neck
20101 Exploration—chest
20102 Exploration—abdomen, flank, or back
20103 Exploration—extremity

All stab/penetrating wounds (large or small) have the potential to precipitate a life-threatening situation. The size of the wound does not reflect proportionally the severity of the wound. Small penetrations sometimes are more lethal than large penetrations. In an ambulatory setting, the focus is on evaluation and stabilization of the injury, providing adequate ventilation if required, and transporting to an appropriately equipped emergency department as quickly as possible when deep injuries and/or involvement of body structures beyond basic lacerations is suspected.

OVERVIEW

➤ Incidence
  ➤ Accounts for 35% of injuries seen in the emergency department
  ➤ Estimated to cause permanent disability in 400,000 individuals in the United States each year
➤ Complications
  ➤ Severance of ligaments, tendons, nerves, muscles, or blood vessels can lead to loss of function.
  ➤ Penetrating trauma in thoracic and abdominal cavities can increase risk of trauma and temporary and/or permanent loss of an organ or its function.
  ➤ Cardiogenic shock
  ➤ Death

HEALTH PROMOTION/PREVENTION

Prevention is focused on eliminating situations that can result in the incidence of penetration wounds. This includes

449

➤ Properly worn seat belts in automobiles with or without airbags
➤ Gun and hunting safety
➤ Avoidance of situations that produce projectile objects
➤ Knowledge of personal safety rules to avoid assault situations

OPTIONS

➤ *Method 1*—penetrating wound without involvement of major body organ
➤ *Method 2*—penetrating wound with involvement of major body organ

RATIONALE

➤ To stabilize the client
➤ To prevent life-threatening complications

INDICATIONS

➤ Penetrating trauma not involving major body organs

CONTRAINDICATIONS

➤ Penetration of major internal organ is suspected. Stabilize and transfer to the emergency department.

PROCEDURE

Stab/Penetrating Wound Stabilization

Equipment

➤ Method 1 only
  ➤ Basin—sterile
  ➤ Povidone-iodine soak—povidone-iodine solution and 0.9% sterile saline mixed 50/50
  ➤ Syringe—20 to 60 mL
  ➤ Two needles—27- to 30-gauge and 18- to 20-gauge
  ➤ 1% lidocaine
  ➤ Scissors—sterile
  ➤ Curved **hemostats**—sterile
  ➤ **Forceps**—sterile
  ➤ Suture—3-0 to 5-0 nylon
  ➤ Culture swab
  ➤ Topical antibiotic—Bactroban or Polysporin
  ➤ Iodoform gauze—$^1/_4$ to 1 inch
➤ Method 2 only
  ➤ Pulse oximeter
  ➤ Oxygen with nasal cannula, mask, or rebreather mask
  ➤ Cardiac monitoring, if available
  ➤ Intravenous solution kits of Ringer's lactate or 0.9% sodium chloride
  ➤ Large-bore intravenous catheters (16- to 18-gauge for adults and 18- to 21-gauge for children)
  ➤ 0.9% sodium chloride irrigation solution—500 mL—sterile

➤ Large abdominal dressings (6 inch × 12 inch or larger)—sterile
➤ Intubation tray—optional but highly recommended
➤ Methods 1 and 2
  ➤ Gloves—sterile
  ➤ 4 × 4 gauze—sterile
  ➤ Adhesive tape rolls (1-, 2-, 4-, and/or 6-inch)

Procedure

METHOD 1—PENETRATING WOUND WITHOUT INVOLVEMENT OF MAJOR BODY ORGANS

➤ If the penetrating wound appears not to involve major organ structures, nerves, tendons, or major blood vessels and appears to meet criteria of deep puncture wound, see Chapters 6 and 22.

METHOD 2—PENETRATING WOUND WITH INVOLVEMENT OF MAJOR BODY ORGANS

➤ Activate the EMS system.
➤ Maintain ABCs of basic life support.
➤ Apply oxygen in as high a concentration as possible.
➤ Monitor oxygen saturation with **pulse oximetry** and cardiac monitoring.
➤ Establish intravenous lines (two) as quickly as permitted.
➤ If *open chest wound*
  ➤ Seal as quickly as possible (see Chapter 87).
➤ If *abdominal injuries*
  ➤ Cover the wound with sterile dressings to prevent further contamination of the wound.
➤ If an *extremity wound* with suspected derangement of ligaments, tendons, and/or severed nerves
  ➤ Cover the wound with a sterile dressing.
  ➤ Splint in functional position.
➤ If time allows and major organ trauma is suspected, insert a **nasogastric** tube and Foley urinary catheter.
➤ Transport as soon as possible.

Client Instructions

➤ Transport to appropriately staffed emergency department as indicated.

B I B L I O G R A P H Y

American Medical Association (1996). *Physicians' current procedural terminology*. Chicago: Author.

Demetriades, D. (1996). Use of emergency medical services for trauma. *Am Fam Physician*, 54(2), 330–335.

Ehni, B. (1991). Treatment of traumatic peripheral nerve injury. *Am Acad Fam Physicians*, 43(3), 445–454.

Peterson, T., and Royer, K. (1991). Motor vehicle crash injuries: mechanisms and prevention. *Am Fam Physician*, 44(4), 804–810.

Rosen, P., et al (1992) (3rd ed.). *Emergency medicine: concepts and clinical practice*. St. Louis: Mosby.

Thelan, L., et al (1994) (2nd ed.). *Critical care nursing*. St. Louis: Mosby.

Gastrointestinal Procedures

89

Anoscopy

MARGARET R. COLYAR

CPT Code

46600   Anoscopy, diagnostic with or without collection of specimen

46606   Anoscopy with biopsy, single or multiple

46608   Anoscopy with removal of foreign body

46614   Anoscopy with control of bleeding, any method

Anoscopy is the direct visualization of the anus using a **speculum**. It is used to screen, diagnose, and evaluate perianal and anal problems.

OVERVIEW

➤ Incidence unknown
➤ Used in
   ➤ Emergency departments
   ➤ Primary care settings
➤ Complications
   ➤ Rectal bleeding
   ➤ Bowel perforation

RATIONALE

➤ To screen, diagnose, and evaluate perianal and anal problems

INDICATIONS

➤ Rectal or anal bleeding or unusual discharge
➤ Perianal or anal pain
➤ Hemorrhoids
➤ Rectal **prolapse**
➤ Digital examination that reveals a mass
➤ Perianal abscess and **condyloma**

CONTRAINDICATIONS

➤ Acute cardiovascular problems—may stimulate the **vasovagal** reaction
➤ Acute abdominal problems

➤ Unwilling patient
➤ Stenosis of the anal canal

☑ *Informed consent required*

PROCEDURE

Anoscopy

Equipment

➤ Anoscope (Fig. 89–1)
➤ Light source
➤ Gloves—nonsterile
➤ Drape—nonsterile
➤ Water-soluble lubricant (K-Y jelly)
➤ Large cotton-tipped applicators—nonsterile
➤ Monsel's solution—to control bleeding
➤ 4 × 4 gauze—nonsterile
➤ Biopsy **forceps**
➤ Container with 10% **formalin**

Procedure

➤ Position the client in the left lateral decubitus position.
➤ Drape the client.
➤ Put on gloves.
➤ Tell the client you are going to touch him or her by the rectum.
➤ Spread the gluteal fold and examine visually.

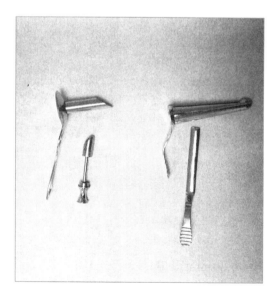

FIGURE 89 • 1 Anoscopes.

➤ Have the client bear down and observe for hemorrhoids or prolapse.
➤ Lubricate your second digit with K-Y jelly and perform a digital examination.
➤ Lubricate the anoscope with K-Y jelly.
➤ Have the client take slow deep breaths to relax the sphincter.
➤ Insert the anoscope slowly and gently into the anus toward the umbilicus.
➤ Remove the obturator.
➤ Visualize the rectal mucosa, noting the vasculature, pectinate line, transitional zone (Fig. 89–2), and drainage.
➤ Remove fecal matter and drainage with a large cotton swab if necessary.
➤ Obtain a biopsy specimen if needed using the biopsy forceps. Place the tissue specimen in a container with 10% formalin.
➤ If bleeding is present, apply Monsel's solution and pressure.
➤ Remove anoscope gently, and observe the mucosa for any injury.

Client Instructions

➤ Slight bleeding is normal after this procedure because of the possibility of an abrasion, tearing of the mucosa or anus, or hemorrhoids.
  ➤ If slight bleeding persists for more than 2 days, notify your health-care provider.
  ➤ To decrease pain and swelling, sit in a tub of warm water for 10 to 15 minutes three times per day.

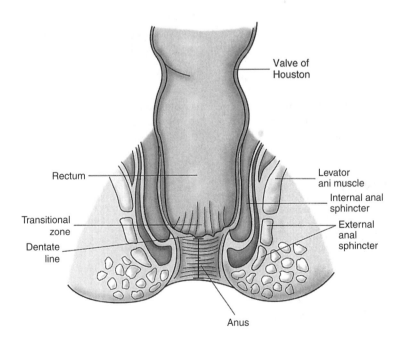

Valve of Houston

Rectum

Levator ani muscle

Internal anal sphincter

Transitional zone

External anal sphincter

Dentate line

Anus

FIGURE 89 • 2 Anatomy of the anus and rectum.

BIBLIOGRAPHY

Pfenninger, J.L., and Fowler, G.C. (1994). *Procedures for primary care physicians.* St. Louis: Mosby.

Wolcott, M.W. (1974). *Ferguson's surgery of the ambulatory patient.* Philadelphia: Lippincott.

Wolcott, M.W. (1988). *Ambulatory surgery and the basics of emergency surgical care.* Philadelphia: Lippincott-Raven.

FLEXIBLE SIGMOIDOSCOPY

90

MARGARET R. COLYAR

CPT Code

45330   Sigmoidoscopy, flexible; diagnostic, with or without collection of specimens by brushing or washing

45331   Sigmoidoscopy, flexible; with biopsy, single or multiple

45332   Sigmoidoscopy, flexible; with removal of foreign body

Flexible **sigmoidoscopy** is a colorectal cancer screening technique that detects 50% to 60% of colon cancers. With flexible sigmoidoscopy, the inner lining of the rectum and the last 2 feet of the distal colon can be visualized; 60-cm sigmoidoscopy is preferred.

OVERVIEW

➤ Incidence unknown
➤ Screening indications
  ➤ Normal clients age older than 50—every 3 to 5 years
  ➤ Annually
    • High-risk clients—age older than 35
    • History of polyps
    • Inflammatory bowel disease
    • Rectal bleeding
    • Constipation or diarrhea—change in bowel habits
    • Abdominal pain
    • Unexplained weight loss

- Anemia
- Family history
➤ Colorectal cancer
  ➤ Second most common cause of cancer death in the United States
  ➤ Appears to be age-related
  ➤ 50% survival rate
  ➤ Causes
    - Inherited
    - Environmental factors (i.e., diet high in fats and low in fiber)
  - Suspicious symptoms
    - Persistent abdominal pain
    - Change in bowel habits
    - Rectal bleeding
    - Positive Hemoccult test
    - Unexplained weight loss or fevers
    - Anemia
➤ Normal versus abnormal findings and when to **biopsy** (Table 90–1)

HEALTH PROMOTION/PREVENTION

➤ Healthy diet—high fiber—20 to 35 g per day
➤ Aspirin 325 mg every day if in high-risk group
  ➤ Contraindicated with aspirin gastritis and gastric ulcers

TABLE 90•1 NORMAL VERSUS ABNORMAL FINDINGS AND WHEN TO PERFORM A BIOPSY

			Biopsy	
DESCRIPTION	NORMAL	ABNORMAL	YES	NO
Adenocarcinoma	✕		✕	
Crohn's colitis		✕	✕	
Diverticula	✕			✕
Diverticulitis		✕		✕
Hyperplastic polyp, rectum	✕		✕	
Lipoma	✕		✕	
Melanosis coli	✕			✕
Multiple colonic polyps		✕	✕	
Proctitis		✕	✕	
Pseudomembranous colitis		✕	✕	
Rectum, first valve of Houston	✕			✕
Rectum, dentate line	✕			✕
Sigmoid colon, valves of Houston	✕			✕
Transverse colon	✕			✕
Tubulovillose adenoma		✕	✕	
Tubular adenoma		✕	✕	
Ulcerative colitis		✕	✕	
Vascular ectasia		✕	✕	
Villose adenoma		✕	✕	

RATIONALE

➤ To screen for colorectal cancer

INDICATIONS

➤ Rectal bleeding
➤ Positive Hemoccult test
➤ Mass on digital examination
➤ Lower abdominal pain and cramping
➤ Change in bowel habits
➤ Foreign body in the rectum
➤ Itching—anal or perianal
➤ Pain—anal or perianal

CONTRAINDICATIONS

➤ Acute abdomen
➤ Diverticulitis
➤ Cardiovascular or pulmonary disease
➤ Ileus
➤ Suspected perforation
➤ Megacolon
➤ Pregnancy
➤ Recent pelvic or abdominal surgery
➤ Coagulation disorders

☑ *Informed consent required*

Bowel preparation needed
➤ Clear liquid diet the night before the procedure
  ➤ May take medications
➤ Fleet enemas until clear 30 to 60 minutes before the procedure
➤ Laxative (bisacodyl) the evening before the procedure

PROCEDURE

Flexible Sigmoidoscopy

Equipment

➤ Flexible sigmoidoscope—60 cm (Fig. 90–1)
➤ Light source
➤ 2 pairs of gloves—nonsterile
➤ Suction
➤ K-Y jelly or 2% lidocaine jelly
➤ 4 × 4 gauze—nonsterile
➤ Absorbent pads—nonsterile

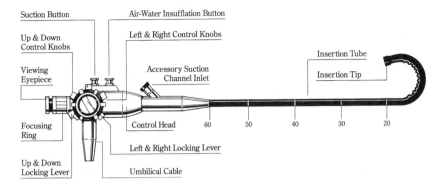

FIGURE 90 • 1 Flexible sigmoidoscope. (Reproduced with permission of Glaxo Wellcome Inc. and the University of Arizona School of Medicine.)

➤ Drape—nonsterile
➤ Culture tubes
➤ Emesis basin
➤ Sigmoidoscopy report sheet (Fig. 90–2)

Procedure

➤ Position the client in the left lateral decubitus position.
  ➤ Right leg flexed at the hip and knee
➤ Put on two pairs of gloves.
➤ Lubricate the second or third digit of the dominant hand.
➤ Perform a digital examination to dilate the sphincter.
➤ Lubricate the anus and the tip of the sigmoidoscope.
➤ Lubricate the distal half of the sigmoidoscope but not the lens.
➤ Remove the top pair of gloves and dispose of them.
➤ Separate the gluteal folds.
➤ Insert the scope gently 8 to 10 cm.
➤ Activate the light, suction, and air.
➤ With the right hand—Advance the scope.
➤ With the left hand—Work the controls on the scope.
➤ Open the colon by insufflating with a small amount of air, and advance the scope gently.
  ➤ Do not use too much air—this causes discomfort.
➤ Advance the scope using one of the following techniques
  ➤ Hook and pullout—used to straighten the colon (Fig. 90–3).
    • Hook mucosal fold, and pull back to straighten the colon.
  ➤ **Dither** and **torque**—used to shorten the colon (Fig. 90–4).
    • Alternate insertion with slow partial withdrawal to pleat the colon.
    • Twist the sigmoid shaft clockwise or counterclockwise with a forward and/or backward motion.
    • Observe for natural landmarks (Fig. 90–5) and abnormalities (Fig. 90–6).

Office
Flexible Sigmoidscopy

Date: _____ Chart #/ID #: _____
Patient Name: _____
Race: _____ Age: _____ Sex: _____
History Abdominal/Gyn surgery?   Yes   No

Bowel Prep Used: Dulcolax Tabs   Golytely   Fleets   Other

Reason for procedure: (circle all that apply)
1. Screening   4. Rectal bleeding   8. Anemia
2. Abdominal pain   5. Guaiac-positive stools 9. Weight loss
3. Change in bowel   6. Constipation   10. Abnormal x-ray
   habits   7. Diarrhea   11. Other: _____
                                               _____
Distance scope inserted: _____ cm

Findings: (circle and diagram)
1. Normal   4. Mucosal abnormality
2. Hemorrhoids   5. Polyp(s) (describe) _____
3. Diverticuli   6. Mass/lesion
                      7. Other: _____

Insertion depth(s) at which abnormality was found: _____ cm
Biopsy performed?   Yes   No

Additional testing needed: Colonscopy?   GI consult?   Barium enema?
Comments and/or pathology report: _____
_____

_____
Signature - Provider

FIGURE 90 • 2 Sigmoidoscopy report sheet.

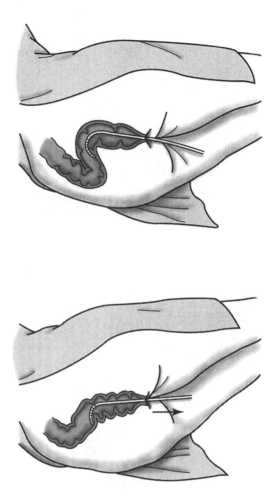

FIGURE 90 • 3 Hook and pullout. Hook the mucosal fold, and pull back to straighten the colon.

> ➤ Take a biopsy specimen of all abnormal areas and put in culture tube for biopsy.
> ➤ Withdraw the sigmoidoscope slowly, reinspecting the mucosa.
> ➤ When in the rectal vault, retroflex the tip of the scope to visualize the distal rectum.
> ➤ Straighten the tip, and gently withdraw the scope.
> ➤ Cleanse, sterilize, and store per manufacturer's instructions.

Client Instructions

> ➤ The following may be expected but will resolve quickly.
> > ➤ Abdominal cramping if a biopsy specimen was obtained

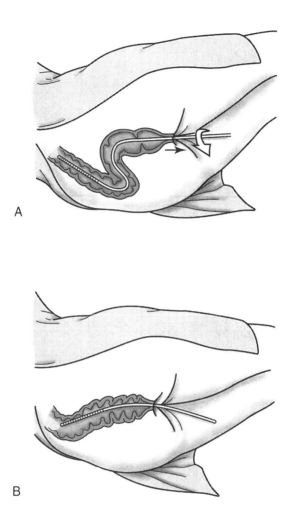

FIGURE 90 • 4 Dither and torque. (A) Pleat the colon by alternating insertion with slow partial withdrawal of the sigmoidoscope. (B) Next, twist the sigmoid shaft clockwise or counterclockwise with a forward and/or backward motion.

- ➤ Feeling of fullness, distention, or flatus
- ➤ No bowel movement for several days
- ➤ Minor bleeding
➤ No special diet is recommended after the procedure.
➤ Watch for signs of infections, such as
- ➤ Elevated temperature
- ➤ Increased or prolonged rectal pain
- ➤ Green or yellow drainage

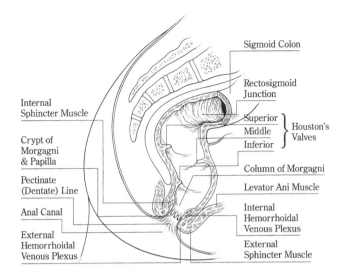

FIGURE 90 • 5 Normal rectal findings. (Reproduced with permission of Glaxo Wellcome Inc. and the University of Arizona School of Medicine.)

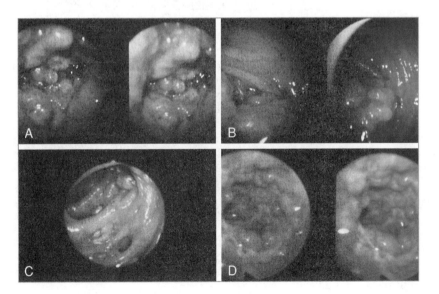

FIGURE 90 • 6 Abnormal rectal findings. (A) Cancer of the rectum. (B) Cancer of the sigmoid colon. (C) Diverticulosis of the sigmoid colon. (D) Crohn's disease of the sigmoid colon. (Reproduced with permission of Glaxo Wellcome Inc. and the University of Arizona School of Medicine.)

BIBLIOGRAPHY

Colodny, C.S. (1996). Procedures for your practice. *Patient Care,* April 15, 151–157.

Dominitz, J.A., et al (1996). Latest approaches to prevention and screening. *Patient Care,* April 15, 124–142.

Reilly, H.F. (1994). Primary care use of the flexible sigmoidoscope to detect colorectal cancer and its precursors. *Primary Care Cancer,* 14(5), 41–45.

91

X-RAY INTERPRETATION— ABDOMINAL

CYNTHIA R. EHRHARDT

CPT Code
Multiple listings based on view ordered

An abdominal x-ray (radiograph) is considered a basic radiologic screening tool when evaluating abdominal disorders. Other, higher technology tools used to evaluate abdominal disorders include computed tomography and magnetic resonance imaging. The ability of the abdominal x-ray to generate high spatial resolution and to visualize various densities within the abdominal cavity can aid in diagnostic evaluation of abdominal disorders but should not be the sole basis for diagnosis. The abdominal x-ray should be correlated with clinical history, physical examination, and additional diagnostic tool results.

OVERVIEW

➤ General principles
  ➢ Adequate knowledge of basic anatomy and physiology is necessary for proper interpretation of the abdominal film.
  ➢ An orderly and systematic approach to interpretation of the abdominal film should be used.

RATIONALE

➤ To obtain visual information about physical anatomy of the abdominal region

➤ To obtain a visual overview of basic pathophysiology of gastrointestinal, vascular, renal, and skeletal systems of the human organism

INDICATIONS

➤ Abdominal trauma
➤ Abdominal pain
➤ Suspicion of abdominal pathophysiology
➤ Ingested foreign body

CONTRAINDICATIONS

➤ Pregnancy (unless shielded)

PROCEDURE
X-ray Interpretation—Abdominal

Equipment

➤ X-ray view box with proper illumination for films
➤ Storage cover for films
➤ Folder storage to prevent bending of films

Procedure

➤ Order flat plate and upright views.
   ➤ If suspicious for free air, order a left lateral decubitus view and chest posteroanterior view.
➤ Place the flat and upright films and left lateral decubitus and chest film (if ordered) on the view box with adequate illumination.
➤ Inspect for the presence of any foreign bodies in the abdominal cavity.
➤ Systematically inspect the abdominal region skeletal system.
   ➤ Identify anatomic skeletal landmarks within the abdominal cavity (lumbar, sacrum, and pelvis) (Fig. 91–1).
      • Determine any aberration.
   ➤ Note the absence or presence of demineralization.
   ➤ Note the lack of continuity or symmetry of skeletal structures that may represent fracture, dislocation, metastases (lytic—low density; sclerotic—high density; and mixed), and calcifications of the lumbosacral spine, illiosacral region, pelvis, acetabulum, and femur region.
   ➤ Note the presence of pathologic calcifications.
➤ Systematically inspect for the soft tissues (Fig. 91–2).
➤ Note the presence or absence of the psoas sign.
➤ *Diaphragm*—Note the presence or absence of an air and/or fluid pattern.
➤ *Liver*
   ➤ Note the homogeneous uniform density of the hepatic shadow.
   ➤ Note the presence or absence of full visualization of hepatic edge.
➤ *Spleen*—The splenic shadow generally is hidden by the gastric bubble and splenic flexure of the colon unless splenomegaly is present.
➤ *Pancreas*—Usually not visible

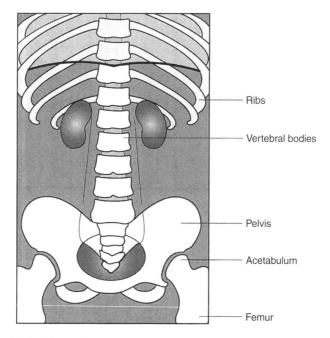

FIGURE 91 • 1 Identify anatomic skeletal landmarks of the abdomen.

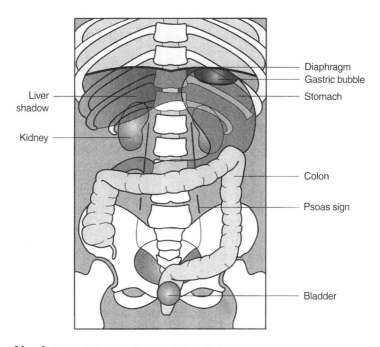

FIGURE 91 • 2 Inspect the soft tissues of the abdomen.

➤ *Renal*—The entire renal shadow outlines generally are not clearly demarcated. It may be difficult to estimate the overall size of the organs.

➤ *Bladder*—If filled, appears as a round homogeneous mass

➤ *Uterus*—Usually not visible; however, can present as an irregular mass if fibroids are present

➤ *Vascular*—Note the presence of any calcifications, widening, or tortuosity of the aorta or renal arteries.

➤ *Gastrointestinal evaluation*

  ➤ *Stomach*—Note that the gastric shadow with presence of gastric bubble usually is located midline to left upper quadrant region (Fig. 91–3).

  ➤ *Intestines*—Air shadow location is scattered in a random, nonspecific pattern throughout the abdominal cavity.

    • Variables, such as age, amount of air ingested, length of small or large intestine, stool concentration, and pathology can cause normal presentations to appear abnormal and vice versa.

    • Abdominal gas pattern location is generally nonspecific (Fig. 91–4).

      • Abnormal concentration of abdominal gas in one location and/or unilateral appearance of the air gas pattern on one side with the absence of any air on the opposite side may suggest *bowel displacement.*

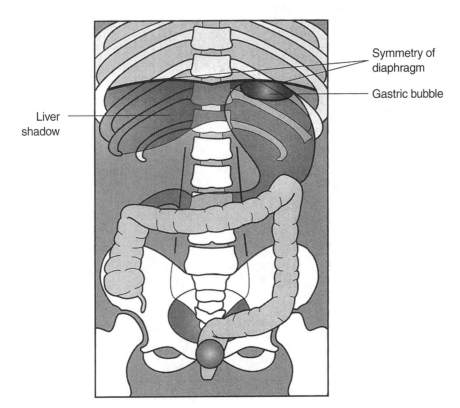

Symmetry of diaphragm

Gastric bubble

Liver shadow

FIGURE 91 • 3 Inspect the stomach for location and presence of gastric bubble.

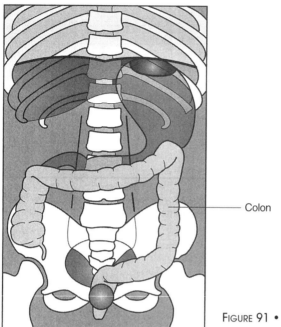

— Colon

FIGURE 91 • 4 The abdominal gas pattern is usually nonspecific in distribution.

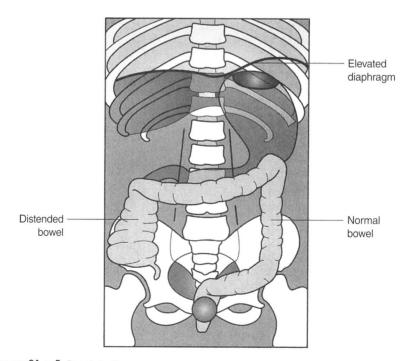

Elevated diaphragm

Distended bowel

Normal bowel

FIGURE 91 • 5 Paralytic ileus.

- Location and concentration of air with accompanying dilated bowel proximally and decreased air shadows distally suggest *paralytic ileus* (Fig. 91–5).
- Localization with the presence of dilated bowel with or without air and/or fluid levels proximally and absence of air shadows distally suggests local obstruction.

➤ *Peritoneum*
  - Note free air in the peritoneal cavity (pneumoperitoneum) (Fig. 91–6). This is usually caused by the disruption of the abdominal wall.

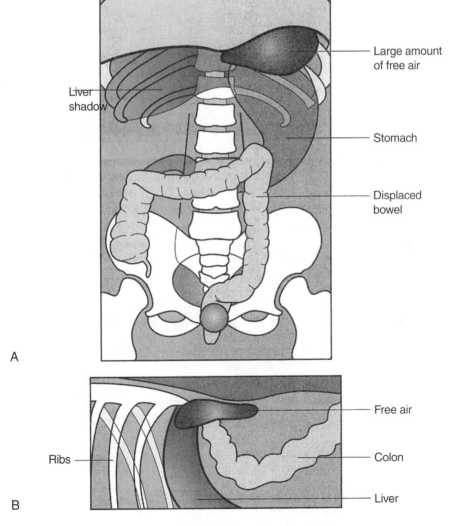

FIGURE 91 • 6 Pneumoperitoneum. *(A)* Upright view; *(B)* left lateral decubitus view.

- Usually seen with left lateral decubitus and chest posteroanterior views; dark air shadows can be visualized in the diaphragm and against the inferior hepatic margin.
> Inspect for intraperitoneal fluid.
- Usually obscures hepatic edges
- Displaces abdominal gas pattern

BIBLIOGRAPHY

Barloon, T., and Weissman, A. (1996). Diagnostic imaging in the evaluation of blunt abdominal trauma. *Am Fam Physician*, 54(1), 205–211.

Spilane, R., et al (1994). Radiographic aspects of pneumothorax. *Am Fam Physician*, 51(2), 459–464.

Stimac, G. (1992). *Introduction to diagnostic imaging*. Philadelphia: Saunders.

Wilson, R., and Walt, A. (1975). *Management of trauma: pitfalls and practice*. Philadelphia: Lea & Febiger.

92

ABDOMINAL PARACENTESIS

MARGARET R. COLYAR

CPT Code	
49080	Peritoneocentesis, abdominal paracentesis, or peritoneal lavage (diagnostic or therapeutic); initial
49081	Peritoneocentesis, abdominal paracentesis, or peritoneal lavage (diagnostic or therapeutic); subsequent

Paracentesis is a procedure in which the abdominal cavity is punctured, using sterile technique. This procedure is not useful with mechanical obstructions or localized abscesses.

OVERVIEW

> Incidence unknown
> Before the procedure
  > Explain the procedure to the client.
  > Measure abdominal girth.
  > Measure vital signs and weight.
  > Have the client void to decompress the bladder.

RATIONALE

➤ To remove excess fluid from the peritoneal cavity for testing
➤ To diminish discomfort caused by ascites

INDICATIONS

➤ Suspected intra-abdominal hemorrhage
➤ Peritonitis
➤ Ascites
➤ To lower intra-abdominal pressure

CONTRAINDICATIONS

➤ Massive bowel dilation—correct with a nasogastric tube (NGT) first.
➤ Widespread adhesions
➤ Bleeding disorders
➤ Previous abdominal surgery

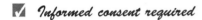 *Informed consent required*

PROCEDURE

Abdominal Paracentesis

Equipment

➤ Antiseptic skin cleanser
➤ 18- or 20-gauge, $1^1/_2$-inch needle
➤ Spinal needle—if client is obese
➤ 25- to 27-gauge, 1-inch needle
➤ Two syringes—10 and 60 mL
➤ 2% lidocaine with epinephrine—epinephrine decreases bleeding and chance of false-positive result
➤ Culture tubes, specimen tubes with and without anticoagulant, blood culture bottles
➤ Microscope slides
➤ Suction bottle—1000 mL
➤ Connector tubing
➤ Three-way stopcock
➤ Drape—sterile
➤ Gloves—sterile
➤ Mask—optional
➤ Gown—optional
➤ Topical antibiotic ointment (Bactroban, Neosporin, or Polysporin)
➤ 4 × 4 gauze—sterile
➤ Tape

Procedure

➤ Ask the client to void.
➤ Cleanse the entire abdomen with antiseptic skin cleanser.

➤ Position the client in an upright position with feet supported on a stool.
➤ Anesthetize the insertion area with 2% lidocaine with epinephrine.
➤ Attach the connecting tubing, stopcock, 60-mL syringe, suction bottle, and 18- or 20-gauge needle (Fig. 92–1).
➤ Insert the needle at a right angle to the skin in the quadrant most likely to yield fluid.
  ➤ If the puncture site is in the upper quadrant, insert the needle lateral to the rectus muscle to prevent organ damage (Fig. 92–2).
  ➤ The most common site is halfway between the symphysis pubis and umbilicus at midline.
  ➤ You will feel the following
    • Firm resistance
    • Then a "give" sensation
➤ If using a spinal needle, remove the obturator and be prepared for drainage.
➤ If no drainage, apply gentle suction with the 60-mL syringe, and advance the needle tip.
➤ Put the specimen in culture tubes and on slides. You should obtain the following
  ➤ Gram's stain
  ➤ Cell count
  ➤ Culture
➤ If the bowel is obviously perforated, remove the needle and apply pressure for approximately 5 minutes. The **perforation** should seal spontaneously.
➤ Apply an absorbent dressing of 4 × 4 gauze covered with tape.
➤ Measure the drainage, describe, and record.
➤ Send specimens to the laboratory.
➤ Monitor vital signs every 15 minutes for 1 hour.

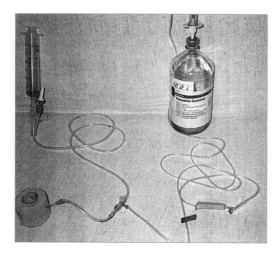

FIGURE 92 • 1 Assemble the connecting tubing, stopcock, 60-mL syringe, suction bottle, and 18- to 20-gauge needle.

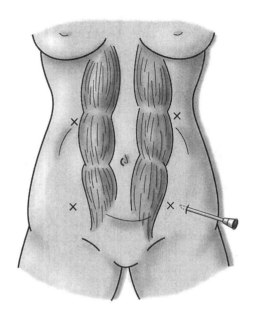

FIGURE 92 • 2 Insert the needle at a 90-degree angle. Use the appropriate puncture sites to prevent organ damage.

Client Instructions

➤ The puncture site may leak slightly for the next 24 hours. Keep it covered with a clean absorbent dressing.

➤ Slight bleeding is expected. Bleeding should stop within 12 to 24 hours.

➤ Because _____ mL of fluid was removed today, there is a chance of low blood pressure and shock. Return to the office immediately if you experience the following
  ➤ Weakness
  ➤ Dizziness or fainting
  ➤ Desire to sleep all the time

➤ Depending on the reason for the fluid developing in your abdomen, it may recur. Notify the office if this happens.

➤ Observe for the following signs and symptoms of infection and return to the office if these occur
  ➤ Fever or chills
  ➤ Increase in pain at the puncture site
  ➤ Nausea and/or vomiting
  ➤ Yellow or green drainage from the puncture site

➤ Your next appointment is _____ .

BIBLIOGRAPHY

Saunders, C.E., and Ho, M.T. (eds.). (1992). *Current emergency diagnosis and treatment.* Norwalk, CT: Appleton & Lange.

Sheehy, S.B., and Jimmerson, C.L. (1994). *Manual of clinical trauma care.* St. Louis: Mosby.

Zimmerman, E. (1976). *Techniques of patient care manual of bedside procedures.* Boston: Little, Brown.

93 GASTRIC LAVAGE

MARGARET R. COLYAR

> **CPT Code**
> 91105   Gastric lavage

Gastric **lavage** is a procedure used to aspirate gastric contents and irrigate the stomach. Gastric lavage also is used to assist in the evacuation of toxic substances that are only partially digested. Toxic substances usually are ingested in suicide attempts or accidents (children).

OVERVIEW

➤ Incidence unknown
>   ➤ Use small-gauge tube (nasogastric route) if
>   • The tube will be left in place after gastric lavage
>   ➤ Use large-gauge Ewald tube (orogastric route) to
>   • Evacuate large particles, such as partially digested pills

HEALTH PROMOTION/PREVENTION

➤ Do not ingest large amounts of medications or toxic substances.
➤ Seek counseling when life circumstances seem overwhelming.
➤ Keep all dangerous substances out of the reach of children.

OPTIONS

➤ *Method 1*—gastric lavage for specimen collection
➤ *Method 2*—gastric lavage for hemorrhage
➤ *Method 3*—gastric lavage for overdose

RATIONALE

➤ To aspirate gastric contents
➤ To collect specimens
➤ To irrigate the stomach
➤ To evacuate toxic substances
➤ To stop gastric hemorrhage

INDICATIONS

➤ Ingested poisons—liquid or solid
➤ Drug overdose

- Gastric bleeding
- Stomach cleansing before endoscopic testing
- Gastric washings for cytology

CONTRAINDICATIONS

- Alkali or acids ingested that may perforate the stomach
- Convulsions
- Ingestion of petroleum products
- Cardiac **dysrhythmias**

PROCEDURE

Gastric Lavage

Equipment

- Method 1 only
  - No. 16 Salem sump NGT
- Methods 1, 2, and 3
  - 60-mL syringe with catheter tip
  - Water-soluble lubricant
  - Glove—nonsterile
  - Towels or absorbent drapes
  - Wash basin—to empty gastric contents
  - Emesis basin
  - Ice water
  - 0.9% sodium chloride
  - Containers for specimens
- Methods 2 and 3
  - Large-bore Ewald orogastric tube
  - Suction machine—optional
- Method 3 only
  - **Antidote**—if needed
    - Call poison control center for appropriate antidote.

Procedure

METHOD 1—GASTRIC LAVAGE FOR SPECIMEN COLLECTION

- Position the client in a Fowler's position (if alert) or left lateral position (if comatose).
- Remove dentures.
- Measure from the bridge of the nose to earlobe to **xiphoid process** and mark with tape (see Chapter 95).
- Drape the client.
- Put on gloves.
- Lubricate the tip of the tube.
- Instruct the client to tilt the head back when the tube is introduced into the nose.
  - *Optional*—Place the NGT in a basin of ice water to stiffen it so that it is easier to insert and does not get coiled on its way to the stomach.

➤ *Optional*—If there is a problem inserting because of nose sensitivity, use a topical anesthetic in the nostril.
➤ Pass the tube through the mouth (Ewald tube) or nose (smaller NGT) into the stomach.
➤ Have the client sip water through the straw to facilitate passage of the NGT.
  ➤ If drinking water is contraindicated, instruct the client to swallow as the tube is advanced.
➤ Insert the tube slowly and gently.
  ➤ If any symptoms of respiratory difficulty are observed (cough, dyspnea, **cyanosis**), the NGT probably is being inserted into the lung. Withdraw immediately and reinsert.
➤ Tape the tube in place.
➤ Check position of the tube with an air bubble and aspiration of gastric contents.
➤ Obtain a specimen of the gastric contents.

METHOD 2—GASTRIC LAVAGE FOR HEMORRHAGE

➤ Position the client in a Fowler's position (if alert) or left lateral position (if comatose).
➤ Remove dentures.
➤ Measure from the bridge of the nose to earlobe to xiphoid process and mark with tape (see Chapter 95).
➤ Drape the client.
➤ Put on gloves.
➤ Lubricate the tip of the tube.
➤ Instruct the client to tilt the head back when the tube is introduced into the nose.
  ➤ *Optional*—Place the NGT in a basin of ice water to stiffen it so that it is easier to insert and does not get coiled on its way to the stomach.
  ➤ *Optional*—If there is a problem inserting because of nose sensitivity, use a topical anesthetic in the nostril.
➤ Pass the tube through the mouth (Ewald tube) or nose (smaller NGT) into the stomach.
➤ Have the client sip water through the straw to facilitate passage of the NGT.
  ➤ If drinking water is contraindicated, instruct the client to swallow as the tube is advanced.
➤ Insert the tube slowly and gently.
  ➤ If any symptoms of respiratory difficulty are observed (cough, dyspnea, cyanosis), the NGT probably is being inserted into the lung. Withdraw immediately and reinsert.
➤ Tape the tube in place.
➤ Check position of the tube with an air bubble and aspiration of gastric contents.
➤ Raise the tube above the client's head.
➤ Take the plunger out of the 60-mL syringe, and use the syringe as a funnel.

➤ Attach the syringe funnel to the tubing, and instill 100 to 200 mL of 0.9% sodium chloride (Fig. 93–1).

➤ Lower the funnel and allow the sodium chloride to flow out into the washbasin, or detach the funnel and attach the tubing to low suction.

➤ Continue this procedure of irrigation and suction until the gastric contents change from red to clear.

➤ Remove the tube if indicated.

METHOD 3—GASTRIC LAVAGE FOR OVERDOSE

➤ Position the client in a Fowler's position (if alert) or left lateral position (if comatose).

➤ Remove dentures.

➤ Measure from the bridge of the nose to earlobe to xiphoid process and mark with tape (see Chapter 95).

➤ Drape the client.

➤ Put on gloves.

➤ Lubricate the tip of the tube.

➤ Instruct the client to tilt the head back when the tube is introduced into the nose.

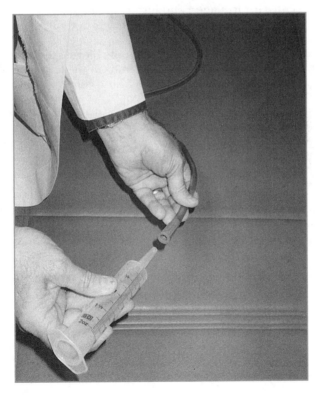

FIGURE 93 • 1 Attach the syringe funnel to the tubing and instill the sodium chloride.

➤ *Optional*—Place the NGT in a basin of ice water to stiffen it so that it is easier to insert and does not get coiled on its way to the stomach.
➤ *Optional*—If there is a problem inserting because of nose sensitivity, use a topical anesthetic in the nostril.
➤ Pass the tube through the mouth (Ewald tube).
➤ Have the client sip water through the straw to facilitate passage of the NGT.
  ➤ If drinking water is contraindicated, instruct the client to swallow as the tube is advanced.
➤ Insert the tube slowly and gently.
  ➤ If any symptoms of respiratory difficulty are observed (cough, dyspnea, cyanosis), the NGT probably is being inserted into the lung. Withdraw immediately and reinsert.
➤ Tape the tube in place.
➤ Check position of the tube with an air bubble and aspiration of gastric contents.
➤ Raise the tube above the client's head.
➤ Take the plunger out of the 60-mL syringe, and use the syringe as a funnel.
➤ Attach the syringe funnel to the tubing.
  ➤ If the poison ingested was liquid, follow the directions of the poison control center for irrigation and instillation of antidote.
  ➤ If the poison ingested was solid, instill 100 to 200 mL of sodium chloride unless contraindicated.
    • Lower the funnel and allow the sodium chloride to flow out into the washbasin, or detach the funnel and attach the tubing to low suction.
    • Irrigate with sodium chloride until gastric contents are clear and no particles are seen.
➤ Instill the appropriate antidote and follow instructions of poison control center.
➤ Obtain several specimens of gastric contents throughout this procedure.
➤ Remove the tube.

Client Instructions

➤ Throat may be sore for 1 to 3 days. Suck on ice chips or throat lozenges.
➤ If the procedure was done to treat overdose or poison ingestion, return to the office in 24 hours for recheck.

BIBLIOGRAPHY

Rakel, R.E. (ed.) (1996). *Conn's current therapy.* Philadelphia: Saunders.
Smeltzer, S.C., and Bare, B.G. (1996). *Brunner and Suddarth's textbook of medical-surgical nursing.* Philadelphia: Lippincott-Raven.

94

INGUINAL HERNIA REDUCTION

MARGARET R. COLYAR

CPT Code

49495   Repair initial inguinal hernia, age younger than 6 months with or without hydrocelectomy; reducible

49500   Repair initial inguinal hernia, age 6 months to 5 years; reducible

49505   Repair initial inguinal hernia, age older than 5 years; reducible

49520   Repair recurrent inguinal hernia, any age; reducible

A hernia is a result of weakness in the abdominal muscle wall through which a bowel segment or peritoneal structure protrudes. Types of hernias include (Fig. 94–1)

➤ Indirect—protrusion of a bowel segment or peritoneal contents through the inguinal ring and down the spermatic cord through the inguinal canal.
  ➤ Often descend into the scrotal area
  ➤ Most common; usually found in men and children
  ➤ Usually **incarcerated** and require surgery
➤ Direct—protrusion of a bowel segment or peritoneal contents through the abdominal wall in an area of muscle weakness
  ➤ More common in elderly

OVERVIEW

➤ Causes
  ➤ Intra-abdominal pressure, such as
    • Pregnancy
    • Obesity
    • Ascites
    • Heavy lifting
    • Coughing

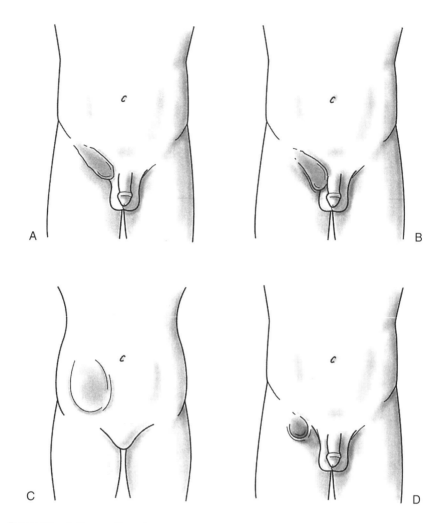

FIGURE 94 • 1 Types of hernias. *(A)* Indirect inguinal hernia; *(B)* direct inguinal hernia; *(C)* direct abdominal hernia; and *(D)* femoral hernia.

> Abdominal wall weakness, such as
  • Inherited
  • Acquired
> Terminology
  > **Reducible**—can be replaced into the abdominal wall with gentle pressure
  > Incarcerated or **irreducible**—trapped bowel that cannot be replaced into the abdominal wall with gentle pressure
  > **Strangulated**—blood supply to herniated bowel is cut off. Signs and symptoms include

- Abdominal distention
- Pain
- Nausea
- Vomiting
- **Tachycardia**

HEALTH PROMOTION/PREVENTION

➤ Maintain normal body weight.
➤ Maintain good physical fitness.
➤ Use proper lifting techniques.
➤ Avoid straining and lifting.
➤ Wear a truss to hold the organs in place if the abdominal wall is sagging.

RATIONALE

➤ To prevent strangulation and incarceration of the hernia

INDICATIONS

➤ Palpable bulging in the abdomen or groin
➤ Discomfort

CONTRAINDICATIONS

➤ If strangulation is suspected, REFER to a surgeon immediately.

PROCEDURE

Abdominal Hernia Reduction

Equipment

➤ Gloves—nonsterile

Procedure

➤ Position the client in a recumbent position or Trendelenburg position with knees flexed to decrease intra-abdominal pressure.
➤ Wait 30 minutes to see if passive reduction occurs.
➤ If passive reduction does not occur, guide the herniated bowel gently through the opening, using fingers flat on the abdomen.
➤ If the client is a child, *follow-up* with a surgeon is necessary for surgical repair.

Client Instructions

➤ If protrusion recurs, lie down on your back to allow passive reduction to occur. If the hernia does not reduce, return to the office.
➤ Bowel obstruction is a possibility with any hernia and can be life-threatening. Symptoms are

- Abdominal distention
- Pain
- Nausea
- Vomiting
- Tachycardia
- If any of these symptoms occur, return to the office or go to the emergency department immediately.

BIBLIOGRAPHY

Ignatavicius, D.D., et al (1995). *Medical-surgical nursing*. Philadelphia: Saunders.

95

NASOGASTRIC TUBE (NGT) INSERTION

MARGARET R. COLYAR

CPT Code	
91105	Gastric intubation and aspiration or lavage for treatment

The NGT is a short, flexible tube inserted through the nose or mouth into the stomach. The NGT is used to remove fluid and gas from the upper gastrointestinal tract. Specimens of stomach contents can be obtained for laboratory analysis. The NGT also can be used to administer medications and feedings. The Levin tube and Salem sump tube are the two most commonly used NGTs. The Levin tube is a single-lumen, clear plastic tube. The Salem sump tube is a double-lumen, clear plastic tube with a blue pigtail.

OVERVIEW

- Incidence unknown

RATIONALE

- To promote healing of the stomach and intestines
- To prevent complications postoperatively
- To obtain specimens

INDICATIONS

- After gastric or abdominal surgery
- Abdominal distention
- Bowel obstruction
- Temporary need for tube feeding
- Obtain specimen of gastric contents
- Medication overdose

CONTRAINDICATIONS

- Seizure activity
- Ingestion of corrosive substances—acids or alkali
- Head or facial trauma

PROCEDURE
NGT Insertion
Equipment

- Glass of water
- Straw
- Towel—nonsterile
- NGT
- K-Y jelly
- Emesis basin
- Ice water
- Gloves—nonsterile
- Tape
- Suction machine
- Syringe
- Stethoscope
- Safety pin—optional

Procedure

- Position the client in a Fowler's position.
- Spread a towel under the chin and down the front of the client.
- Measure the distance the tube is to be passed using the following procedure
  - Place the tip of the tube on the bridge of the nose and stretch the tube to the ear lobe and from the ear lobe to the bottom of the **xiphoid process**.
  - Mark the tube with a piece of tape.
- Lubricate the first 4 inches of the NGT with K-Y jelly.
- Occlude the client's nostrils one at a time to determine **patency**.
- Instruct the client to tilt the head back when the tube is introduced into the nose.

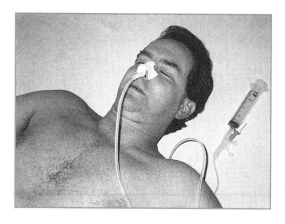

FIGURE 95 • 1 After insertion of the NGT, fasten the tube to the client's nose securely with tape.

➤ *Optional*—Place the NGT in a basin of ice water to stiffen it so that it is easier to insert and does not get coiled on its way to the stomach.
➤ *Optional*—If there is a problem inserting because of nose sensitivity, use a topical anesthetic in the nostril.
➤ Have the client sip water through the straw to facilitate passage of the NGT.
  ➤ If drinking water is contraindicated, instruct the client to swallow as the tube is advanced.
➤ Insert the tube slowly and gently.
  ➤ If any symptoms of respiratory difficulty are observed (cough, dyspnea, cyanosis), the NGT probably is being inserted into the lung. Withdraw immediately and reinsert.
➤ When the tube is inserted to the area marked on the tape, stop.
➤ Fasten the tube to the client's nose (Fig. 95–1).
➤ Position the blue pigtail above the stomach to avoid siphoning of gastric contents.
➤ Check placement by aspiration of gastric contents and instilling 10 to 20 mL of air into the tube.
  ➤ Listen with a stethoscope for the air bubble (gurgle) just below the xiphoid process and in the left upper quadrant of the abdomen.
➤ Obtain a specimen if needed, or attach the tube to low intermittent suction (80 to 120 mL) as necessary.

Client Instructions

➤ Take nothing by mouth while the NGT is in place.

B I B L I O G R A P H Y
Ignatavicius, D.D., et al (1995). *Brunner and Suddarth's medical-surgical nursing*. Philadelphia: Saunders.

PERCUTANEOUS ENDOSCOPIC GASTROSTOMY (PEG) TUBE REINSERTION

96

MARGARET R. COLYAR

CPT Code

43750   Percutaneous placement of gastrosto-
        my tube
43760   Change of gastrostomy tube

A **percutaneous** endoscopic gastrostomy (PEG) tube usually is used to administer feedings and medications and extends from the external abdomen directly into the stomach. Reinsertion of the tube is necessary when the client or caregiver inadvertently dislodges it.

OVERVIEW
➤ Incidence is unknown.
➤ Two types of surgery are used (Fig. 96–1).
  ➤ Permanent gastrostomy with **stoma**
➤ PEG

RATIONALE
➤ To promote continuous nutrition and medication to the client

INDICATIONS
➤ PEG tube is dislodged.

CONTRAINDICATIONS
➤ Newly inserted tube—within 4 to 5 days
➤ No obvious **fistula** opening

☑ *Informed consent required*

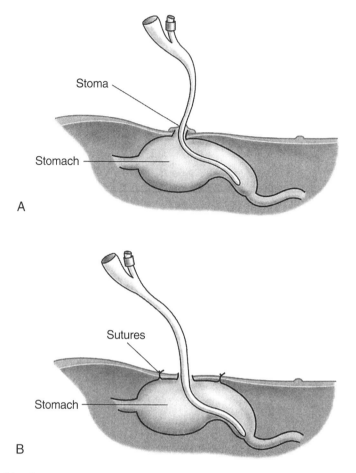

FIGURE 96 • 1 Two types of surgery for PEG tube insertion are permanent gastrostomy with (A) stoma and (B) percutaneous endoscopic gastrostomy.

PROCEDURE

PEG Tube Reinsertion

Equipment

➤ Foley catheter tube—same size as tube dislodged with one size larger balloon
➤ Topical skin cleanser
➤ Drape—sterile
➤ K-Y jelly
➤ Gloves—sterile
➤ Scissors—sterile
➤ 10-mL syringe with Luer-Lok

➤ 50- to 60-mL syringe with catheter tip
➤ 0.9% sodium chloride—enough to fill the balloon
➤ 4 × 4 gauze—sterile
➤ Tape catheter plug

Procedure

➤ Position the client in the supine position.
➤ Cleanse the stoma or insertion site with topical skin cleanser.
➤ Open the Foley catheter on the sterile drape.
➤ Put on gloves.
➤ Check the balloon by inflating with the Luer-Lok syringe filled with sterile saline, then deflate.
➤ Lubricate the tip of the catheter tube with K-Y jelly.
➤ Insert the tube 3 to 6 inches into the previous tube site (Fig. 96–2), using sterile technique.
  ➤ Watch the client's face for signs of pain.
  ➤ Stop if unable to advance the tube or the client is in pain.
➤ Aspirate stomach contents with 60-mL catheter-tipped syringe through big port of the tube (Fig. 96–3)
➤ If gastric contents are obtained, inflate the balloon with the appropriate amount of sterile saline.
➤ Pull back the tube gently until resistance is met (Fig. 96–4).
➤ Insert a catheter plug into the large port of the PEG tube.
➤ Cut a slit halfway through the 4 × 4 gauze.
➤ Apply the slit 4 × 4 gauze dressing around the newly inserted tube (Fig. 96–5).
➤ Tape the tube securely to the abdomen.

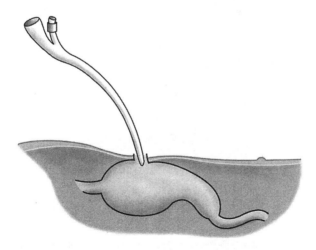

FIGURE 96 • 2 Insert 3 to 6 inches of the catheter into the old PEG tube site.

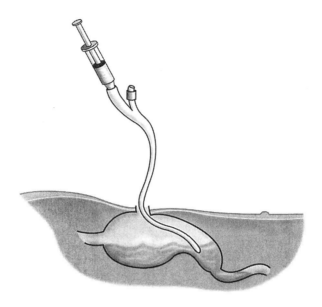

FIGURE 96 • 3 Aspirate stomach contents with a 60-mL catheter-tipped syringe to ensure proper placement.

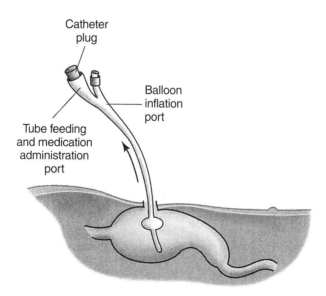

FIGURE 96 • 4 Inflate the balloon and gently pull back on the PEG tube until resistance is met. Plug the large port with a catheter plug.

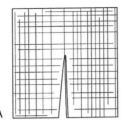

A

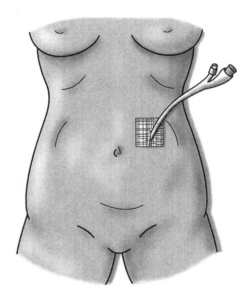

B

FIGURE 96 • 5 *(A)* Cut a slit in the 4 × 4 gauze and *(B)* secure it around the PEG tube.

Client Instructions

➤ Keep the tube taped securely to the abdomen to prevent the tube from becoming dislodged.
➤ Observe for signs and symptoms of infection, such as
  ➤ Increase in pain after 24 hours
  ➤ Increase in temperature
  ➤ Redness or swelling
  ➤ Yellow or greenish drainage
  ➤ Foul odor
➤ If any signs or symptoms of infection are found, return to the office.
➤ Give acetaminophen (Tylenol) every 4 to 6 hours as needed for pain.
➤ Return to the office if complications occur.

BIBLIOGRAPHY

Gutt, C.N., et al (1996). Experiences with percutaneous endoscopic gastrostomy. *World J Surg*, 8, 1006–1008, 1108–1109.

Penfield, A.J. (1995). Twenty-two years of office and outpatient laparoscopy: current techniques and why I chose. *J Am Assoc Gynecol Laparoscopy*, 3, 365–368.

Zacherl, A., et al (1997). Office laparoscopy under local anesthesia. *Minimal Invasive Surgical Nursing*, 2, 73–78.

Zimmerman, E. (1976). *Techniques of patient care manual of bedside procedures*. Boston: Little, Brown.

97

THROMBOSED HEMORRHOID REMOVAL

MARGARET R. COLYAR

CPT Code

46221   Hemorrhoidectomy, by simple ligature

46230   Excision of external hemorrhoid tags and/or multiple papillae

46320   Enucleation or excision of external thrombotic hemorrhoid

46935   Destruction of hemorrhoids; any method, external

External hemorrhoids that have **thrombosed** (formed a clot), usually after defecatory straining, may or may not need removal. If pain is not severe and the clot is small, removal is not necessary.

OVERVIEW

➤ Incidence unknown
➤ Recurrence rate—2% to 5%
➤ Signs and symptoms include
  ➤ Constant anal pain
  ➤ Sensation of sitting on a marble
  ➤ Itching
  ➤ Purple mass at the anus (Fig. 97–1)

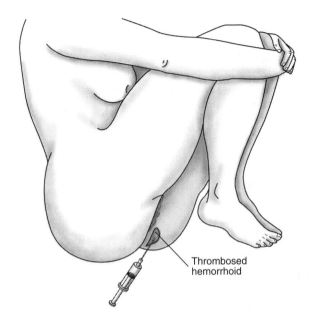

FIGURE 97 • 1 Thrombosed hemorrhoid. Infiltrate with lidocaine around the hemorrhoid.

RATIONALE

➤ To prevent necrosis, pain, and infection

INDICATIONS

➤ Thrombosed hemorrhoid that is painful

CONTRAINDICATIONS

➤ Small thrombosed hemorrhoid that is not causing pain
➤ Immunocompromised client
➤ Bleeding disorders
➤ Pregnancy
➤ Rectal prolapse

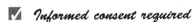 *Informed consent required*

PROCEDURE

Removal of Thrombosed Hemorrhoid

Equipment

➤ Antiseptic skin cleanser
➤ Gloves—sterile

- ➤ 27-gauge, $1^1/_2$-inch needle
- ➤ 1% or 2% lidocaine with epinephrine
- ➤ No. 11 scalpel
- ➤ Curved scissors—sterile
- ➤ Hemostats—sterile
- ➤ Cautery, silver nitrate sticks, or Monsel's solution
- ➤ 4 × 4 gauze—sterile
- ➤ Tape—3 inch
- ➤ Tape—1 inch

Procedure

- ➤ Position the client side lying with thrombosed side down.
- ➤ Separate buttocks, and tape (using 3-inch tape) to side of table to keep area exposed.
- ➤ Cleanse the area with antiseptic skin cleanser.
- ➤ Drape the client.
- ➤ Put on gloves.
- ➤ Infiltrate around the hemorrhoid with 1% or 2% lidocaine with epinephrine.
- ➤ Using the No. 11 scalpel, make an elliptical incision around the vein (Fig. 97–2).
- ➤ Evacuate all of the clot.
- ➤ Explore the cavity for clots, and break down any septa (pockets) with the hemostats.
- ➤ Leave the cavity open.
- ➤ Pack with dry gauze and secure with 1-inch tape.

Client Instructions

- ➤ To decrease pain, do the following
  - ➤ Apply ice packs to wound intermittently for 24 hours.
  - ➤ Take acetaminophen every 4 to 6 hours as needed.
- ➤ Leave packing in for 24 hours, then remove gently.
  - ➤ Minor bleeding is expected.
- ➤ To promote healing
  - ➤ Soak wound in pan or tub of warm water for 20 to 30 minutes three to four times per day for 1 week.
- ➤ To prevent recurrence
  - ➤ Avoid prolonged sitting and straining to stool.
  - ➤ Include in your daily diet
    - • Fruits, vegetables, and bran
    - • Four to five glasses of water
- ➤ Return to the office in 4 weeks.

BIBLIOGRAPHY

Pfenninger, J.L., and Surrell, J. (1995). Nonsurgical treatment options for internal hemorrhoids. *Am Fam Physician, 52*(3), 821–834.

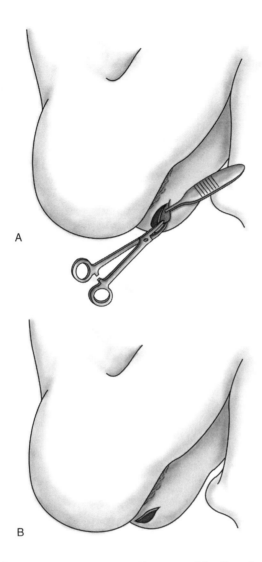

A

B

FIGURE 97 • 2 *(A)* Make an elliptical incision around the thrombosed hemorrhoid and *(B)* remove.

Rakel, R.E. (ed.). (1997). *Conn's current therapy.* Philadelphia: Saunders.

Tierney, L.M., et al (eds.) (1995) (34th ed.). *Current medical diagnosis and treatment.* Norwalk, CT: Appleton & Lange.

Zaines, G., et al (1994). Office treatment of hemorrhoids. In Pfenninger, J.L., and Fowler, G.C. (eds.). *Procedures for primary care physicians.* St. Louis: Mosby.

GLOSSARY

A

Acetone • A colorless, volatile, inflammable liquid, miscible in water, useful as a solvent, and having a characteristic sweet, fruity, ethereal odor.

Acrochordon • A small outgrowth of epidermal and dermal tissue. SYN: skin tag.

Actinic keratoses • Horny, keratotic, premalignant lesions of the skin caused by excess exposure to sunlight.

Alignment • To put in a straight line.

Allen's test • Objective test to ensure patency of the ulnar artery.

Amblyopia • Reduction or dimness of vision, especially where there is no apparent pathologic condition of the eye.

Angioma • Form of tumor, usually benign, consisting principally of blood vessels or lymph vessels.

Ankyloglossia • Abnormal shortness of the frenulum of the tongue. SYN: tongue-tie.

Anoscope • Tool used to visualize the anus directly.

Antecubital • In front of the elbow; at the bend of the elbow.

Antidote • A substance that neutralizes poisons or their effects.

Approximate • To place or bring objects close together.

Arrhythmia • Irregularity or loss of rhythm, especially of the heartbeat. SYN: dysrhythmia.

Arthrocentesis • Puncture of a joint space by using a needle.

Arthropods • Crustaceans, insects, myriapods, and arachnids.

Asymmetric • Lack of symmetry.

Atrioventricular (AV) node • A tangled mass of Purkinje fibers located in the lower part of the interatrial septum from which the AV bundle (bundle of His) arises.

Atrophy • A decrease in size of an organ or tissue.

Audiogram • An objective measuring tool for the detection of hearing problems or hearing loss.

Auricular • Relating to the auricle of the ear.

Avulsion • A tearing away forcibly of a part or structure.

B

Bartholinitis • Inflammation of one or both of Bartholin's glands at the opening to the vagina.

Basal cell carcinoma • A malignancy of the skin that rarely metastasizes. A lesion with whitish borders around a central depression.

Benzoin • A solution applied to the skin to prepare the site for application of adhesives.

Biochemical • Chemical changes accompanying the vital functions of plants and animals.

Biopsy • Excision of a lesion or small piece of living tissue for microscopic evaluation by punch, shave, curettage, or elliptical excision.

Bradycardia • Slow heartbeat less than 60 beats/min.

Bronchospasm • Abnormal narrowing with obstruction of the lumen of the bronchi due to spasm of the peribronchial smooth muscle.

Bundle branches • Part of the ventricular conducting system that carries current down the right and left sides of the interventricular septum.

Bundle of His • The uppermost portion of the ventricular conducting system. It emerges from the AV node and divides into the right and left bundle branches.

C

Cautery • A means of destroying tissue by electricity, freezing, heat, or corrosive chemicals.

Cellulitis • A spreading inflammation of cellular or connective tissue.

Cervical cap • Helmet-shaped, rubber device that fits over the cervix to provide a nonsystemic, nonhormonal, and reversible method of contraception.

Cervicovaginal • Pertaining to the cervix and the vagina.

Chemosis • Edema of the conjunctiva about the cornea.

Circumcision • Surgical procedure in which the prepuce of the penis is excised.

Coagulopathies • A defect in the blood-clotting mechanisms.

Collateral circulation • Circulation of small anastomosing vessels, especially when a main artery is obstructed.

Colposcopy • Examination of the vaginal and cervical tissues by using a colposcope.

Condyloma acuminatum • Wart in the genital and perianal areas. The virus that causes the wart is usually sexually transmitted.

Confrontation • A method employed in determining the extent of visual fields in which the patient's visual field is compared with that of the examiner.

Costophrenic • Pertaining to the ribs and diaphragm.

Crepitus/Crepitation • A crackling sound heard in certain diseases.

Cryogenic • Producing or pertaining to low temperatures.

Cryoglobulinemia • Presence in the blood of an abnormal protein that forms gels with low temperatures. Found in association with pathologic conditions such as multiple myeloma, leukemia, and certain forms of pneumonia.

Cryoprobe • Device for applying cold to a tissue.

Cryosurgery • Technique of exposing tissues to extreme cold to produce well-demarcated areas of cell injury and destruction. The tissue usually is cooled to less than $-20°C$.

Curettage • Scraping of a cavity.

Curette • A spoon-shaped scooping and scraping instrument for removing foreign matter from a cavity.

Cutaneous • Pertaining to the skin.

Cyanosis • Slightly bluish, grayish, slatelike, or dark purple discoloration of the skin caused by the presence of abnormal amounts of reduced hemoglobin in the blood.

Cycloplegics • Medium that produces paralysis of the ciliary muscles.

Cystocele • A bladder hernia that protrudes into the vagina.

D
Decubitus view • Lying down, flat.
Defecatory • Evacuation of the bowels.
Deflection • The deviation from 0 shown by the indicator of a measuring instrument.
Depolarizations • Electrical stimulus of the heart muscle causing heart cells to contract.
Dermabond • Skin closure adhesives used over flat areas of the body that do not require increased potential for tension to the repair site (i.e., over joints).
Dermatofibroma • A nonmalignant skin fibroma (a fibrous, encapsulated, connective tissue tumor).
Dermis • The skin.
Desiccation • The process of drying up.
Diaphragm • Contraceptive barrier device that consists of a soft latex rubber dome supported by a round metal spring on the outside of various sizes.
Digital block • Nerve block accomplished by injecting anesthetic agents between the web of the fingers or toes.
Diphasic • Having two phases.
Disseminate • Scatter or distribute over a considerable area.
Dither • A technique during the sigmoidoscopy procedure.
Doppler • Ultrasound instrument used to detect arterial blood flow.
Dorsal • Pertaining to the back.
Dysmenorrhea • Pain in association with menstruation.
Dyspareunia • Occurrence of pain in the labial, vaginal, or pelvic areas during or after sexual intercourse.
Dysplasia • Abnormal development of tissue.
Dysrhythmias • Abnormal, disordered, or disturbed cardiac rhythms.

E
Edema • A local or generalized condition in which the body tissues contain an excessive amount of tissue fluid.
Effusion • Escape of fluid into a part.
Electrocardiogram (ECG) • Tool to assist with diagnosis or ruling out a myocardial infarction, potentially life-threatening arrhythmias, and many other cardiac problems.
Electrode • A medium intervening between an electrical conductor and the object to which the current is to be applied.
Endocervix • The lining of the canal of the cervix uteri.
Endoscopy • Inspection of the body organs or cavity by use of the endoscope.
Enucleation • To remove the eyeball surgically.
Epistaxis • Onset of nasal hemorrhage with or without trauma.
Epithelialization • The growth of skin over a wound.
Erythema migrans • An annular erythema occurring after an insect bite, especially that of the tick infected with the spirochete that causes Lyme disease.
Eschar • A slough, especially one occurring after a cauterization or burn.
Exocervix • Outside the cervix.

Extra-articular • Outside a joint.
Extra-articulation • Amputation of a limb through a joint; excision of a part of a joint.

F

Fascia • A fibrous membrane covering, supporting, and separating muscles.
Fasciitis • Inflammation of any fascia.
Felon • Infection or abscess of soft tissue of the terminal joint of a finger.
Fenestrated • Having openings.
Fibrillation • Irregular heartbeat from multiple foci.
Field block • Method of anesthetizing a small area by injecting anesthetic solution around the lesion to block the nerves supplying the operative field.
Fistula • An abnormal tubelike passage from a normal cavity or tube to a free surface or to another cavity.
Flail chest • A condition of the chest wall due to two or more fractures on each affected rib resulting in a segment of ribs that is not attached on either end; the flail segment moves paradoxically in with inspiration and out with expiration.
Fluoresce • To emit light when exposed to ultraviolet rays.
Fluorescein • A red, crystalline powder, used for diagnostic purposes and for detecting foreign bodies in or lesions of the cornea of the eye.
Fluorescence • The emission of light of one wavelength, usually ultraviolet.
Flutter • Regular sawtoothed beat from single ectopic focus.
Foci • Locations.
Forceps • Pincers for holding, seizing, or extracting.
Formalin • Aqueous solution of 37% formaldehyde.
Fornix • Any body with vaultlike or arched shape.
Fossa • A furrow or shallow depression.
Frenotomy • Division of any frenum, especially for tongue-tie.
Frenulum • A small frenum.
Frenulum linguae • Fold of mucous membrane that extends from the floor of the mouth to the inferior surface of the tongue along its midline.
Furuncle • Abscess of hair follicle or sweat gland; a boil.

G

Ganglion cyst • Cystic tumor developing on a tendon or aponeurosis; sometimes occurs on the back of the wrist.
Gastrostomy • Surgical creation of a gastric fistula through the abdominal wall.
Gluteal • Pertaining to the buttocks.
Granuloma • A granular tumor or growth, usually of lymphoid and epithelial cells.

H

Heimlich valve • Plastic one-way valve used for chest drainage.
Hemoccult • Hidden blood.
Hemolysis • The destruction of red blood cells with the liberation of hemoglobin, which diffuses into the surrounding fluid.
Hemolytic • Pertaining to the breaking down of red blood cells.

Hemopneumothorax • Blood and air in the pleural cavity.
Hemosiderin • An iron-containing pigment derived from hemoglobin from disintegration of red blood cells.
Hemostatic agent • Any drug, medication, or blood component that stops bleeding (e.g., ferrous subsulfate or aluminum chloride).
Hemostats • Devices that arrest the flow of blood.
Hemothorax • Blood or bloody fluid in the pleural cavity caused by rupture of blood vessels as a result of inflammation of the lungs in pneumonia or pulmonary tuberculosis, malignant growth, or trauma.
Hemotympanum • Blood in the middle ear.
Herniated • Having a protrusion or projection of an organ or a part of an organ through the wall of the cavity that normally contains it.
Hidradenitis • Inflammation of a sweat gland.
Holter monitor • Portable ECG machine with a memory.
Hyperpnea • An increased respiratory rate or breathing that is deeper than that usually experienced during normal activity.
Hyperresonance • Increased resonance produced when the area is percussed.
Hypertrophy • Increase in size of an organ or structure that does not involve tumor formation.
Hypospadius • Placement of the penile os on the underside of the penis.

I

Iatrogenic • Caused by treatment or diagnostic procedures.
Impregnated • Saturated.
Incarcerated • Imprisoned, confined, constricted, as an irreducible hernia.
Indurated • Hardened.
Infarction • Formation of an area of tissue in an organ or part that undergoes necrosis after cessation of blood supply.
Infiltrate • To pass into or through a substance or a space.
Inspissated • Thickened by evaporation or absorption of fluid.
Intercostal • Between the ribs.
Interphalangeal • In a joint between two phalanges.
Introitus • An opening or entrance into a canal or cavity, as the vagina.
Inverted • Turned inside out or upside down.
Iodoform • Gauze.
Irreducible • Not capable of being reduced or made smaller, as a fracture or dislocation.
Ischemic • Local, temporary deficiency of blood supply arising from obstruction of the circulation to a part.
Ischiorectal • Pertaining to the ischium and rectum.
IUD (Intrauterine Device) • Device inserted through the cervix and retained in the uterus to prevent pregnancy.

K

Keloid • Scar formation in the skin after trauma or surgical incision.
Keratoacanthoma • A papular lesion filled with a keratin plug that can resemble squamous cell carcinoma.

L

Laceration • An injury to the integument system usually associated with trauma and resulting in the disruption of integrity.

Latrodecism • Abdominal rectus muscle spasm.

Latrodectism • The toxic reaction to the bite of spiders of the genus *Latrodectus* (i.e., black widows).

Lavage • Washing out of a cavity.

Lentigo • Small brown macules or yellow-brown pigmented areas on the skin sometimes caused by exposure to sun and weather.

Leukoplakia • Formation of white spots or patches on the tongue or cheek; may become malignant.

Ligament • A band or sheet of strong fibrous connective tissue connecting the articular ends of bones, serving to bind them together to facilitate or limit motion.

Limb leads • On ECG, these measure electrical waves of depolarization and repolarization, moving up and down and left and right in a vertical or frontal plane. The electrodes for these measurements are placed on the arms and legs.

Loculated • Divided into cavities.

Lordotic • Abnormal anterior convexity of the spine.

Lumbar puncture • Diagnostic procedure involving introduction of a hollow needle in the subarachnoid space of the lumbar portion of the spinal column.

M

Maceration • Process of softening a solid by steeping in a fluid.

Macroglobulinemia • Presence of globulins of high molecular weight in serum.

Manubrium (sterni) • The upper segment of the sternum articulating with the clavicle and first pair of costal cartilages.

Melanoma • A malignant, darkly pigmented mole or tumor of the skin.

Menorrhagia • Excessive bleeding at the time of a menstrual period, in number of days and/or amount of blood.

Metacarpophalangeal • Concerning the metacarpus and the phalanges.

Metaplasia • Conversion of one kind of tissue into a form that is not normal for the tissue, characterized by small, waxy, globular, epithelial tumors that are umbilicated and contain semifluid caseous matter or solid masses.

Midclavicular line • Vertical line extending from the midpoint of the clavicle.

Molloscum contagiosum • The usual mildly contagious form of molloscum that affects mainly children and younger adults.

Mosaicism • Abnormal chicken wire, cobblestone, or tile floor pattern.

Multifocal • Concerning many foci.

Mydriatic • Any drug that dilates the pupil.

N

Nasogastric • Concerning the nose and stomach.

Nebulizer • An apparatus for producing a fine spray or mist.

Necrotic • Pertaining to death of areas of tissue or bone surrounded by healthy parts.

Neuralgia • Pain along a nerve pathway.
Nevi • Congenital discoloration of circumscribed areas of the skin from pigmentation.
Nulliparous • Having never been pregnant.

O

Oblique view • Slanting, diagonal.
Obturator • Anything that obstructs or closes a cavity or opening; two muscles on each side of the pelvic region that rotate the thighs outward.
Occipital nerve block • Diagnostic and therapeutic injection with or without steroid along the occipital nerve of the posterior skull.
Orbiculus oris • Circular muscle surrounding the mouth.
Organomegaly • Enlargement of visceral organs.
Orogastric • Concerning the mouth and stomach.
Orthopnea • Respiratory condition in which there is discomfort in breathing in any but erect sitting or standing position.
Ossicular • Pertaining to one of the bones of the inner ear.
Osteomyelitis • Inflammation of bones, especially the marrow, caused by a pathogenic organism.
Oximetry • Method of determining the amount of oxygen in the blood.

P

P wave • On ECG, represents atrial depolarization and contraction. Usually occurs before the QRS complex.
PMI • Point of maximal impulse.
P-R interval • On ECG, includes the P wave and the straight line connecting it to the QRS complex. It measures the time from the beginning of atrial depolarization to the start of ventricular depolarization.
Papanicolaou (Pap) smear • A study for early detection of cancer cells.
Paracervical • Pertaining to tissues adjacent to the cervix.
Paronychia • Acute or chronic infection of marginal structures about the nail.
Parous • Having been pregnant.
Patency • The state of being freely open.
Percutaneous • Effected through the skin.
Perforate • To puncture or to make holes.
Perforation • The act of making a hole, such as that caused by ulceration.
Perianal cyst • A cyst located around or close to the anus.
Perichondrium • Membranes of fibrous connective tissue around the surface of cartilage.
Peritoneal • Concerning the peritoneum.
Phalanx • Any one of the bones of the fingers or toes.
Pilonidal cyst • A cyst in the sacrococcygeal region, usually at the upper end of the intergluteal cleft.
Pneumothorax • Collapsed lung.
Polychromatic • Multicolored.
Porokeratosis plantaris discreton • A rare skin disease marked by thickening of the stratum corneum in linear arrangement, followed by its atrophy.

Porphyria • A group of disorders that result from a disturbance in porphyrin metabolism, causing increased formation and excretion of porphyrin or its precursors.

Prolapse • A falling or dropping down of an organ or internal part, such as the uterus or rectum.

Properitoneal • In front of the peritoneum.

Proteolytic • Hastening the hydrolysis of proteins.

Pruritus • Severe itching.

Punctation • Abnormal stippled appearance.

Purkinje fibers • Atypical muscle fibers lying beneath the endocardium. They form the electrical impulse–conducting system of the heart.

Pyoderma gangrenosum • A purulent skin disease.

Q

Q wave • On ECG, first downward stroke of the QRS complex.

QRS complex • On ECG, represents beginning of ventricular contraction; usually lasts less than 0.12 second.

R

R wave • On ECG, first upward stroke of the QRS complex.

Reducible • Able to be restored to the original position.

Repolarization • Resting or relaxation phase of the heart muscle.

S

S wave • On ECG, downward deflection of the QRS complex after the R wave.

ST segment • On ECG, flat piece of baseline between the QRS complex and the beginning of the T wave. It measures the time from the end of ventricular depolarization to the start of ventricular repolarization.

Sebaceous cyst • A cyst filled with sebum from a distended oil-secreting gland.

Seborrheic keratoses • Pigmented, raised, warty, and slightly greasy lesions, usually on the trunk, hands, and face.

Septa • Tissue pockets.

Septicemia • Presence of pathogenic bacteria in the blood.

Sigmoidoscopy • Colorectal anal screening technique using lighted tube to visualize the inner lining of the rectum and the distal colon.

Sinoatrial nodes • Dominant pacemaker cells in the heart located high up in the right atrium.

Slough • To shed or cast off dead tissue cells.

Speculum • A retractor used to separate the walls of a cavity to allow for visual examination.

Spicule • A sharp body with a needlelike point.

Squamous cell carcinoma • A form of epidermoid carcinoma, principally of squamous cells.

Stenosis • Constriction or narrowing of a passage or orifice.

Steri strip • Noninvasive skin closure device.

Stoma • A mouth, small opening, or pore.

Strabismus • Disorder of the eye in which the optic axes cannot be directed to the same object.

Strangulated • Constricted so that air or blood supply is cut off, as a strangulated hernia.

Subcutaneous emphysema • Pathologic distention by gas or air beneath the skin.

Subungual • Situated beneath the nail of the finger or toe.

Suturing • A procedure used to repair lacerations of the skin. Suturing may involve the use of suturing material or use of Dermabond.

Syncope • A transient loss of consciousness caused by inadequate blood flow to the brain.

T

T wave • On ECG, repolarization of the ventricles.

Tachycardia • Abnormal rapidity of heart action, usually defined as a heart rate greater than 100 beats/min in adults.

Tamponade • Pathologic condition resulting from accumulation of excess fluid in the pericardium.

Telangiectasia • A vascular lesion formed by dilation of a group of small blood vessels.

Tenaculum • Sharp, hooklike, pointed instrument with slender shank for grasping and holding a part, as an artery.

Tendon • Fibrous connective tissue serving for the attachment of muscles to bones and other parts.

Tensile • Strong.

Thrombosed • Coagulated; clotted.

Torque • A force producing rotary motion.

Transformation zone • Area of columnar epithelium and squamous metaplasia in the vagina or on the cervix.

Tympanometry • Procedure for objective evaluation of the mobility and patency of the eardrum and for detection of middle ear disorders and patency of the eustachian tubes.

Tympanostomy • Incision of the tympanic membrane.

U

Ulceration • Suppuration occurring on a free surface, as on the skin or on a mucous membrane, to form an ulcer.

Unifocal • Having one focus.

Unna's boot • Compression and paste bandage used to treat ulcers caused by venous insufficiency.

V

Vasectomy • Sterilization technique for men.

Vasovagal • Concerning the action of stimuli from the vagus nerve on blood vessels.

Vector • On ECG, the average direction of electrical flow within the heart.

Venipuncture • Puncture of a vein for any purpose.

Venous insufficiency • An abnormal circulatory condition characterized by decreased return of the venous blood to the trunk of the body.

Verruca vulgaris • Common wart, usually on the back of hands and fingers, but may occur anywhere on the skin.

Vitreous humor • Clear, watery gel filling the cavity behind the lens of the eye.

Volar • Palm of the hand or sole of the foot.

W

Wood's light • Tool that emits ultraviolet rays used to detect fluorescent materials in skin and hair diseases.

X

Xiphoid process • Lowest portion of the sternum.

INDEX

Note: Page numbers of figures are in *italics,* page numbers of tables are indicated by *"t".*